A Textbook of
CLINICAL NUTRITION

A Textbook of
CLINICAL NUTRITION

Dr. Luxita Sharma
Associate Professor and Head
Dietetics and Applied Nutrition
Amity University, Haryana

ISBN: 978-93-55810-24-3

Edition: 2022

Printed at: Shree Maitrey Printech Pvt. Ltd., Noida

Preface

"Healthy does NOT mean starving yourself EVER. Healthy means eating the right food in the right amount".

– Karen Salmansohn

Clinical Nutrition is the backbone of Nutrition Sciences. Nutrition is an old age subject which enlightens about balanced diets and their role in maintaining health free from diseases. Therapeutic Nutrition is advancing day by day in curing the disorders through food therapy. Hospitals are now looking to dietetics department for proper planning and preparation of diets. The dietetics department is looking after the patients to treat ailments while they are admitted in the hospitals as well as when the patient is discharged.

Therapeutic Nutrition is a science to plan, prepare and prescribing diets to patients suffering from various diseases of heart, liver, kidneys, gastrointestinal system, etc. Nutrition is a progressing entity and the researches are being published at a large scale everyday. The students studying nutrition should be aware of the trends in nutrition science and they should be encouraged to look into the new researches to implement the outcome in the management of ailments.

This book is written after referring new researches and also the latest trends are included for each and every ailment. This book will enlighten the readers about the new trends in nutrition and also the researches that are authentic to treat the ailments in the patients. The topics are included in detail that are not mentioned in the traditional books of the nutrition or that are very much prevalent in the market or industry but are often ignored. The students when pass out from a particular course are often clueless of the various new developments in nutrition science. For example, the various diets such as keto, paleo, Mediterranean, etc., are very much popular among the celebrities and sportspersons but nutrition students are often unaware of this content. So as an academician, I feel a great need of teaching these topics in the textbooks of Nutrition and Dietetics.

This book will have the answers to the queries of nutrition and dietetics students for major issues and topics. The theory should be properly understood to practise nutrition. The teaching and learning outcomes would be justified through this book in the subject of Clinical Nutrition.

Dr. Luxita Sharma

Contents

Preface *v*

1. Classification of Diets and Nutritional Assessment Tools **1**
1.1 Hospital Diets and Enteral, Parenteral Nutrition 1
1.2 Techniques of Nutritional Assessment 12
1.3 Nutritional Interpretation of Medical and Laboratory Data 17
Questions *20*

2. Obesity **23**
2.1 Definition 23
2.2 Aetiology of Obesity 25
2.3 Assessment of Obesity 26
2.4 Complications during Obesity 29
2.5 Management of Obesity 33
2.6 Recent Trends in Diets of Obesity 39
Questions *59*

3. Cardiovascular Disorders **61**
3.1 Definition 61
3.2 Atherosclerosis 62
3.3 Angina Pectoris 63
3.4 Hyperlipidemia/Hyperlipoproteinemia 64
3.5 Congestive Heart Failure 64
3.6 Myocardial Infarction (Heart Attack) and Heart Stroke 65
3.7 Cerebrovascular Disease 66
3.8 Peripheral Vascular Disease 66
3.9 Aetiology of Cardiovascular Disorders 67
3.10 Dietary Management of the Disease 69
3.11 Hypertension 72
3.12 Relationship between Omega Three Polyunsaturated Fatty Acids and Omega Six Polyunsaturated Fatty Acids 76
Questions *88*

4. Diabetes Mellitus **89**
4.1 Introduction 89
4.2 Types of Diabetes 90
4.3 Other Factors that Cause Diabetes Mellitus 95
4.4 Signs and Symptoms 96
4.5 Emergencies or Sudden Complications of Diabetes Mellitus 97
4.6 Metabolism of Carbohydrates, Proteins and Fats in Diabetes Mellitus 97
4.7 Assessment of Diabetes Mellitus 102
4.8 Insulin and Types of Insulin 102
4.9 Hypoglycaemic Drugs 107
4.10 Management of Diabetes Mellitus 112
4.11 Glycaemic Index and Glycaemic Load 122
4.12 Conclusion 131
Questions *134*

5. Gastrointestinal Disorders and Gastrointestinal Surgeries **137**

A. Dietary Management in Gastrointestinal Disorders

5.1 Peptic and Duodenal Ulcer 137
5.2 Constipation 149
5.3 Diarrhoea 158
5.4 Dumping Syndrome 162
5.5 Gluten Intolerance (Celiac Disease) 168
5.6 Gastro-Oesophageal Reflux Disease (GORD) 174
5.7 Hiatus Hernia 179
5.8 Dyspepsia 180
5.9 Foods to Improve Digestive System 183
5.10 Inflammatory Bowel Disease (IBD) 188
5.11 Diverticulitis 196

B. Dietary Management in Gastrointestinal Surgeries

5.12 Hernia 206
5.13 Haemorrhoids 207
5.14 Bariatric Surgery 210
5.15 Lactose Intolerance 219
Questions 222

6. Renal Disorders **223**
6.1 Human Kidney 223
6.2 Nephrotic Syndrome 233
6.3 Glomerulonephritis 233
6.4 Renal Calculi (Kidney Stones) 237
6.5 Dialysis 246
6.6 Water and Electrolyte Balance in Kidney Disorders 248
6.7 Other Treatments 257
Questions *282*

7. Liver Disorders **283**
7.1 Cirrhosis 283
Questions *296*

8. Inborn Errors of Metabolism **299**
8.1 Phenylketonuria 299
8.2 Galactosemia 312
8.3 Maple Syrup Urine Disease 323
8.4 Glycogen Storage Disease 330
8.5 Cystic Fibrosis 332
Questions *334*

9. Hormonal Disorders **337**
9.1 Polycystic Ovarian Syndrome (PCOS) 337
9.2 Thyroid Disorders 345
Questions *349*

10. Cancers **351**
10.1 Types and Dietary Management 351
10.2 Aetiology of Cancer 352
10.3 Dietary Management 354
10.4 Types of Cancers 355
Questions *371*

11. Nutrition in Bone and Joint Disorders **373**
11.1 Gout 373
11.2 Arthritis 378
11.3 Osteoporosis 382
Questions *385*

12. Nutrition in Febrile Conditions **387**
12.1 Introduction 387
12.2 Metabolism in Fevers 388

12.3 Role of Various Nutrients during Infections 389
12.4 Acute Fever Typhoid 391
12.5 Tuberculosis 395
Questions *401*

References **403**

Index **405**

1

Classification of Diets and Nutritional Assessment Tools

1.1 HOSPITAL DIETS AND ENTERAL, PARENTERAL NUTRITION

1.1.1 Therapeutic Modifications of Normal Diet

Therapeutic diet is also known as adaptation of the normal or regular diet. The modification in the normal diet depends on the disease, the nutritional status of the patient, the severity of the problem as well as the metabolic changes involved.

Therapeutic diets are made to maintain or to provide good nutrition to the patient. So, it is known as the modified version of basic nutrition which has been altered according to the patients or their disease condition.

1.1.2 Objectives of Therapeutics Diets

(a) The achievement of good nutritional status is the main objective of planning therapeutic diets.

(b) The nutritional deficiencies are present in the diseased body so first of all they should be corrected by proper planning of diets. In severe malnutrition or undernutrition cases the immediate intervention of enteral and parenteral nutritional support is to be provided.

(c) Rest is another form of therapy that is foremost recommended by the physicians with drugs/medications and diet planning. Rest to the body leads to the healing of the diseased condition as well as if any damage is caused to the organs.

(d) The food intake should be adjusted to the body needs and its ability to metabolize the nutrients.

(e) The body weight should be measured and a pattern of weight gain or weight loss should be maintained so that adequate diet could be planned and prescribed.

Points to be remembered while planning therapeutic diets:

(a) To make change in consistency in fluid as well as in soft diet.

(b) To reduce or increase the energy needs.

(c) To reduce or increase the bulk in the diet.
(d) To include or exclude certain allergens from the diet.

Changes in normal diet mainly occur due to:

- Disease.
- Metabolic condition.
- Injury or other disorder.
- To correct the deficiencies which have occurred.
- Rest given to certain organs or certain part of the body that helps for the metabolism of diseases.
- Change in the body weight whenever necessary.

1.1.3 Therapeutic Adaptation of Normal Diet

Normal diet may be modified according to the disease or the status of the patient. Therapeutic and operations are:

(a) The change in consistency of the food is according to the patient's health like soft, liquid, solid or normal. For example, for ulcers the solid food is prohibited and the bland or soft diet is recommended. In diabetes and hypertension normal consistency of diet may be recommended.

(b) There is the modification of energy intake according to the disease. For example, obese patient would be recommended low-energy diet and underweight patient would be recommended high energy diet.

(c) Modification in the nutrition like low sodium diet, high or low protein diet, moderate fat diet and high and low carbohydrate diet according to the disease. For example, sodium diet is restricted in hypertension, fat is restricted in the liver disorder, simple carbohydrate is restricted in the diabetes mellitus.

(d) The modification in the content of fibre. For example, in diarrhoea low fibre is recommended and in constipation high fibre is recommended.

(e) Bland diet is recommended in the gastrointestinal disease. It is the chemically, mechanically and thermally bland.

(f) The removal of certain foods from the diet to which the patient is allergic.

(g) Adjustment of the frequency of feeding in some diseases–the patient may not be able to eat large amount of food so it is recommended to eat small amount of food at certain hours.

(h) There is modification of the mode of feeding like patient who cannot take food orally, special type of feeding method is used like parenteral or enteral feeding.

Balanced diet is recommended for all age groups. The word "balanced" means having different elements in correct proportion and in terms of food it means the diet which sufficiently meets the daily nutritional needs. The recommended dietary allowances as laid down by Indian Council of Medical Research (ICMR) defines the nutrient requirements of different age groups. The food pyramid has already given different food groups and their amount to be ingested daily. Therefore, to achieve daily balanced diet, it is necessary to eat the foods from different food groups. It will help to reach a state of equilibrium. The state of equilibrium means the adequacy of nutrient balance in the body and it is also called nutritional homeostasis. Now this we are talking about the eating of healthy food with no restrictions and everything could be included in daily diet. Therapeutic modifications of diet or a modified diet is defined as any diet which could be altered, i.e., by including and excluding certain types of nutrients such as carbohydrates, proteins, fats, minerals and vitamins. The therapeutic modifications are done to manage certain bodily conditions such as obesity, hypertension, diabetes mellitus and so on or any mineral or vitamin deficiencies. There are many factors which are to be considered before altering the daily diet as per the need of the body.

The factors which should be considered before the modification of a diet are as follows:

(a) Demographic details: Before planning or changing the daily diet of the patient the details regarding the age, sex and location should be noted down. This will help a dietician to understand the recommended dietary allowances (RDAs) for the patient and the prescription of the type of diet. The location of the patient will determine the type of diet to be given because then only the diet will be followed. The availability of the food should be considered while planning diets. For example, a north Indian should be given the north Indian food products while people belonging to north-east region should be given their local foods such as green vegetables, fruits, steamed foods, etc. The next detail to be considered while planning of diet includes the socio-economic status of the patient. The diet should not include the food products that are not affordable for the patient. The diet should be given much wider options and variety with low cost so that it is available for all. The local foods are easily available and are also cost effective. And above all our body accepts and digests the food that it is habitual of receiving since birth. The patient's social circle, and the type of food eaten by the family matters while planning diets. The collection of the above details of the patient is helpful for effective preparation of the modified diets.

(b) **Medical history:** Nutritionist should always procure the details of the medical history of the client because the past ailments are necessary to be known for future preparations. Genetics is one of the major factors that contributes to many diseases. For example, if one of the parents is suffering from diabetes mellitus or obesity then the chances of developing the disease becomes 80-90 per cent. Therefore, it is important to know the past history or the family history of the diseases of the patient. The patients could also be made cautious also about the diseases which are caused due to genetics after knowing the history. The patients can take precautionary measures such as regular monitoring of the biochemical parameters, controlled dietary intake and also exercising at least for some time daily. These measures can easily combat the development of metabolism and cure ailments present in the family.

(c) **Dietary history:** The dietary history of a patient involves 24-hour dietary recall of past seven days. This gives brief details of the dietary habits and eating preferences of the patient. The eating habits should be checked and analyzed. After this the diet for the patient should be planned as per the guidelines. The nutrient calculation needs be altered according to RDAs and diseases. The diets are modified with changes in the nutrients as per the ailment such as a high fibre and low carbohydrate diet for diabetic patient, a low protein diet in renal disorders, a low sodium diet for hypertensives, etc.

1.1.4 Types of the Therapeutic Diets

Therapeutic diets are defined as the planning of a day's diet by controlling and recommending the intake of some particular foods. The therapeutic diets are always modified according to the need of the person or as prescribed by the physician or dietician. Diet therapy aims for the recovery from the illness and prevention of the disease. The normal or regular diets are modified and are called therapeutics diet. The diets are modified according to following parameters.

1.1.5 Modified Diets

1.1.5.1 Normal Diets

Normal diet is recommended for the patients who are permitted to eat food without any restriction of certain amount of food and its content. It is also known as regular diet, general or full diet.

The energy is provided approximately 1600 to 2000 kcal 60 to 80 gm protein. 50 to 60 % of carbohydrate and 10 to 15% of fats.

(a) It is the diet which is nutritionally balanced as it contains the food from all groups.

(b) It is based on the usual meal pattern. It shows better acceptability in the patient.

(c) It easy to evaluate and modify according to the patient.

Foods allowed: All foods are recommended which are eaten by the patient.

Foods to be restricted:

- Fried foods like rolls, paranthas, etc.
- Fatty foods like pastries, cakes, etc.
- Spices, pickles and condiments
- Strongly flavored vegetables like onion, garlic, etc.

Diet modifications according to consistency: These diets are planned for gastrointestinal (GI) disorders. Low residue diets are recommended. Fibre is restricted in most of the stomach and intestinal diseases. It is the diet for the patient who is unable to tolerate solid food and it is given in the post-operative or febrile states. This diet is free from mechanical and chemical irritants and is required to easily digest the food. Nutritional adequacy depends upon the liquid which is recommended in the food.

The solid food is not given in GI diseases. The diets included in this category are of three types:

(a) Clear fluid diet.

(b) Full fluid diet.

(c) Soft diets or low residue diets

(a) **Clear fluid diets** are defined as the diets which are in liquid state at room temperature. These can be clear liquids and full fluid diets. Clear liquids are provided in febrile, post-surgeries, diarrhoea, vomiting, after heart attack, acute infections of stomach or intestines and before some X-rays of digestive tract. The foods which are allowed in this category are plain water, soup broths, carbohydrates mixed with electrolytes such as glucose water with salt, clear sodas, fruit juices without pulp such as grape juice, apple juice, cranberry juice which are more energy giving, weak tea or coffee with no cream or milk added in them and sports drinks which are available in the market as well. These diets are provided for short periods of time.

It is the diet which contains only clear liquids. It is the diet which is used in the acute diarrhoea patient. Also used in the post-surgery patient to furnish non-gas forming liquid and nourishment. During surgery when there is a intolerance of food shown by nausea, vomiting, diarrhoea, anorexia, nutrients have to be restricted. In this condition clear liquid diet is prescribed to prevent dehydration and maintain water and electrolyte balance.

Clear fluid diet is mainly composed of carbohydrates, water and some electrolyte. It can normally provide 400 to 500 kcal energy and 5 gm protein, negligible amount of fat and 100 to 120 grams of carbohydrate in 24 hours.

So, it is a nutritionally inadequate diet therefore it is used only for a short period of time. If it is continued for the longer period of time supplementation of the protein, minerals and vitamins are recommended.

Foods allowed

- Strained fruit juices.
- Weak tea or coffee without milk or cream.
- Carbonated beverages.
- Clear soups and broths.
- Whey water, coconut water, barley water
- Fruit juices, gelatin
- Glucose water, lime water, and honey.

Foods avoided: All the solid foods are restricted.

(b) **Full fluid diet** comprises clear liquids with addition of milk and small amounts of fibre. These diets are prescribed to the patients with esophageal problems or swallowing and chewing issues. Small amounts of fibre are given with clear liquid foods. Full fluid diet is well planned in terms of calories, protein and fats and is energy giving as well but it could be deficient in vitamins and minerals. It also does not meet the daily requirements of fibre. All kinds of clear diets are included in full fluid diet. The food products given in full fluid diets are thin cereal and pulse gruels (hot or cold), vegetable juices or purees, strained cream soups, nutritional supplements in the form of shakes, tablets or powders, Bournvita, Horlicks, Proteinex, milk powder, all milk based beverages as custard, puddings, ice cream, milk shakes, egg nog, frozen yoghurt, corn starch puddings, carbonated beverages, tea, coffee, sugar sherbets, hard candy, plain gelatin, plain added sugar or butter, cream or oil to various recipes as stated above This is the transitional diet between a clear liquid diet and soft diet. This diet is free from irritating condiment and spices as well as cellulose. Full fluid diet includes all fruits which are liquid at room temperature.

This diet is given to patients who are unable to chew or swallow solid foods in the surgery or other gastrointestinal disorders.

Full fluid diet is a nutritionally adequate. It contains 1500 to 2000 kcal energy, 55 to 65 gm protein with adequate amounts of vitamins and minerals–except for fibres.

So it is recommended for a longer period as compared to clear fluid diets. For maintaining full diet to a longer period of time careful planning is required. Supplementation of proteins, vitamins and minerals is required to maintain the nutritional value.

Foods allowed:

- Strained fruit and vegetable juices and purees.
- Cream soups and broths.
- Refined and strained cereal and pulses gruels.
- Plain gelatin deserts, plain ice cream, soft custards and cornstarch puddings.
- Milk and milk based beverages like eggnog, malted milk, etc.
- Butter, cream, oil are added to food in moderate amount.
- Tea, coffee and carbonated beverages.
- Sugar, honey, salt and mild flavouring foods.

(c) **Soft diets or low residue diets** as the name indicates are soft to chew and light to digest. It is soft in fibre content also. Soft diets are given for stomach disorders or the patients having problems in digestion. The conditions of abdominal surgeries, gastroenteritis, diverticulitis or inflammatory bowel require soft diets. Low residue diets consist of fruits and vegetables without peels, ground tender meats so that connective tissues could be reduced. The coarse, fibrous or meat products with tough connective tissue, fruits, vegetables, nuts, coconut are avoided in soft diets. All high fibre foods such as peas, beans, lotus stem, ladyfinger, apple, pears, tomato, beans should be avoided completely. The soft diet is meshed or cooked in pureed form to serve the purpose. This kind of diet fulfils the nutritional requirements of the patient. The food products such as refined cereals as rice, bread with milk or butter, sooji kheer, pasta, vermicelli, poha, pulses soup with added soft pectin vegetables such as potato, meshed cereal-pulse combination, boiled eggs, curd, cottage cheese, bananas, papaya, butter, cream, vegetable oils, salt and sugar but moderately, pureed vegetables cooked properly, all types of gourds could be given in soft diet. This type of diet is soft in texture and bland in taste as restriction of sugar, salt and spices is imposed while planning and preparation.

It is the diet which is soft in consistency. It is the transitional diet between normal diet and full fluid diet. It is easy to chew, easily digestible foods are present, made in a simple method, and it is nutritionally adequate.

Diet planned for the patience whose digestion and mechanical ease in eating or both are disrupted. This diet is prescribed in gastrointestinal disorder or in the surgery. The energy is 1800 to 2000 kcal and 55 to 65 gm of protein, moderate amount of carbohydrate and fat are recommended.

Foods allowed:

- Washed pulses as such in the form of soup and in combination with vegetables and cereals.
- Rice and its products semolina bread biscuit, etc.
- Eggs and lean meat like fish and chicken.
- Milk and its products such ad curd cottage cheese, etc.
- Soft fruits like mango, banana, papaya, etc. The fruits are eaten after removing the seeds and skin.
- Starchy and low fibre vegetables like spinach, potato, bottle gourd, tori, etc.
- Fruits and vegetables in the form of juice, soup, etc.
- Fats like butter, cream, vegetable oil, etc.
- Salt and sugar in moderate amount.

Foods restricted

- Raw vegetables and fruits.
- High fibre vegetables like tomato, beans, etc.
- Whole grain cereal and its products like cracked wheat and aata.
- Whole pulses and split pulses with husk.
- Fried foods, fatty and tough meats.

- Bakery products.
- Dry fruits and nuts.
- Highly flavoured and spiced foods and pickles.

1.1.5.2 Dietary Modifications According to Change in Nutrients

Diet is modified through alterations in the nutrient intake due to various deficiencies or illnesses. Change in the composition of diet is made so that the availability of nutrients could be made to the unwell or healing body.

(a) **Diet modifications according to energy intake - high calorie diet:** The energy level needs to be increased in certain conditions of diseases. The disorders in which increased levels of calories are needed are hyperthyroidism, weight loss in conditions like fevers (short and long duration), protein energy malnutrition, burns, sepsis and infections. The calories are increased and this helps the patient to recover and maintain the homeostasis. In high calorie diets carbohydrates 400-450 gm, proteins – 1-1.5 gm per kg body weight and fats 50 gm on the basis of per day could be prescribed for an adult. The modifications are done on the basis of RDAs as recommended by ICMR.

(b) **Low calorie diet:** These kind of diets are controlled in carbohydrates, proteins and fats as these nutrients are energy giving foods. But these diets should be planned in such a way that the vitamins and minerals need to be kept in consideration. The deficiency disorders occur frequently when the energy dense foods are restricted. The calories are reduced to 1200,1500 or 1800 calories depending on the diseases to be treated. The calories are never be reduced below a level of 1000 calories. In some cases if it is done so then supplements of B-complex vitamins and minerals should be recommended. Four to five servings of fruits and vegetables are to be given when the person is on low calorie diets. Low calorie diets are given in diabetes mellitus, heart diseases, gout, arthritis, obesity, hypertension, gall bladder diseases and pre-operative stages.

(c) **High fibre diet:** Fibre is known as potential nutrient for maintaining the health of intestines or colon. The ailments of constipation and high lipid levels can be managed by high fibre diet. Fibre is also useful in reducing weight and serum triglycerides. The fibre intake can be increased to 15-20 gm/day for adults. Whole grains, fruits and vegetables with peels are prescribed to increase the fibre content.

(d) **Low fibre diet:** The diet comprises foods that can be completely absorbed or leaves no residue thus no faecal formation. This can lead to low vitamin and mineral content. The diet includes soft and full fluid diets also. The diseases in which they are given are discussed above already.

(e) **High protein diet:** These diets include high in plant and animal proteins that are used to build up muscles and increase lean body mass. High protein diet of 1.5-2 gm/kg body weight per day is prescribed in fever, burns, severe weight loss, post-surgical conditions, diarrhoea, elderly, alcoholics, dialysis, peptic ulcers and cancers.

(f) **Low protein diet:** Low protein diet in which the proteins are reduced to 0.5-0.8 gm/kg body weight/day. Low proteins are given in conditions as acute and chronic renal failure, hepatic encephalopathy, acute and chronic glomerulonephritis, metabolic errors and in some liver disorders. In these diseases proteins cannot be metabolized properly so the nitrogenous waste products are accumulated in the blood. Ammonia and urea are metabolic products of proteins and they are not excreted by the body in the diseases mentioned above especially in renal failure cases. Low protein diets of 18-22 gm per day are also prescribed in patients suffering from in-born errors of metabolism that are caused by lack of enzymes of urea cycle.

(g) **Low fat diet:** These diets consist of 15-30% of lipids per day which has 7-10% of saturated fats and rest are MUFA & PUFA. Low fat diets are given in cardiovascular disorders such as hyperlipidemia, atherosclerosis, myocardial infarction, gall stones, obesity and hypertension. Cholesterol content of diet is also controlled till 300 mg. Fat is never completely omitted from the diet as it is required by our body for various functions such as absorption of fat soluble vitamins and providing cushions to organs.

(h) **Adequate electrolyte diet:** There are body conditions such as heavy workers in tropical climate, chronic diarrhoea, weaning diarrhoea, excessive heat and AIDS patients who require sodium and potassium in their diet. The deficiency of electrolytes can disturb acid-base balance of the body and even may lead to death. So it is very important to maintain the Na-K levels in the body. Chlorine is also an equally important mineral and not to be ignored. The orange juice with glucose and salt added is mostly provided to the patients. It is also helpful in deficiency conditions. Further glucose solution and oral rehydration therapy are given to such patients.

(i) **Low sodium diet:** The mineral content is considered especially sodium in diseases such as hypertension, congestive heart failure, liver, renal, hypothyroidism and obesity also. These diseases aften cause water retention or oedema in lower parts of the body. The four levels of sodium restriction are 250, 500, 1000 and 2400 mg. The diet includes kempners rice diet (rice cooked in fruit juices without salt) which was earlier given to severe hypertensive patients. The treatment of oedema and high blood pressure depends on sodium intake in daily diet.

(j) **Food allergy diet:** Certain foods cause allergic reactions in some individuals after consumption–leading to rashes, hives, discomfort, diarrhoea, etc. In such conditions elimination of that specific food from the diet solves the problem. For example, elimination diet (where all the suspected foods are eliminated from the diet and are again reintroduced in order to identify the allergen food such as wheat allergy diet or peanut allergy diet).

1.1.6 Enteral Nutrition

This is also known as 'tube feeding' as it is done by passing a tube into the stomach or duodenum through the nose called–nasogastric feeding. When the tube is inserted into the duodenum or jejunum directly by surgical operations it is called gastrostomy or jejunostomy feeding. For short-term feeding, i.e., 3 to 4 weeks, nasogastric, nasoduodenal or nasojejunal tubes are generally administered whereas for a long-term feeding gastrostomy or jejunostomy is performed. Different types of elemental feeds are:

(a) **Natural liquid foods:** Skim or whole milk or cooked strained cereal grains can be given. Vegetable oil or cream and non-fat dry milk are also incorporated to increase the calorie and protein levels. Many convalescing patients are often depressed and lack appetite get benefits from these appetising foods of high nutrient density.

(b) **Blenderized feeding:** Normal foods are blended to make thin liquids which can easily pass through the nasogastric tube. Blenderized food can be prepared using starch, milk or milk powder, curd, egg, soya flour, refined oil, etc. These feeds are better tolerated and are also cheaper than commercial formulas.

(c) **Amino acid diet:** It has no advantage over polymeric diet containing undigested protein and fat for patients having normal intestinal function. The administration of these has also been questioned due to its high osmolarity which may lead to diarrhoea. Whole protein diets are a better option for normal intestinal function patients since the whole protein achieves nutritional balance quicker and is less expensive. Amino acid diets are required in certain cases of critical illness, e.g., glutamine is conditionally essential during inflammation or injury.

(d) **Fatty acid diet:** This diet is required to overcome the essential fatty acid deficiency. Here, essential fatty acids provide 4% of the total calories.

(e) **Feeding modules:** There are certain concentrated sources of one nutrient, e.g., Pro-mix (protein), Lipomul (fat) and Polycose (carbohydrate). They are added to the formula diets in order to fulfil a deficient component or to yield a small quantity as well as nutrient dense mixture (especially for patients in whom fluid intake has been restricted).

1.1.7 Parenteral Nutrition

It is also known as intravenous feeding. In parenteral nutrition a sterile nutrient dense solution (such as glucose, synthetic amino acid mixture, fat emulsion, commercially prepared trace element containing solution like Addamel, etc., is infused intravenously. These are originally developed in order to provide nutrition to the patients who are capable of digesting and absorbing the nutrients. When parenteral nutrition is infused directly into the peripheral vein, it is known as peripheral parenteral nutrition (PPN), which is for a short-term use, i.e., less than 10 days. And when higher concentration solutions are administered for a longer time period using central venous access, it is known as total parenteral nutrition (TPN).

1.2 TECHNIQUES OF NUTRITIONAL ASSESSMENT

Nutritional needs and the status of each and every individual is something, that requires to be assessed at regular intervals. There are a number of processes and proceedings to check the nutritional status or perform nutritional assessment, but the simplest among them includes serial weight measurement. A nutritional assessment procedure is completed in four detailed processes. It is quoted as "ABCD", and includes all the essential steps required for the complete screening and tests to detect the current nutritional status of the individual.

The nutritional assessment is done by the following four steps:

1. Anthropometric measurements of body composition.
2. Biochemical measurements of serum protein, micronutrients and metabolic parameters.

3. Clinical assessment of altered nutritional requirements and social or psychological issues, that could affect adequate intake.
4. Measurement of dietary intake.

The nutritional assessment also includes collection of patient's medical history, any critical diseases or metabolic disorders that he/she is suffering from, the dietary practices followed by the individual, treatment he/she is going through currently to treat any ailment and situations regarding food security.

The assessment of a person on the basis of nutrition is mandatory because it can provide us with the information if the person is having optimal nutritional status, which is basically the condition or state of body in accordance with the ideal amount of each and every nutrient and conditions related with overall body weight. This could act as a technique or major factor in prevention of diseases, treating them and promotion of awareness related to health and nutrition.

It is also regarded that if the body weight is less by 10 per cent or more than the usual body weight, it is in most of the cases, related to certain adverse conclusions and development of certain metabolic disorders and could result in prolonged hospitalization. On the other hand, in the individuals who are lean or healthy, the loss of 35 per cent or more of body weight from the ideal structure could result in death of the individual. Not only this, nutritional status also destroys the body's immunological system or weakens it and faintly affects the body's response to various medications and therapies related to health.

The dietitians and other healthcare facilities are in a practice of checking the nutritional status of their patients because it helps:

(a) To detect and identify people, who are prone or are at risk of developing health problems related to malnutrition. This also helps to prevent them from becoming malnourished.
(b) In identification of clients who are already malnourished and help them by providing proper treatment according to their health conditions.
(c) To keep track of growth in child and development of individuals going through adolescence.
(d) To detect the cases in which an insight is needed to identify if the person is suffering from any medical complications, which could have affected the body's capacity to utilize nutrients supplied through the diets.

(e) In detection of certain procedures and practices which can adversely increase the chances of the person suffering from malnutrition and from certain infections.

(f) In spreading knowledge and passing information about nutrient related counselling of individuals.

(g) In the establishment of correct, to-the-point and appropriate nutrition diet and care plans, that are customizable for each and every patient according to his disease conditions and the level of criticality.

The data related to the nutritional assessment and also classifying the specific nutritional requirements that are needed by different individuals are the tools to determine each and every essential element that could possibly be the part of nutritional assessment, counselling of patients related to some specific health conditions and their solutions and also the support as per the person and his/her needs.

The choice of whether a person needs to be nutritionally assessed depends on the nutritionist and the medical team. Most of the times, seeing the physical state of the patient, the dietitian could determine if he/she is suffering from any malnutrition related metabolic disorders and then a detailed nutritional assessment is performed. The screening could be done by nutritionist and other trained health-care providers in facilities for health care. In highest vicinity, these tests are done during monitoring growth or home care and also during certain meetings or gatherings related to health. A normal or simple screening on the basis of nutritional status could be accompanied by certain measures and techniques which include bilateral pitting oedema, measurement of weight and mid-upper arm circumference (MUAC). Also, another important part of this study is to know the current status regarding the diseases he/she has suffered from or is suffering from and his/her appetite and hunger conditions. Problems associated with certain diseases that can affect the digestibility are also questioned about.

The screening related to nutritional assessment is quite tough and trained professionals are required for carrying out these processes who are in line with national polices related to health. Also certain special materials are required for solving the problems related to counteracting upon problems. Proper guidance and screening support should be given on the basis of whom to screen, how and what are the things to be kept in mind while screening and, of course, the time interval of carrying out such nutritional assessment. Also support for incentives are to be given to the health personnels to perform accurate and consistent screening of nutritional assessment of the individuals. The proceedings and processes related to these screenings in community service centers and government health clinics are done with the correct precision and while following all the steps to get an exact result. The errors can affect the community.

Even after following all the proceedings and processes minutely, the professionals cannot go for each and every individual as per the need of the hour.

The client's nutritional status should be the ultimate priority in conditions like:

(a) Children whose age is below 2 years and are not breastfeed.

(b) Pregnant women and those who are lactating till six months.

(c) If people are found to have unintentional weight loss.

(d) People who have been counselled with specific diet for treatment of malnutrition.

(e) People who are suffering from certain metabolic disorders and can be helped by following certain specific diets.

(f) People who are suffering from certain specific chronic disorders such as AIDS, tuberculosis, etc.

1.2.1 ANTHROPOMETRIC ASSESSMENT

Making assessment on the basis of anthropometry includes various measuring entities such as size, weight and body proportions. Weight, height, mid upper arm circumference (MUAC), head circumference and skinfold thickness.

The BMI (body mass index) and weight- for- height ratios are some of the vital measurements needed for carrying out the anthropometric studies and are presented as indexes. These indexes have a special system for recording their values. This value comes out by carrying out the process of median marker. There are a number of measurement techniques used in this process but it should be maintained that the client is assessed with same measurement techniques every time, to avoid any sort of complications or varying values.

1. **Weight:** The primary and most important step while carrying out the anthropometric readings is weighing. It requires a digital or an analogue measuring scale, that can measure weight of at least 120 kg, with the perfection of nearest 100 gm. Weight should be measured accurately as any fault in the findings could result in despaired conclusions in the process of screening.
2. **Length and height:** Measurements related to height or length are taken with the help of measuring tapes with centimetre markings or

height boards. The height of children who are less than two years old are measured as per their length. Children who are more than two years old are measured according to their height.

3. **Weight-for-height:** This is the index that is used to measure the nutritional status for children whose age is between birth and 59 months. It does a comparison of the subjected child with the standard child growth chart given by WHO.
4. MUAC is generally measured in millimetres to make it more accurate. MUAC is a standard measuring unit for pregnant women and lactating women till 6 months.
5. **BMI:** Body mass index is by far the most trusted measuring technique used by the dieticians, as it is easy to calculate and time saving. It can be used easily and is based on the ratio of weight-to-height. This measurement technique is also used to identify malnourished adults, pregnant women and children as well.

1.2.2 Biochemical Assessment

Biochemical assessments stand for all those parameters which are related to blood and other bodily constituents. It checks the level of various nutrients in an individual's blood, urine or stools. These tests are done in specified labs and are performed by trained technicians. The results from these tests serve the medical professionals with vital information related to medical problems and help in determining the cause for certain changes in the appetite or nutritional status of the patients.

1.2.3 Clinical Assessment

This part in the process of nutritional assessment is mainly and primarily concerned with the bodily or physical signs and symptoms in close relation to nutritional deficiencies such as bilateral pitting oedema, muscle wasting, emaciation, loss of hair, and changes in hair colour. Medical history of the concerned person is also mandatory. This history confirms the current status of the individual and his/her past records in dealing with metabolic disorders and or any other diseases.

1.2.4 Dietary Assessment

Assessment of foods to be taken and the intake of fluid is one of the vital and most important part in the process of carrying out nutritional investigations. It provides information on various dietary needs, their quantity and quality. Also, if there is any change in the structure of appetite of a particular individual, the accompanied food allergies and intolerances.

These results are compared with all the preloaded values as per the regularly rechecked recommended dietary allowance (RDA). This, in turn, helps to counsel and discuss the benefits of following some particular diets in diseases, especially those related to metabolic disorders. The counselling part helps the patients to deal with the conditions of malnutrition and help them fight such situations with utmost dedication.

(a) **24-hour recall:** The process was mainly developed or designed to assess and quantify the regular dietary intake of a mass of people over a time period of 7 days. However, this is well equipped to be used as an assessment tool to gather the nutritional data of an individual. In this process, the patient is asked to remember all sorts of foods and liquids or fluids consumed in the last 24 hours. The method is flexible enough to be used with customization to demonstrate different states of a patient suffering from various ailments and especially those suffering from malnutrition.

The time period for this recall method starts from when the person wakes up and ends when the person goes to sleep.

(b) **Food frequency questionnaire:** This method is designed to assess the quality of food products taken, rather than the quantity or the nutrition provided by those products. This method, as the name suggests, focuses on the frequency in which a person is taking his/her foods in a day. This method is quick and less expensive but its results are not as accurate as the 24-hour recall.

(c) **Food group questionnaire:** This is another method of dietary assessment in which the patient is shown pictures or models of various foods in different food groups and then they are questioned on whether they have consumed any of those products or food groups in their previous meals.

1.3 NUTRITIONAL INTERPRETATION OF MEDICAL AND LABORATORY DATA

Moreover, this method uses a number of laboratory dietary and medical data to analyze and calculate the amount of nutrition present in the body of the person and malnutrition he or she is suffering from. Biochemical tests are performed for levels of nutrients and biological fluids which precisely consist of blood in urine–one of the major factors in determining the nutritional needs of a person. Dietitian or trained medical staff can get a lot of information and accurate results when the nutritional assessment or interpretation is based on the findings from a lab. However, the metals or minerals which are to be found by a lab need not be correlated with clinical or dietary findings. Results from lab are also costly which many of the patients can't afford. As far as accuracy is concerned assessments are more dependable when they are calculated by laboratory details.

1.3.1 Objectives

There are two primary functions of every test which is done for carrying out the process of nutritional assessment.

It is used in the process of detecting nutritional deficiencies which an individual particularly suffers. If he or she shows any clinical signs of diseases which could be metabolic disorders, perfect remedies for medications for certain modifications in his or her diet could be taken.

It helps in the process of enhancing studies with dietary assessment. A specific population group which should be pinpointed on the basis of nutritional problem that they are facing. The models that could be used on them in suggesting the process that will decrease their suffering.

Basically, laboratory investigation, is of little practical use. But the findings confirm the accuracy of nutritional needs a person requires. Often it is seen that lab values can be done on a large scale and could suggest a signal of certain acute or chronic deficiencies or problems which the patient doesn't look like to be having when they are counselled about their diet or from the medical history.

1.3.2 Methodology

Laboratory tests that are done for assessing the nutritional status of the patient are generally of two types: measuring the exact level of nutrients that are circulating in the fluid (blood, urine) and functional tests.

The first process is very accurate and helps in finding or identifying the presence of any nutritionally affected problems in a person. The second, pays more attention on the severity level of the detected nutritional deficiency. The basic functional tests which are performed, scale in the presence or absence of certain enzymes in the body and their effect. For instance, the enzyme thiamine and its deficiency can be detected by testing the constituents of urine. But if the measurement of the enzyme transketolase could be detected in the patient's body, that will be a more accurate indicator. The current status and severity could be thus determined with the exact calculations.

There are also certain cases in which a number of other kinds of laboratory tests are required. They are special and unique in their characteristics, specific to the demand and are sophisticated in their own way. Microbiological assay is one of such cases which is performed in special conditions and circumstances by experienced lab technicians.

1.3.3 Planning of a Laboratory Assessment

Laboratory test performed on the basis of finding out certain nutritional needs of a patient should be accurate and precise. Medical practitioner should we very careful on what test should be done and what not to be done for finding out certain values that are needed for the nutritional status and for assessing the patient. Medical practitioner should also be concerned about the health of the patient and if there are certain symptoms and which show that he/she is going through a nutritional deficiency. For such patients the nutritional assessment should be based on the signs and symptoms on their faces or bodily apprehensions. The laboratory tests and the data should be nurtured carefully.

For instance, if a person is suffering from diabetes and he is also showing certain signs for obesity, then it is almost clear that only tests determining his blood sugar level are enough to determine the current status of diabetes. For obesity we can go for his body mass index test. We can avoid various laboratory tests. There is also a category of patients who are not able to perform many tests as they can't afford such tests. As a dietitian one should understand the economic status of the patient and only then plan a laboratory assessment. There are also certain standards given by certain medical institutions, WHO and ICMR, according to them evaluation test should be planned.

1.3.4 Precautions in Laboratory Evaluations

They are certain precautions which should be taken before carrying out any lab tests or assessments. A large number of biological tests which are performed in a lab can vary in a number of ways. Some are very accurate and others may not be so accurate to a certain extent. One should be clear about the fact that lab tests could be different from each and every other lab depending on the equipment they are using. For example, urine infections for urinary excretion are much more defective from the sense of accuracy level than test including the amount of plasma levels in the body. However, the nutrition level of an individual may change from time to time. Nutrition level of a patient was saying something seven days ago and if the test is done once more after a week, the nutrition level may change or show varied results.

1.3.5 Laboratory Assessment for Individual Nutrients

There are some specific descriptions of certain nutrients such as protein, vitamins, carbohydrates and certain minerals on which the laboratory assessments are done.

(a) **Protein:** If there is deficiency of protein in the diet especially the serum protein or albumin protein, then it can cause many problems along with nutritional deficiencies. To calculate the amount of protein, laboratory tests are done on the basis of the total protein and serum protein present in the body. This gives an accurate result of the current status of the person and whether he/she falls under the malnutrition category or normal category.

(b) **Vitamins:** To check the number of vitamins present in the body there are various tests which are performed. These are divided into two categories: for the water-soluble vitamins and for the fat-soluble vitamins. Water-soluble vitamins and the presence of vitamin C are measured by laboratory test.

Fat-soluble vitamins in the body test are solely based on the constituent of the vitamins and their quantity in the serum. Example: for finding out the amount of vitamin A and beta carotene in the body, the amount of carotene is checked upon by the lab and also for vitamin D serum level is a game changer.

(c) **Minerals:** There are various minerals in our body along with certain micronutrients. Some of the most important minerals are iron, magnesium, potassium sodium and calcium. These tests are carried out by taking a blood sample and screened under certain machinery. Iron is calculated by the amount of iron metal present in the body and especially in the blood. In case of anemia, the amount of blood iron decreases as there is a deficiency of iron in the body. Search minerals are calculated by the amount of their natural component present in the blood serum or the blood. The amounts of sodium, potassium and other micronutrients are also calculated using a simple blood test.

QUESTIONS

1. What are the different types of diets?
2. Write short notes on:
   (i) Soft diet
   (ii) Liquid diet
   (iii) Full fluid diet
3. Describe enteral feeding.
4. What is total parenteral feeding? What are its disadvantages over tube feeding?
5. Differentiate between enteral feeding and parenteral feeding.

6. Write brief notes on:
   (i) Refeeding syndrome
   (ii) Elemental diet
   (iii) Tube feeding
7. What are the different techniques used for nutritional assessment?
8. How can the medical and laboratory data help in establishing the nutritional requirement of the patient?
9. Mention two situations in which TPN is given along with a sample regimen for an adult.
10. Differentiate between pre- and post-operative diets.

2

Obesity

2.1 DEFINITION

Obesity is accumulation of fat in the body due to eating more food than needed. In clinical terms, obesity is defined as the state where there is elevation of the body weight above the normal and an excess of adipose tissue leading to 20% or more increase in the ideal body weight. This condition arises when the calories consumed are more than the calories expended.

Calorie consumption > Calorie expenditure = Overweight/obesity

Calorie consumption = Calorie expenditure = Normal weight

Calorie consumption < Calorie expenditure = Underweight

Whereas overweight is a condition where the ideal body weight increases by 10 to 20%. Therefore overweight and obesity are relative terms but not synonyms. The ideal weight of an individual depends on age, height, gender and the body frame.

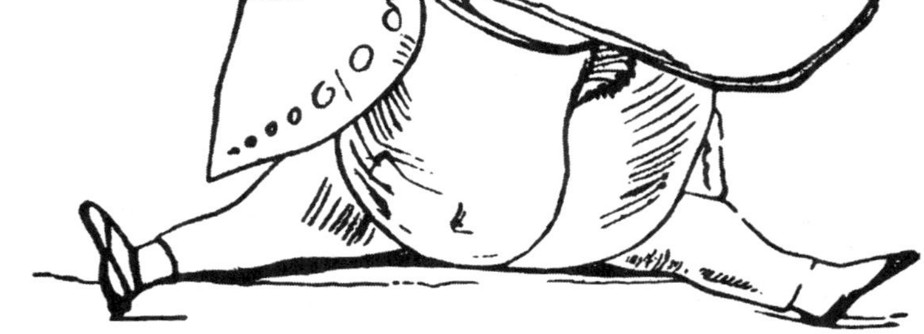

Table 2.1: Statistics by WHO, Global Health Observatory (2016)

Age group	Overweight		Obesity	
	Men	Women	Men	Women
Adulthood	39%	39%	39%	39%
Childhood and adolescence	18%		18%	

According to BMI: **(WHO)**

- 18.5-24.9 Normal
- 25-29.9 Grade I obesity
- 30-40 Grade II obesity
- >40 Grade III obesity

2.1.1 Body Composition

The concept of body composition came into existence when a lot of queries rose regarding the definitions of weight. Are they adequate to adjudge about a person's overweight or obese status. The weight we usually measure using a weighing scale is not just the weight of the fat in the body instead it's the sum total of the fat and lean body mass (LBM).

Body fat comprises essential fat and total fat:

- **Essential fat** is required for normal functioning of the body and is present in muscles, bone marrow, heart, lungs, liver and nervous tissue.
- **Storage fat** is the adipose tissue (energy reserve) present beneath the epidermis/hypodermis and around the body organs internally.

Fat is very important for our body even though there are many myths about its usage in the body. This prenotion makes people to avoid consuming it without knowing the repercussions of the same. The total body fat (essential and non-essential fat) for optimal health is 10-25% of the body weight for a normal adult male and 18-30% of the body weight for a healthy adult female.

Distribution of fat in the body is referred to as adiposity. It is different for both men and women and is controlled genetically.

- Excess of subcutaneous truncal fat (abdominal fat) is called android fat distribution and the resultant body structure is "apple shaped", common in men.
- Excess of gluteo-femoral fat (hip-thigh fat) is called gynoid fat distribution and the resultant body structure is "pear shaped", common in women. After menopause women are at risk of android fat.

2.2 AETIOLOGY OF OBESITY

Genetic (biological), behavioural and environmental factors are responsible for obesity. It is interplay of both involving variables.

Genetic factors: It influences 80-90% a person's chance of becoming obese, if both the parents are obese. Mutation in the human receptor gene for B3 in adipose tissue increases the chances of obesity. The genes influencing obesity are ASIP, CPE, LEP, LEPR, TUB and POMC in mammals.

Age and sex: These are not compulsory factors for obesity as there is no age for obesity and in either sex. Studies conducted at Nutrition Foundation of India have shown that females have greater chances of becoming overweight than males.

Tryptophan deficiency: Tryptophan is an essential amino acid, that is, it cannot be synthesized by our body, it must be taken in diet. Serotonin is formed by combination of tryptophan with tryptophan hydroxylase, i.e., tryptophan is the precursor of serotonin. Low intake of tryptophan in diet can lead to decrease in levels of serotonin. This further leads to hunger and increased intake of carbohydrates.

Eating habits: Poor eating habits can lead to obesity.

- Non-inclusion of fruits and green leafy vegetables in diet.
- Consuming sugar or sugar added beverages every day.
- Business meetings in which lunches and dinners are a practice
- Habit of overeating.
- Frequent consumption of food outside home increases chances of becoming obese as these foods are usually high in calories.
- Due to busy schedule or tight jobs force people to rely on precooked or instant mixes and processed foods which are high in calories.
- Personnel who work in different shifts, whose body clock is disturbed, may overeat.
- Nibbling between meals is a potential cause of obesity which is commonly seen in housewives.
- Those people who have habit of eating fast tend to consume more food.

Physical activity: People who lead sedentary life are prone to obesity because they have positive energy balance as input of energy is more than the expenditure. Though there is no age for obesity but it is more common in middle age when the person is less active but the relative consumption of food has still not decreased. Obesity can also be seen in scholars who have the habit of studying more than playing, who do not participate in school games and who use vehicles for commuting.

Stress: It is seen that people who are under stress, anxiety, depression, pain, gratification take more calories as food is one of the many stimulants of endorphin, "feel good" neurotransmitter. According to a study, children consume more fatty foods and empty calories as their life is more stressful. Deprivation of sleep can also increase the appetite.

Endocrine factor: Obesity is associated with hypothyroidism, diabetes, hypogonodism, PCOD (polycystic ovaries) and Cushing's syndrome. Obese people have low metabolism generally due to genetics and hormonal disbalance. The metabolism is generated by our endocrine glands. Any difficulty in their functioning directly affects our metabolism, for example, failure of anterior pituitary gland to secrete hormone is the cause for juvenile obesity while over secretion of adrenal gland is the cause of Cushing's syndrome–in this fat is usually deposited on the trunk leading to obesity. Decrease in the secretion of thyroid gland causes hypothyroidism, metabolism slows down causing obesity. Obesity is common at puberty, pregnancy and menopause.

Trauma: Damage to hypothalamus after head injury can lead to obesity as it is not able to regulate appetite, hunger or satiety.

2.3 ASSESSMENT OF OBESITY

Recently relative weight has become the most popular and convenient obesity indicator. "Relative obesity" is calculated by dividing an actual weight by ideal weight according to an individual's height, age and sex. A relative weight is more than 20 per cent or more than the average weight. The most common clinical tool to define obesity is increase in body weight that has been used since years. The Metropolitan Life Insurance company in 1959 developed a tool based on body weight for height standards. It is still being used, although it is not an accurate measure of obesity. Therefore, height-weight tool is very popular till now also. The doctors generally used these height weight tools that was before 1980 and it was different for males and females. The table indicated weight prescription for age group which changed with increase in the inches of height. Now the tables used only show the weight parameter rather than the body composition in detail.

Discovery of body mass index (BMI): In 1832 a Belgian statistician named Adolphe Quetelet came up with the Quetelet Index of Obesity, which measured obesity by dividing a person's weight (in kilograms) by the square of his or her height (in metres). BMI since long is said to be an international standard for obesity dimension. Body mass index closely relates to the grades of obesity, while height and weight prediction could not explain the degree of obesity in a patient. A BMI range of 25 to 29.9 is well thought out to be said as obese. The International Obesity Task Force (2002) proposed a different classification of obesity for Asians.

Table 2.2: IOTF – proposed classification of BMI

BMI kg/m^2	Classification
< 18.5	Under weight
18.5 – 22.9	Normal weight
23.0 – 24.9	At risk for obese
25.0 – 29.9	Obese I
> 30	Obese II

*Table taken from mentioned in my thesis

There is a separate category for grades of obesity as grade I,II, III and the range is between 30-40 kg/m^2. The morbid obese person BMI is more than 40 kg/m^2.

In general obesity can be arranged as upper truncal obesity and lower truncal obesity otherwise called 'apple shaped obesity' and 'pear shaped obesity', individually. There is high pervasiveness rate of coronary illness (CHD) in every single hefty individual whose weight record (BMI) are >25

Android obesity: Android is a type of obesity which is compared to the state of an apple. The shoulders, face, arms, neck, chest and upper bit of the stomach area are enlarged. The stomach and lower body (legs, thighs, hips, stomach) give a more solid appearance when compared to the proportions of the upper body. Although most common in males, it's also sometimes seen in females too, especially during the age of menopause or in cases of any hormonal imbalances.

Gynoid obesity: In this sort the lower portion of the body has the additional fats. This sort of obesity is additionally basic to both genders, however, females are more prone to it. Gynoid kind of obesity is like pears. The substance is to some degree fat in the mid-region, thighs, backside and legs. The face and neck generally give a typical appearance. In certain people, the cheeks might be drawn as well. As these people get old their body gets a stooping stance and the spine is never erect because of the substantial weight of hips and thighs. The essential organs influenced for the most part are the kidneys, uterus, digestive tracts, bladder and bowls. In some individuals, however, they may not show either of the two types of obesity but their entire body may have equal and excess fat distribution.

On the basis of body composition

Our entire body is mainly divided into two important components: body fat and fat-free mass. The fat is usually stored inside muscle tissues, and is known as subcutaneous fat, or around organs (instinctive fat). Some fat is essential for general well being. It is called essential fat and secures the inner organs, stores fuel for vitality, and manages imperative body hormones.

Waist circumference: Waist circumference is another parameter to measure Obesity. It basically estimates the amount of fat deposited around waistline. Waist circumference is the extent that counts the quantity of plump fat within the skin and contained by the abdominal area. In men the waist circumferences greater than 102 centimetres (40 inches) and in women it should be greater than 88 centimetres (35 inches).

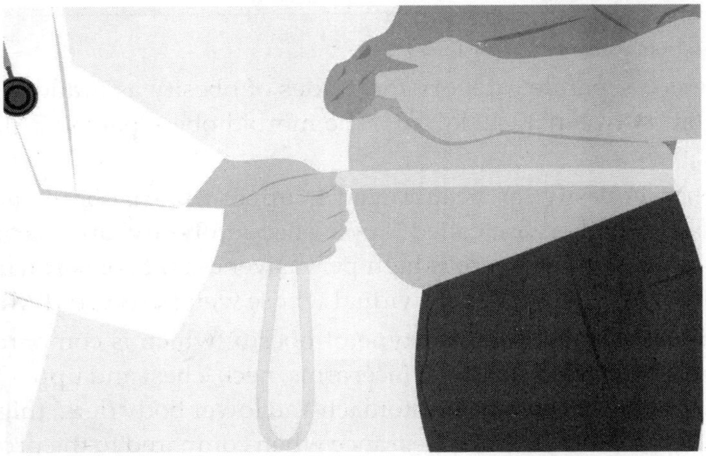

Waist -hip ratio: This is also calculated to measure obesity. If it is greater than 1 then it's a dangerous situation in men and same is the case with women if it is greater than 0.85, such individuals are more prone to metabolic diseases.

Skinfold thickness: The prime location of fat deposition is beneath one's skin so skinfold thickness measurement can guide us regarding the fat accumulated in the abdomen, highs, arms, etc. Therefore, the skinfold thickness is measured from four parts, i.e., triceps, biceps, subscapular and suprailiac regions. The thickness which is more than 80 cm is categorized as obese.

2.3.1 Assessment for Children

2.3.1.1 Head and Chest Circumference

During the infancy period the head size is proportional to brain size and is seen as rapid development of brain. Hence, this method is mostly used to detect any malnutrition (PEM, obesity, etc.) amongst children. Expanded head is the point at which the deliberate separation around the most largest part of the skull is bigger than anticipated for the kid's age and foundation.

An infant's head is normally around 2 cm bigger than the chest. Between a half year and 2 years, the two estimations are about equivalent. Following 2 years, the chest measure increases. Flexible fibreglass is used for measurement.

Head circumference is measured using the tape around the head over the supraorbital ridges of the frontal bone in front and the most protruding point of the occiput on the back of the head.

2.3.2 Dietary Assessment

Dietary assessment indicates relative dietary inadequacies, which is helpful in planning health education activities, assessing an individual's dietary pattern, making any necessary lifestyle or dietary changes, etc. The evaluation of dietary admission in youngsters audits past dietary admission, analyzes factors influencing current admission, decides macronutrient and micronutrient prerequisites and the capacity to meet them, and recognizes dangers for healthful issues. Key regions that ought to be investigated incorporate the accompanying: craving, articulation of appetite, and fullness after a meal

2.4 COMPLICATIONS DURING OBESITY

2.4.1 Cardiovascular Disorder/Hyperlipidemia

Obese people with BMI 30 or higher are prone to not only atherosclerosis but they also develop hypertension and incidences of varicose veins. More than one lakh excess cases of CHD can be attributed to increased obesity burden. Excess body fat and abdominal obesity lead to development of CHD in Asian Indian adults. Obesity and coronary heart diseases often coexist. Insulin resistance and hyperinsulinemia are associated with all types of heart diseases. The disorders of obesity to coronary artery diseases are directly proportional as the BMI increases so the lipid levels in human body.

2.4.2 Sleep Apnea

While sleeping a transitory cessation in breathing is increasingly identified in obese children and adolescents.

2.4.3 Physical Disabilities/Stress and Strain on Joints

Due to excess weight load on the body and inner organs obese people suffer from various physical disabilities. The bone joints in lower extremities carry extra load in obese people and it leads to complications such as arthritis, gout or pain in joints. The extra load around stomach put a load on spinal cord and pain in lower back is also common due to obesity.

2.4.4 Osteoarthritis

It is caused due to excess weight on joints. It is a degenerative disease of weight bearing joints leading to various disabilities. In middle aged women the most affected joint are the knees. It is a kind of arthritis which is characterised by the breakdown of cartilage which is the flexible but tough connective tissue that covers the ends of the bones at joints. The arthritis is almost an irreversible degenerative disorder which deteriorates joints to extreme levels as well.

2.4.5 Metabolic Disorders

In simple obesity insulin resistance is found specially in muscles and there is hyperinsulinemia because of impaired insulin uptake by receptors in target tissues. Gall stones are commonly formed in obese individuals due to high plasma cholesterol. Atherosclerosis develops in the presence of excess cholesterol levels in plasma leading to intima of arteries. Gout (uric acid) is common in obese people.

2.4.6 Obstetrical risks

Obese women during pregnancy have greater chances of obstetrical risk because of hypertension, diabetes and post-partum infection. Restriction of weight gain in these women causes complications during pregnancy.

2.4.7 Cancer

Certain cancers like colon, rectum and prostate in men; uterus, biliary tract, breast and ovary in women, digestive tract diseases like gallstones, reflux, esophagitis and skin disorders are more common in obese people. There are many reasons for the development of cancer due to obesity. The fat tissue deposited in the body has an adverse effect on the body. The fat tissue produces excess amount of oestrogen which is dangerous and is linked with the development of breast, endometrial and other cancers. The insulin resistance or hyperinsulinemia is also a reason which promotes tumor. The development of breast cancer is more in women who have more fat percentage and this condition is more prevalent in post-menstrual stage. The menopause hormone therapy is necessary for the women to avoid the risk of developing cancers. In women the other type of cancer is endometrial cancer which is the cancer of lining of uterus. The obese and overweight women are more prone to endometrial cancer due to high level of estrogen production by fat tissues present excessively in them. Thus, two measures are abdominal fat, waist-hip ratio or waist circumference is predictor of colon cancer. An obese individual is two times more likely to develop esophageal cancer than a healthy person.

2.4.8 Gastrointestinal Disturbances

Obesity is associated with increased risk for gastro-esophageal reflux disease (GERD) symptoms such as erosion esophagitis. These include increased incidences of hiatal hernia as well as abdominal wall hernias and gall bladder diseases. Obese people have higher output of cholesterol in the bile. So their bile is constantly in danger of forming gall stones.

2.4.9 Gall Bladder Disease

The solid material often gets deposited in the gall bladder. It is in the form of clumps and is mostly made up of cholesterol and bilirubin. There could be symptoms such as pain, nausea, vomiting and indigestion. These symptoms together indicate the presence of symptomatic gall stones and sometimes there are no symptoms and are called asymptomatic or silent gall stones. These stones cause excessive pain in the gall bladder when they get stuck in the bile duct. Bile is the fluid made by the liver and secreted by gall bladder in small intestine for the purpose of digestion. Through the liver the bile also helps to eliminate excess cholesterol from the body. The excess cholesterol is excreted out of the body along with the bile. The three most common causes of gall stones development are: when bile becomes saturated by cholesterol which means more fat is present than it can be digested by the bile leading to the formation of residues of cholesterol left in the bile. The second reason is imbalance of proteins in human body and cholesterol crystallization. The last reason is decrease in secretion of bile for fat digestion due to loss of contractions of the gall bladder. Since the gall stones are generally made of cholesterol hence it can be concluded that if the person is obese then obviously his high cholesterol level leads to formation of gall stones.

2.4.10 Polycystic Ovarian Disease

The female body produces hormones like estrogen, progesterone, gonadotropin, follicle stimulating hormone and luteinizing hormone along with these hormone androgens is also produced but in small amount. When the levels of androgen increase to a greater extent in females this leads to PCOD or PCOS. In PCOS there is excess facial hair and body hair, irregular menstruation, acne, heavy periods, dark and velvety skin. Obesity sleep apnea, heart diseases, diabetes, mood swings and endometrial cancer are among the associated conditions of PCOS. The most common cause of PCOD is the role of obesity. The excess of adipose tissue in obese women creates a condition where both androgen and oestrogen are in excess which leads to inhibition of follicle stimulating hormone by negative feedback of estrogen.

2.4.11 Respiratory Disorders

Obesity is considered to be one of the causes of respiratory disorders like dyspnea, obstructive sleep apnea, chronic obstructive pulmonary disease, asthma and aspiration related pneumonia. The increase in fat causes physical exertion in patients which causes breathlessness. The obesity has unconstructive physiologic possessions on the lungs which acts as burden and causes inflammation. The increased weight is the cause of decreasing lung volumes and problems in breathing arise. The elevated BMI lowers forced expiratory volume, forced vital capacity, decrease in residual volume and total lung capacity.

2.4.12 Chronic Obstructive Pulmonary Disease

Sedentary lifestyle and increased pollution brought about by industrialization pose major challenges for prevention of both obesity and chronic respiratory diseases such as chronic respiratory diseases such as chronic obstructive pulmonary disease (copd), asthma and obstructive sleep apnea.

Prevention of COPD is directly proportional to reduction of obesity and hence the lung function is improved. Increased levels of systemic inflammation had been earlier reported in relation to excessive fat mass in COPD patients. Interleukin (IL)-6 and leptin plasma levels are very rapidly increased in obese Individuals. Diet is already linked to improve the ill effects of COPD. The factors influencing COPD are the lack of oxygen in tissues, atrophy, changes in basic metabolism and caloric intake, the process of cell degeneration with old age, faulty dietary habits and malnutrition. One research showed that the hormone leptin elevates in obesity as fat cells are more in body and it has direct link in developing asthma in such patients.

The weight loss strategies can definitely be helpful in letting go the respiratory problems. Many patients report a positive change in their lifestyle and respiration after losing weight. They reported that they can walk and exercise more comfortable after achieving weight loss. It is very obvious that when body does not have to carry extra load and make extra efforts for the movement, the respiratory system also works more effectively.

2.5 MANAGEMENT OF OBESITY

2.5.1 Treatment

Obesity requires long-term treatment as it is a chronic disease. Even a 5% to 10% loss from initial weight reduces the comorbidities of obesity thus improving diabetes, dyslipidemia and even sleep apnea. The problem with the weight management is not losing it but maintaining that weight is the challenge in obesity.

- Strategies for management of obesity are:
    1. Diet therapy
    2. Physical exercise
    3. Stress management
    4. Pharmaco therapy
    5. Behaviour therapy
    6. Weight loss surgery

Apart from these strategies it is very important to maintain the lost weight for long this is where weight maintenance programme comes into play. It is the most important part of any weight management programme.

The goals of treatment are:

- To bring about a slow and steady weight loss.
- To maintain a good nutritional status.
- To bring about lifestyle modifications so as to maintain desirable body weight.
- To maintain the weight loss.

To achieve these dietary modifications need to be made suitably.

2.5.2 Diet Therapy

Very low calorie diet <800 kcal: Much weight is initially lost on very low calorie diets, more weight is usually regained. Rapid weight reduction does not teach behavioural changes. A very low calorie diet leads to increased risk for developing gallstones. Very low calorie diets (400 to 800 kcal/day) can be safe in extreme obese individuals (>50% overweight) when under the care of physician and registered dietician.

Reducing diet: The beginners for weight loss therapy should focus on the reduction of 10% calories per day. And after following this diet for three months at least further reduction of calories should be carried out. The person enters in negative energy balance by reduction of 500-1000 calories per day as per RDA. An ideal reduction of 500 grams to 1 kg per week is approved and is safe. Due to utilization of carbohydrate and water store in body usually 3 kg are lost in first 3 months; this loss should not be misunderstood with the loss of body fat. The calories reduction in diet should provide adequate amount of protein, vitamins and minerals as they also play an important role.

2.5.2.1 Energy

The equation of weight loss is a 1000 kcal deficit equals 1 kg body weight per week and reduction of 500 kcal per day for week reduces ½ kg per week.

1 g fat = 9 kcal

1 g body fat = 7.7 kcal

Therefore, 500 g body fat = 500 x 7.7 = 3850 kcal

According to this per day reduction in calories should be : 3850/7 = 550 kcal for reducing ½ kg per week and for 1 kg approximately 1000 kcal should be reduced per day from the RDA.

There should be not drastic or complete reduction in energy as it leads to hunger, frustration, weakness, eating disorder, inadequacy of other nutrients and nervous exhaustion.

Energy requirements

Table 2.3: ICMR, recommended dietary allowances

Activity	Energy requirements (kcal/kg ideal weight/day)		
	Obese	Normal	Underweight
Sedentary	20–25	30	35
Moderate	30	35	40
Heavy	35	40	45–50

2.5.2.2 Protein

Protein intake is higher than normal as it helps in maintaining a good nutritional status and gives satiety. 0.8–1 g/kg/day is given. Approximately 20% of energy should be from protein. It is important for tissue repair and for specific dynamic action. High biological value proteins should be given including milk, eggs, whole pulses and lean meats.

2.5.2.3 Fats

Low to no fat diet should be given to reduce the calorific value of the food. 20% or less of the total energy should be from fats. Emphasis must be on unsaturated fats. Some amount of fat is important to make the food palatable and acceptable. However, foods rich in fats like nuts and oil seeds should be strictly avoided and fried foods must be restricted. Skim milk should be the preference.

2.5.2.4 Carbohydrates

Approximately 60% of the energy should be from carbohydrates. Complex carbs should be preferred such as starches and dietary fibres. Simple carbohydrates should be restricted like sugar as it gives empty calories. Foods rich in carbohydrate content like potatoes and rice are restricted. Fruits rich in carbohydrates like banana should be avoided.

2.5.2.5 Vitamins

Due to reduction in fats it is possible that the fat-soluble vitamins which are A, D, E, K may not be absorbed therefore supplementation of vitamin A and D may be needed for proper functioning of the body. Fruits should be included in ample amounts in diet. Vitamin C should be taken as it converts cholesterol into cholic acid which is excreted through urine. Intake of 200-300 mg ascorbic acid per day reduces cholesterol.

2.5.2.6 Minerals

Calcium should be increased as researches suggest that calcium-rich diet helps in keeping a check on weight and may reduce overall levels of body fat specially in women. Sodium (as common salt) intake should be reduced as it is helpful in weight reduction, excess intake of salt predisposes to retention of fluid.

2.5.2.7 Fluid

Intake should be increased to keep the body hydrated and full. Water should be consumed before meals as it gives early satiety, reducing the portion size.

2.5.2.8 High fibre

High fibre diet is preferred as:

- It is low in calories
- Provides sufficient amounts of vitamins and minerals
- Gives feeling of fullness
- Reduces blood cholesterol
- Automatically cuts down fat and calories
- Gives early satiety

British Nutrition Foundation has proved that intake of high fibre diet is the best way of reducing weight without side effects. It is the least expensive and least torturous way than medical treatment for weight loss.

Glycemic index: Low GI foods should be given. They may benefit in controlling weight in two ways

- By promoting early fullness.
- By promoting fat oxidation with the help of stored carbs.

When high GI foots are consumed, rise in glucose and insulin concentration increase carbohydrate oxidation through rate limiting enzymes.

2.5.2.9 Diet and feeding pattern

- High protein foods, fibrous fruits and vegetables, whole grains, cereals and pulses should be given for satiety and cut down food intake.
- Salt should be restricted.
- Fluid intake to be increased either in the form of drinking water or beverages, sweetened beverages to be restricted.
- Bulking agents like Isabgole or psyllium husk may be used as they are harmless and provide bulk to the food.
- High fat foods like chocolates, ice cream, cheese, butter, samosa, mathris, parantha, poori, potato chips, pastries, etc., should be restricted.
- Alcohol may be permitted in limited amount but the amount should be adjusted according to the total calories. Each gramme of alcohol provides 7 kcal.
- High carbohydrate foods such as bakery products or starchy products as rice, potatoes, sweet potatoes, jams, jelly, marmalades, honey etc should be restricted.
- To reduce the intake of food serving size can be reduced, small size plates can be used.
- Small and frequent meals should be given. No meal should be skipped.
- Feasting should be avoided specially at the time of festival and while attending parties.
- Red meat should be avoided. Fatty portions of chicken should be discarded.
- Cooking methods should be modified, boiling, poaching, steaming, pressure cooking with no added fat should be used as a method for cooking.

Criteria for weight reducing diets

- Deficiency in energy (hypo calorie)

- Adequacy in other nutrients (protein, vitamins, minerals, water)
- Sufficient bulk for satiety
- Easy to cook
- Easy to follow when eating out
- Time effective
- Cost effective
- According to the nature of eating
- Must modify dietary behaviour

2.5.3 Physical Exercise

Low calorie diet with moderate level of exercise is effective in losing weight. The problem with obese people is that they lead sedentary life which makes them lethargic; many adults do not want to exercise due to this reason. Their level of fitness is so low that they cannot sustain moderate level of exercise intensity for very long. However, this will change as one continues to exercise regularly. Aerobic exercise increases energy expenditure and is ideal for weight loss and long term weight maintenance. Exercising not only helps reducing body fat but also preserves lean body mass and partially prevents the decrease in basal energy expenditure. It helps to regulate appetite, increase BMR and reduces set point level. Physical activity in over weight and obese people improves cardio respiratory fitness. Best exercise for an obese person is walking.

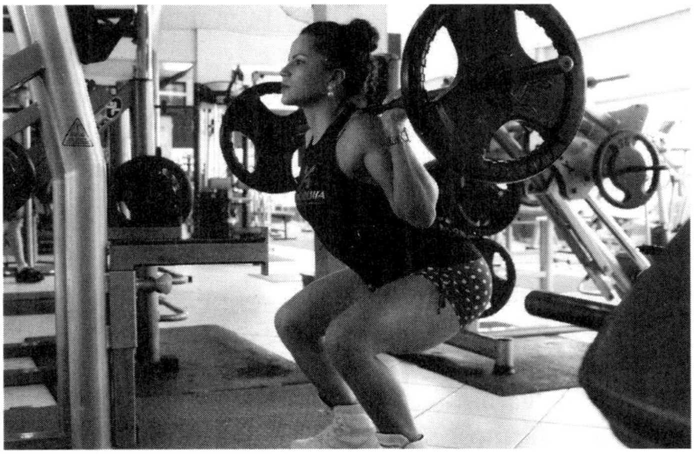

2.5.4 Stress Management

Many patients have reported that the reason for their obesity is stress related overeating. In the treatment of obesity it is very important to manage stress as it is the major reason for relapse and overeating. People should be taught how to deal and reduce stress. Most common methods include meditation, listening to their favourite music, deep breathing, deep muscle relaxation, physical exercise and outdoor playing. These techniques provide a distraction to the stressful event.

2.5.5 Pharmacotherapy

Drug therapy may also be used for weight loss along with diet and physical exercise for patients with BMI 30 and with no concomitant comorbidities or complications. These drugs should be given along with lifestyle modification. Continual assessment of drug therapy for safety is necessary. New drugs like sibutramine and orlistat combined with phentermine are given by health assistants for weight management but these drugs have side effects too. Orlistat inhibits digestion of fat by 30% and also reduces absorption of some fat soluble vitamins therefore it becomes necessary for the patients to take vitamin supplements. Most commonly observed adverse events are faecal urgency, oily evacuation and increased defecation. While sibutramine enhances satiety and increases thrombogenesis, improves lipid profile and increases energy expenditure. Side effects include lethargy, constipation, nausea, insomnia. It should only be used with combination with reduced diet. The medications should only be followed under medical supervision.

2.5.6 Behaviour therapy

Changes in eating behaviour are required to maintain long term weight loss. Menu planning and planning exercise schedules should be taught to the patients. Actual behaviour record should be maintained. This therapy not only helps in behaviour change but also helps to provider to make specific suggestions for problem solving. Stress management along with behaviour management helps in both losing and maintaining weight.

2.5.7 Surgery

For patients with Grade III obesity (BMI is >40) which makes it very difficult for them to lose weight, bariatric surgery remains the only option. Patients with BMI between 35-40 range are also considered for the bariatric surgery.Surgery uses various surgical interventions for the treatment of obesity out of which the most common is to reduce the volume of stomach using gastric bypass and gastroplastry. This reduces the capacity of the stomach to as little as 30 mL. It is beneficial for early satiety, in turn, reducing the food intake. Approximately 65% of excess weight is lost within 5 years of bariatric surgery and most complications resolves in about 80% of the cases.

Weight loss is drastic as compared to other medical treatments. Vomiting is the common risk and the patients are at risk of nutritional deficiencies and dumping syndrome. Excess fat from the skin is removed using plastic surgery only to the individuals who have isolated deposits of fat in abdomen and thigh areas but the root cause of the obesity is not treated. For these patients it is necessary for them to have social support. Continuous contact with the therapist, involvement of the family and friends is very helpful in achieving the goal. Most successful programmes employ a multidisciplinary approach to weight loss along with hypocaloric diet, behaviour modification, aerobic exercise, pharmacological therapy and social support.

2.6 RECENT TRENDS IN DIETS OF OBESITY

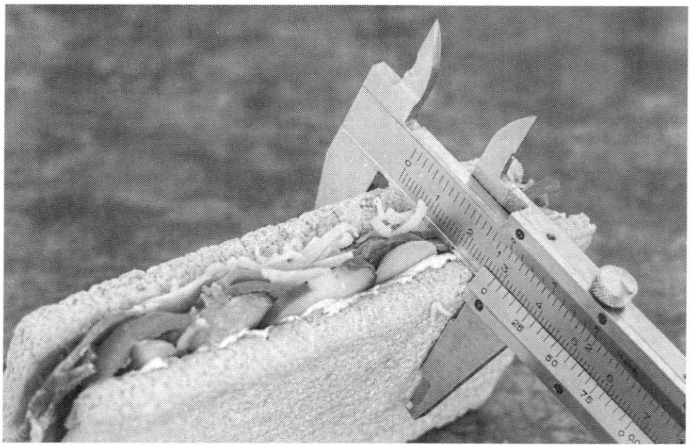

2.6.1 Hypocaloric Diets

Generally, one of the most used and effective diet therapy plans to treat obese patients are the hypocaloric diets. These diets are of various types, starting from reducing the regular diet intake from around 500 calories to as high as 1000 calories less than the normal intake limit.

The diets are planned on a customized pattern and vary from person to person. The diets in which 500 kcals are reduced can decrease the weight by around 0.5 kg/week and diets which are 1000 kcal less than the normal can reduce as much as 1 kg/week. The diets have a lot of worldwide popularity depending on their types. Some of them are protein rich, others are solely dependent on the fat intake. But they are most effective when coupled with regular light exercises. There are also various new concepts being integrated into diet planning for the sake of treating and inspiring obese patients. Weight watchers' diet and Ornish diets are a very positive and new approach in the field of treating obesity. People who are practical and are quite passionate about losing weight are the most successful ones. A person who can imbibe the good qualities and control his/her cravings for junk foods(pizza, burgers, momos, chowmeins, pastas, noodles, fried foods and various such other food products made from maida) with strict diet follow-ups and the least number of cheat days in a month; can reach their goal more easily and within a short time. Willpower is an important tool to maintain such a strict diet schedule and physical regime.

2.6.2 Ketogenic Diets

The keto diet is a very popular diet nowadays and it breaks the myths of regular diets followed in weight loss, that is, to follow low carbs and low fat diet. In keto diet there are phases in which we increase the fat content of the diet and making carbohydrates very low in daily diet. The main aim of this diet is to change the metabolic pathway of the body from carbs to ketones by attaining ketosis. Once the carbohydrates are strictly restricted in the diet, the insulin level of the body also lowers as its functioning load decreases. Brain starts supporting ketones as its main foods. Providing high proteins is also a form of keto diet but it reduces the production of ketones. The amount of carbohydrates given are counted to each gramme to be ingested. The cereal intake is almost nil to very low and the vegies with carbohydrate stores are also counted before ingestion. The carbohydrate intake is as low as 50 gm per day but can also be restricted further to 20-30 gm. The ketogenic diets are very disciplined and strict diet regimes are to be followed with availability of only a few selected items in the diet. The food products mainly included in this diet are meat and meat products in boiled or grilled form, cheese, fishes, milk and milk products, nuts and berries. The dietary schedule for ketogenic diets are basically to increase the fats in diet, and proteins are given in moderation with very low carbohydrates or sometimes only a diet with 20 gm of carbs is planned.

If we have to give an explanation for what a ketogenic diet actually is, we can say it is a diet with maximum fat sources, sufficient protein sources and less carbohydrate sources. But there are some parameters you have to consider before starting this diet.

The diet was named so because as a result of this diet there will be increase in the production of ketone bodies in the body. Hence the name, ketogenic diet. Basically, ketone bodies are three molecules that are soluble in water - acetoacetate, beta-hydroxybutyrate and acetone which is a spontaneous breakdown of the former two molecules - and they contain ketone group in them. These are produced by the liver from fatty acids while fasting, or diets with low carbohydrates or as a result of starvation and the many more reasons to add to this list.

Why does liver produce ketone bodies? As a result of all the reasons listed above, liver undergoes intense gluconeogenesis, i.e., producing glucose from sources other than carbohydrates. After this happens, along with the newly formed glucose, the additional uninvited guests, ketone bodies, are also released in to the bloodstream. These ketone bodies are characterized by a specific smell, like that of a fruit or of nail polish remover, which can be identified by the person's breathe.

Now the formulation of ketone bodies happens in a healthier rate of 1 mg/dL in every human being and they are utilized by the extrahepatic tissues. So when the rate overreaches the above-mentioned level, their level in the blood rises - ketonaemia - and then is succeeded by the excretion of ketone bodies through urine called ketonuria. Both these conditions together are defined as ketosis. This ketosis is the desired achievement by being on a ketogenic diet.

Ketogenic diet is primarily used for treating children with epilepsy and sometimes adults with epilepsy. The ketosis effect generated by ketogenic diet is believed to be helpful in controlling the occurrence and severity of seizures in epileptic patients.

2.6.3 Atkins Diet

Basically, this diet restricts carbohydrate sources and influences on high protein intake. It encourages intake of all kinds of rich sources of protein but restricts or discourages the intake of carbohydrate rich foods. It also allows moderate amount of fat because both fats and proteins require more time for getting completely digested. This results in reduction in development of food cravings. The diet is mainly focused towards the intake of food items rich in fibres, lean protein and healthy fats as constituent of daily diet.

The diet is divided into two major stages: induction stage and the balancing stage

In the induction stage the carbohydrate intake is kept as low as 20 gm per day. The regular diet mainly consists of protein rich foods. Next comes the balancing stage, where the intake of carbohydrate sources is increased to around 50 gm per day. It has also been proven by many researches that the people who mainly consumed veg foods rich in plant fats and proteins showed a better result than those who readily consumed non-veg meats and poultries for protein intake. The diet is very helpful and fruitful with respect to weight loss. The diet also has shown to increase HDL cholesterol, blood sugar level and triglycerides. Atkin's diet is solely based on the principle that the body will use the stored amount of fat as energy resource in the absence of carbohydrates and thus help in weight loss.

This diet has been a miracle and helpful in kids with drug-refractory forms of epilepsy, and performs kidney protection functions.

But following Atkin's diet for a longer time period can be dangerous too as it can cause several health-related problems. Constipation is one of the most common physiological problem faced by an individual due to lack of carbohydrates in the diet and hence levels of fibre deteriorate. Higher than normal intake of fats can also lead to increase in the cholesterol level which can lead to cardiac diseases.

2.6.4 The Pritikin Diet

Founder of Pritikin diet was Nathan Pritikin, and the concepts of the diet were revised by his son Robert Pritikin. The grounds on which the foundation of Pritikin diet is laid are food high in fibre and low in fat content. Grains, vegetables and fruits are plant based foods and are high in fibre and low in fats, hence, are given in this diet. Robert focuses more on the calorie density rather than just calories. According to him, the major culprit is not calories but the density with which they are provided. The idea is to focus more on low calorie dense foods. This can be explained more easily by taking the example of broccoli and chocolate chips. One pound each of raw broccoli and chocolate chip contains 130 calories and 2,140 calories respectively. Thus, we need to choose more wisely.

Restricted food groups of this diet include processed food, red meat and alcoholic beverages. Initially just like some other new concepts, this diet was also turned down by many other scientists. But, eventually with time, its concepts are used extensively to cure many nutrition related ailments. Diet is categorised under fad diets. Just like any other thing, it has both advantages and disadvantages. Disadvantages include very less availability of options, excessive hunger and flatulence.

2.6.5 The Ornish Diet

The basic concept of this diet is to eat vegetarian food items which include fruits, vegetables, whole grains and cut down intake of refined carbohydrates, protein sources which comes from animals and fats. It is mainly used by the cardiac patients to fight against chronic and acute heart diseases. But is also useful in weight loss.

Ornish diet aims for the psychological factors along with the diet which makes it helpful in obesity. A person is asked to go through simple yoga plans or meditation while following Ornish diet. Some of the training exercises such as stretching and resistance exercises are also commonly followed with this diet. With increase in the consumption of fruits, vegetables and fibre rich food items and decreasing refined flour in one's diet, the food intake is lowered. Since satiety value of fibre rich food items is much higher, so it takes much more time for their emptying.

This diet hardly has any side effects, since it cuts around all the unhealthy food products from the food items but not taking animal protein can reduce the micronutrient and vitamin levels in the body.

2.6.6 The Mediterranean Diet

Mediterranean diet is known as one of the most healthy diets or we can say that it is healthy as a biological process in which the food is consumed rather than taking it as a diet inside the regular sense of the word. This kind of diet is found in the countries surrounded by the Mediterranean sea. There is a researcher named Francesco Visioli who wrote two books on the topic which brings the title of"Mediterranean diet". From various reports it was found that people whose eating regime was in accordance to the Mediterranean diet have seen significant reduction in the risk of diabetes, cardiovascular, neuro-degenerative, malignant growth ailments and even death. This diet also helped in increased weight loss in contrast with other diets.

People in Mediterranean countries (particularly Italy and Spain) have found that close-by adherence to a standard Mediterranean eating routine is connected with lower weight and a lower weight record. Despite having very few records of diet's claim of weight reduction, are search group at the Harvard School of Public Wellbeing in 2007, reported that a Mediterranean diet is a suitable method to manage weight for certain people.

A critical clarification behind its practicality is the wide arrangement of wonderful substances permitted on the eating routine along with ethnic recipes. These substances make it easier and dynamically simple for people to stay on the eating routine for broad stretches of time.

The Mediterranean diet is a demonstrated type/form of this classic dietary pattern. The main thing to focus on is described "daily physical activity" along with the consumption of food having four coverings on a regular basis over it.

The other food stuffs like poultry, fish, eggs and sweets are taken in another segment of the pattern. Like for example; these are the foods that can be eaten in a week or on weekly basis.

The red meat among all the foodstuffs is placed on the very top of the pattern of Mediterranean diet because it is not allowed to be eaten more than once in a month.

Another important point that is included in the Mediterranean diet is the increased levels of breads, whole grains and other cereals, various fruits and vegetables including the green vegetables, beans, potatoes, nuts and seeds.

2.6.7 Paleo Diet

Paleo diet is one such diet that has a direct link to our history. Because this diet is derived from our very own Paleolithic era. This particular age was long enough to continue from 2.6 million years ago to 12,000 years ago. This was similar to the Pleistocene epoch. We can say that this specific geographic dimension had many radical changes that made an important impact on the human social aspects.

In this age, there was formation of tools made from stones. All the hominies created small groups of them and started surviving by doing fishing, gathering plants and hunting or scavenging animals.

A time when humans were still using wood and bone tools, Paleolithic age made its distinguished entry by the use of leather and vegetable fibres. But there are only sayings, because of the kind of nature of those materials; those items could not be preserved to any great lengths. By the upper Paleolithic, humankind took a step forward. They developed from the genes of Homo habitis–the members who used simple stone tools and evolved into modern humans in respect to anatomically and behaviourally. And by the end of paleo era, artifacts were formed and one more thing was invented–God. All the blind rituals that are still followed were also started to be practised in this era.

Moving forward with keeping in details of Paleolithic era, this diet was devised to enable resemblance with our very own hunter-gatherer ancestral feeding regime, and basically what they ate all those thousand years ago.

Since, there are no steady resources from all around the world came to the conclusion that they had more of whole foods. The perks of consuming whole food based diet makes one lead a physically active life and also have most probably lower chances of acquiring less of lifestyle diseases and heart diseases, which are very old like obesity, diabetes and heart diseases.

There are claims, that this is a prominent weight loss diet and improves your health.

2.6.7.1 Conclusion

It is the most difficult part when it comes to losing weight as there are many incidences where people regain the weight they actually lost. To avoid this following points should be kept in mind:

- If more weight loss is needed only then any further attempts should be made after 6 months.
- Adjusting to reduce body weight is difficult which increases the chances of regaining weight until a proper weight maintenance programme is followed indefinitely.
- Preventive diets generally supply 1500 to 1800 kcal.
- Weight maintenance programme should always be a combination of diet therapy, physical exercises and behaviour therapy.
- Eat whole grain cereals and legumes and pulses, wheat porridge, wheat bread, oats to integrate fibre in daily diet.
- Salads should be added to daily diet and dressings should be of lemon.
- Polyunsaturated and monounsaturated fatty acids should be a part of daily diet. The oils recommended are olive/ soya bean/ canola/ rice/bran/mustard oil.
- Change in oils should be made so that all fatty acids are provided to the body.
- Avoid full cream or whole milk and use toned/ skimmed milk
- Limit the amount of salt intake and sodium rich foods such as papad/ achaar/chutneys should be less in consumption.

2.6.8 Eating Disorders

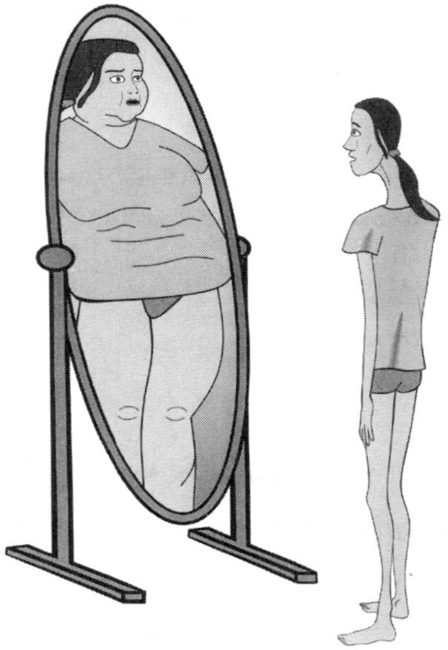

2.6.9 Anorexia Nervosa

Anorexia nervosa is a turmoil which makes eating very troubling. It makes individuals fanatically on edge to keep up or on the other hand lessen their body weight through unbending control of their calorie admission. Individuals with anorexia nervosa regularly have a very misshaped view of what they look like and keep on feeling the need to get more fit in any event, when they are slim to such an extent that their well-being is intensely in danger. They have an exceptional dread of putting on weight and feel that their incentive as an individual is straightforwardly influenced by their body shape.

2.6.9.1 Who has Anorexia Nervosa?

Current appraisals propose that up to 1% of ladies in the UK between the ages of 15 and 30 experience the ill effects of anorexia nervosa. Young ladies under 15 can likewise be influenced and it appears that anorexia nervosa is turning into an expanding issue in these more youthful kids. A few ladies more than 30 likewise have anorexia nervosa, in spite of the fact that the condition by and large first happens sooner than this. 90-95% of individuals with anorexia are ladies, however it is significant to understand that it is a condition which can happen in youngsters as well as ladies. There is likewise proof to recommend that in the more youthful age gathering (7-14 years) up to 25% of cases are young men. It is hard to pass judgment on careful quantities of individuals who have anorexia nervosa the same number of cases are not revealed or not analyzed. A few people experience a considerable lot of the manifestations of the condition yet would not be officially analyzed. This might be on the grounds that their weight has not fallen underneath the level identified by dietary issue specialists (normally 15% beneath 'typical' body weight) or on the grounds that they don't fit the symptomatic models in some other manner.

Individuals with this subtype place extreme limitations on the sum and sort of nourishment they devour. This can show in various manners including a few or the entirety of the accompanying:

- Restricting certain nutritional categories
- Counting calories
- Skipping dinners
- Obsessive guidelines and inflexible reasoning

2.6.9.2 Binge Eating / Purging Subtype

People with this subtype additionally place serious limitation on the sum and kind of nourishment they devour. Notwithstanding this the individual will show cleansing conduct and may likewise take part in voraciously consuming food. Voraciously consuming food includes eating a lot of nourishment and feeling a 'loss of control'.

2.6.9.3 What Causes Anorexia Nervosa?

The name 'anorexia' is confounding as actually it signifies 'loss of craving'. Individuals with anorexia nervosa don't lose their hunger, they despite everything feel hungry, yet dread weight gain such a lot of that they lose the capacity to eat a typical eating regimen. A few people assign anorexia nervosa to media and style and obviously the two of them have their impact. Numerous individuals who don't adjust to the goals introduced by the design business and the media feel that they have to eat less. For certain individuals this presents no issue while for other people, it can transform into anorexia nervosa. The media can likewise sustain issues for individuals who have an eating issue as it is exceptionally hard to split away from consuming less calories cycle in the event that you are continually being given pictures of attractive slim models such a lot of that they lose the capacity to follow a typical eating routine.

Anorexia nervosa can offer them a method for deferring a portion of the physical signs that they are turning out to be ladies. Young ladies with anorexia nervosa don't have such evolved bosoms or hips as different young ladies of their age since they have pretty much nothing muscle to fat ratio. They may likewise defer the beginning of their periods. This can be consoling for young ladies who don't feel prepared for these physical advancements. Individuals who have anorexia nervosa frequently feel that they are underachievers in scholastic or work life. This is normally not the case and proof has indicated that numerous individuals with anorexia nervosa are in truth extremely high achievers. They are, be that as it may, individuals who set themselves guidelines which are essentially difficult to accomplish and leave them with sentiments of insufficiency. For individuals with little confidence, their eating issues may appear to be the main thing about them which is uncommon or unique. Their capacity to feel hungry but decline to eat can feel like an extraordinary ability that the vast majority can't accomplish and can give a genuine feeling of pride. For individuals who have low confidence and who can see for all intents and purposes no other region in their lives where they are effective, this can out of nowhere offer them a feeling of direction. Anorexia nervosa can likewise be a method for adapting to troublesome feelings. The measure of time and vitality spent contemplating nourishment and weight reduction can leave almost no space to manage any different feelings. Anorexia nervosa can hence go about as a sort of defensive boundary against the challenges and enthusiastic weights of regular daily existence. Understand that anorexia nervosa can fulfil a few needs and not to anticipate that somebody should surrender it without having their requirements met in some other manner.

2.6.10 Bulimia Nervosa

Bulimia nervosa, also called basically bulimia, is a dietary issue described by gorging followed by purging. Binge eating alludes to eating a lot of nourishment in a short measure of time.

2.6.10.1 Indications

Bulimia signs and indications may include:

- Being engrossed with your body shape and weight.
- Living in dread of putting on weight.
- Rehashed scenes of eating strangely a lot of nourishment at a time.
- Feeling lost control during gorging – like you can't quit eating or can't control what you eat.
- Driving yourself to regurgitation or practising an excessive amount to shield from putting on weight in the wake of gorging.
- Utilizing intestinal medicines, diuretics or douches in the wake of eating when they're not required.
- Fasting, limiting calories or keeping away from specific nourishments between gorges.
- Utilizing dietary enhancements or home grown items too much for weight reduction.

2.6.10.2 Non-cleansing Bulimia Nervosa

This subtype is substantially less normal, since it just happens in 6-8% of cases. There are individuals who don't depend on heaving or other compensatory strategies for this sort after pigging out. They don't utilize intestinal medicines, oedemas, and so on. Right now bulimia nervosa, the principal strategy used to shed pounds is the presentation of exceptional physical exercise, just as falling back on fasting and eating less junk food. These extensive stretches of starvation are the reason for pigging out once more, as the individual encounters an insatiable yearning that can't rule. Once more, after this gorge scene, the young lady will feel regret and blame, denying herself of nourishment again or doing physical exercise in an over the top way. These techniques for weight control are extremely inadequate in killing the measure of calories expended in a solitary gorge from the body. Extreme physical exercise and consequent fasting likewise normally happens in the laxative subtype of bulimia nervosa, albeit optionally. The results that this subtype of bulimia nervosa creates are considerably less complemented than the laxative subtype.

2.6.10.3 Bulimia Nervosa Laxative

The extraordinary larger part of individuals who present bulimia nervosa are arranged in the laxative sort, which is portrayed by the nearness of retching and utilization of intestinal medicines or douches after voraciously consuming food. The objective of these individuals is to dispose of at the earliest opportunity the most elevated conceivable extent of nourishment ingested, to end the uneasiness that makes them feel that they will put on weight. They likewise present nonsensical musings about the working of the lifeform.

For instance, a few young ladies initially eat a nourishment of a trademark shading, for example, a red tomato, and they demand proceeding to upchuck until the regurgitation is a similar shading (since it was the main nourishment eaten and implies that there is never again nothing in the stomach). This and other totally incorrect data are transmitted day by day through informal organizations and pages about anorexia and bulimia. In spite of the fact that these pages are mistreated and consistently edited, they return with another name and with a similar goal: to transmit data that they think about honest, to make rivalries to see who loses more weight in a brief timeframe, to help each other, and so forth.

Then again, in spite of the fact that this sort of anorexia nervosa has similitudes with a kind of anorexia nervosa-laxative subtype-in this kind of bulimia nervosa the young ladies are not underweight. Actually, in bulimia nervosa-in the two sorts the young ladies are in ordinary weight or have some kind of overweight.

This subtype is the one that creates the best negative impacts, both according to the desolates endured by the lifeform and the practices and musings that appear: It is seen that these young ladies want to be slim, which drives them to get fixated on getting in shape. There is likewise an increasingly genuine real contortion or, what is the equivalent, they see a more noteworthy distinction between their genuine outline and that before the mirror. Also, it is discovered that eating designs are more abnormal than on account of non-cleansing bulimia nervosa. At long last, it is discovered that it is increasingly basic to discover mental clutters related with this subtype, particularly those identified with the state of mind - for example, discouragement-and those that incorporate over the top considerations.

2.6.10.4 Nutritional Management

Energy : The level of energy intake is adjusted to meet individual's weight requirements and if a decrease is required then 2000 kcal should be reduced daily.

Protein: It is advisable that a slightly higher than normal protein should be given as it gives a feeling of satiety and also helps to maintain a good nutritional status. 20% of the total calories should come from protein.

Fat: It should provide only 20% or less of total energy and the maximum fat given should be the unsaturated one.

Carbohydrates: 60% of the total energy should come from carbs and the maximum should be from the complex ones as they are slow to digest and do not raise the blood glucose level. Simple carbs should be taken in a limited amount. Dietary fibre is important to provide bulk and satiety.

Minerals and vitamins: Fruits are vegetables should be amply included in the meals as they provide more of vitamins and minerals and also provide bulk to the diet and relieve constipation.

2.6.10.5 Diet Plan for Bulimia Nervosa

Calories = 1800 cal

Carbs = 300 g

Protein = 90 g

Fat = 40 g

Food exchange		Energy	Carbs	Protein	Fat
Milk	3	510 kcal	36 g	21 g	30 g
Meat	2	160 kcal	-	14 g	12 g
Pulse	2	200 kcal	34 g	14 g	-
Cereals	10	700 kcal	150 g	20 g	-
Veg A	2	40 kcal	7g	2 g	-
Veg B	2	80 kcal	14 g	4 g	-
Fruits	2	45 kcal	10 g	-	-
Fats	1	45 kcal	-	-	5 g
Sugar	2	20 kcal	5 g	-	-
TOTAL		1800 kcal	256 g	75 g	47 g

Meal Pattern							
Food exchange	**Early morning**	**Breakfast**	**Mid morning**	**Lunch**	**Tea time**	**Dinner**	**Post Dinner**
Milk	-	1	-	1	-	-	1
Meat (lean)	-	-	-	-	2	-	-
Pulses	-	-	-	1	-	1	-
Cereals	-	2		3	2	3	-
Veg A	-	1	-	-	-	1	-

Veg B	-	-	-	1	-	1	-
Fruits	1	-	1	-	-	-	-
Fat	-	-	-	½	-	½	-
Sugar	-	1	-	-		-	1

Meal	Food exchanges	Food items	Amount	Menu
Early morning	Fruit	watermelon	303 g	Watermelon
	milk	milk	250 mL	
Breakfast	Cereal	bread	2	Cucumber sandwich with milk
	Veg a	cucumber	140	
Mid morning	fruit	apple	75 g	Apple
	milk	curd	258 g	Roti with curd, dal, rice and lady finger
Lunch	pulse	dal	30 g	
	cereal	rice	19 g	
	veg b	onion	56 g	
	fat	olive oil	5 g	
		roti	2	
	meat	egg	80 g	
Tea Time	cereal	bread	2	Egg sandwich
	pulses	dal	30 g	Roti with bitter gourd, rice and dal
	cereal	roti	2	
Dinner	veg a	bitter gourd	83 g	
	veg b	onion	56 g	
	fat	olive oil	5 g	
		rice	19 g	
Bed Time	milk	milk	250 mL	Milk

CASE STUDIES

1. TO PLAN A PRITKIN DIET FOR A FEMALE MODEL, 25 YEARS OLD

Personal Information

Sex: Female

Age: 25 years old

Lifestyle: Heavy

Guidelines:

- This diet includes fibre rich foods and unprocessed grains.
- Water intake should be higher than normal.
- Includes lots of green vegetables and whole grains.
- Avoid fried foods

Nutritional Requirements

Energy: 2300-2400 kcal

Carbohydrates: 280-300 g/day

Protein: 90-100 g/day

Fats: 40-50 g/day

Food Exchange List

Food exchange	Number of exchanges	Energy (kcal)	Protein (g)	Carbohydrates (g)	Fats (g)
Milk	3	510	24	36	30
Meat/fish	2	105	21	-	1.5
Pulse	4	400	28	68	-
Cereal / Starch	11	770	22	165	-
Vegetable A	4	80	4	14	-
Vegetable B	2	80	4	14	-
Fruit	3	135	-	30	-
Fat	3	135	-	-	15
Sugar	1	20	-	5	-
Total		2235	103	332	46

Food Distribution Table

Exchange	Total no.	Before workout	After workout	Breakfast	Mid-morning	Lunch	Evening (before workout)	Evening (after workout)	Dinner
Milk	3	-	1	1	-	0.5	-	0.5	-
Pulse	2	-	-	-	0.5	1	-	-	0.5
Lean meat	4	-	1	-	-	2	-	-	1
Cereal/ Starch	11	2	2	2	-	3	-	-	2
Veg A	4	-	1	-	-	2	-	-	1
Veg B	2	-	-	-	-	1	-	-	1
Fruit	3	1	-	1	-	-	1	1	-
Fat	3	-	-	1	-	1	-	-	1
Sugar	1	-	-	0.5	-	-	-	-	0.5

Diet Plan

Early morning: Jeera water/lukewarm lemon water with honey along with 8 almonds

Before workout: Banana and 2 slices of toast with fat free nut butter

After workout: Whole wheat bread chicken sandwich and boiled broccoli and plain yogurt

Breakfast: Oats porridge/daliya porridge with small bowl of vegetable upma and an apple

or

Vegetable poha/vegetable stuffed baked pockets along with blueberry smoothie/soyamilk

Mid-morning: Coconut water with sprout salad

Lunch: Sweet potato with black chana salad and 1 bowl of brown rice pulao with chicken and saute mushroom, peas and spinach along with plain yogurt

or

Whole wheat flour chapatti with saute green vegetables and mushroom and peas salad along with yogurt

Evening: Green tea with papaya

Late evening (after workout) : Pumpkin seeds/flaxseeds with an orange

Dinner: Brown rice pulao along with cucumber salad and raita along with stir fry beans and roasted chicken ½ cup

or

1 stuffed whole grain chapatti with big bowl of any dal (boiled) and cucumber

Bed time: 1 glass of toned milk with flaxseeds (2 tsp)

2. TO PLAN AN ORNISH DIET FOR A MAN, 35 YEARS OLD

Personal Information

Sex: Male

Age: 35 years old

Lifestyle: Moderate

Guidelines

- Eat all the beans, legumes, fruits, grains, and vegetables you need to feel full.
- Eat low- or non-fat dairy products such as milk, cheese, and yogurt in moderation. Only 10 per cent of your calories should come from fat.
- Avoid meats (red and white), oils and products containing oils, including avocados, olives, nuts, seeds, full-fat dairy, and sugar.
- Exercise for at least 30 minutes five times a week or 60 minutes three times a week.
- Manage stress with yoga and meditation and by spending time with your loved ones.

Nutritional Requirements

Energy: 2500-2700 kcal

Carbohydrates: 300-390 g/day

Proteins: 100-120 g/day

Fats: 40-50 g/day

Food Exchange List

Food Exchange	Number of Exchanges	Energy (kcal)	Protein (g)	Carbohydrates (g)	Fats (g)
Milk	3	510	24	36	30
Meat/fish	3	105	21	-	1.5
Pulse	4	400	28	68	-
Cereal/starch	15	1050	30	225	-
Vegetable A	4	80	4	14	-
Vegetable B	2	80	4	14	-
Fruit	3	135	-	30	-
Fat	4	180	-	-	20
Sugar	2	40	-	-	-
Total		2580	111	387	51

Food Distribution Table

Exchange	Total no.	After exercise	Breakfast	Mid-morning	Lunch	Evening	Dinner
Milk	3	1	0.5	0.5	-	-	1(bed time)
Meat	3	-	-	-	2	-	1
Pulse	4	-	1	0.5	1	0.5	1
Cereal/ starch	15	-	5	-	4	1	4
Veg A	4	-	1	-	2	-	1
Veg B	2	-	-	-	1	-	1
Fruit	3	1	-	1	-	1	-
Fat	4	-	1	-	1	-	1
Sugar	2	-	1	-	-	1	-

Diet Plan

Early morning: Luke warm water with 4 almonds and 4 wallnuts

Breakfast: Whole grain stuffed chapatti (2) along with yogurt and 1 apple

or

Daliya porridge with fruit salad and 2 slice of whole wheat bread

Mid-morning: Fat free yogurt/clear chicken soup (200 mL)

Lunch: Baked potato stuffed with fat free cheese with spinach and broccoli and fresh fruit with fat free cream and steamed brown rice

Evening: Cinnamon tea/green tea along with roasted chana/puffed rice

Late evening: Salted lassi

Dinner: Egg whites and white chana salad with spinach and mushroom along with peanut Butter multi-grain bread toast and fat free yogurt

3. TO PLAN AN ORNISH DIET FOR A FEMALE, 28 YEARS OLD

Personal Information

Sex: Female

Age: 28 years old

Lifestyle: Moderate

Guidelines

- Eat all the beans, legumes, fruits, grains, and vegetables you need to feel full.

- Eat low- or non-fat dairy products such as milk, cheese, and yogurt in moderation. Only 10 per cent of your calories should come from fat.
- Avoid meats (red and white), oils and products containing oils, including avocados, olives, nuts, seeds, full-fat dairy products and sugar.
- Exercise for at least 30 minutes five times a week or 60 minutes three times a week.
- Manage stress with yoga and meditation and by spending time with your loved ones.

Nutritional Requirement

Energy: 2000-2200 kcal

Carbohydrates: 300-350 g/day

Proteins: 80-90 g/day

Fats: 40-50 g/day

Food Exchange List

Food Exchange	Number of Exchanges	Energy (kcal)	Protein (g)	Carbohydrates (g)	Fats (g)
Milk	3	510	24	36	30
Meat	2	70	14	-	1
Pulse	2	200	14	34	-
Cereal / Starch	14	980	28	210	-
Vegetable A	3	60	3	10.5	-
Vegetable B	2	80	4	14	-
Fruit	2	90	-	20	-
Fat	3	135	-	-	15
Sugar	2	40	-	-	-
Total		2165	87	324	46

Food Distribution Table

Exchange	Total no.	After exercise	Breakfast	Mid-morning	Lunch	Evening	Dinner
Milk	3	1	1	-	-	-	1(bed time)
Meat	2	-	-	-	1	-	1
Pulse	2	-	-	0.5	0.5	-	1
Cereal/ starch	14	-	4	-	5	1	4

Veg A	3	-	-	-	2	-	1
Veg B	2	-	-	-	1	1	-
Fruit	2	1	-	1	-	-	-
Fat	3	-	1	-	1	-	1
Sugar	2	-	1	-	-	1	-

Diet Plan

Early morning :Luke warm water with 5 almonds and 2 wallnuts

After walking : Whole wheat bread (2 slices) with fat free nut butter

Breakfast : Oat-banana smoothie with multi-grain flour pancakes and fat free yogurt

Mid-morning : Papaya with coconut water

Lunch : Chickpea salad with dressing and vegetable stuffed chapatti with dal and fat free curd

Evening : Green tea with handful of makhana

Late evening : Carrot juice

Dinner : Brown rice with baked potato and saute vegetables along with fat free yogurt

Bed time : 1 glass of skim milk with flaxseeds

4. TO PLAN A MEDITERRANEAN DIET FOR A FEMALE, 40 YEARS OLD.

Personal Information

Sex: Female

Age: 40 years old

Lifestyle: Sedentary

Guidelines

- Eat natural foods like fruits, vegetables, whole grains and nuts
- Make olive oil your primary source of dietary fat
- Reduce the consumption of red meat
- Eat little or moderate amount of fish and white meat (weekly)

Nutritional Requirements

Energy: 2000 kcal

Carbohydrates: 220-240 g/day

Proteins: 70-90 g/day

Fats: 30-40 g/day

Food Exchange List

Food Exchange	Number of Exchanges	Energy (kcal)	Protein (g)	Carbohydrates (g)	Fats (g)
Milk	3	510	24	36	30
Meat	2	70	14	-	1
Pulse	2	200	14	34	-
Cereal / Starch	14	980	28	210	-
Vegetable A	3	60	3	10.5	-
Vegetable B	2	80	4	14	-
Fruit	2	90	-	20	-
Fat	3	135	-	-	15
Sugar	2	40	-	-	-
Total		2165	87	324	46

Food Distribution Table

Exchange	Total no.	After exercise	Breakfast	Mid-morning	Lunch	Evening	Dinner
Milk	3	1	1	-	-	-	1 (bedtime)
Meat	2	-	-	-	1	-	1
Pulse	2	-	-	0.5	0.5	-	1
Cereal/ starch	14	-	4	-	5	1	4
Veg A	3	-	-	-	2	-	1
Veg B	2	-	-	-	1	1	-
Fruit	2	1	-	1	-	-	-
Fat	3	-	1	-	1	-	1
Sugar	2	-	1	-	-	1	-

Diet Plan

Early morning: Vegetable sandwich with whole grain bread along with sprout salad and grapes and greek yogurt

Mid-morning: Avocado/apple

Lunch: Sweet potato salad/cucumber salad along with multi-grain aata chapatti and dal along with broccoli

Evening: Pumpkin seeds along with green tea

Late evening: Small bowl of corn chat

Dinner: Brown rice along with stir fried beans and onions along with fat free yogurt

Bed time: 1 glass of skimmed milk with sunflower seeds/flaxseeds.

QUESTIONS

1. Define obesity. Write about its causes and risk factors associated with it.
2. Describe different assessment techniques for obesity.
3. Describe the dietary management of obesity.
4. How is obesity responsible for:
   (i) CHD
   (ii) Cancer
   (iii) PCOD
   (iv) Metabolic disorders
5. Compare Mediterranean diet and Paleo diet.
6. What is ketogenic diet? Plan a ketogenic diet plan for a male obese patient.
7. What are Atkins and Pritkins diets. Describe their similarities and differences.
8. How are chronic obstructive pulmonary disease and obesity related? Kindly describe briefly.
9. What effect does hypocaloric diets have incidences of obesity and also on its management?
10. What is bulimia nervosa? What are its symptoms. Describe its dietary management.
11. Differentiate between bulimia nervosa and anorexia nervosa.
12. Plan a day's diet for 40 years old male of 80 kg weight and height of 160 cm suffering from diabetes mellitus.
13. Write short notes on:
    (i) Atkins diet
    (ii) Pritkin's diet
    (iii) Ketogenic diet
    (iv) Ornish diet

3

Cardiovascular Disorders

3.1 DEFINITION

Cardiovascular disease (CVD), in general, is the diseases of the heart and blood vessels. Mostly seen form of cardiovascular disease is coronary heart disease (CHD) which is caused by atherosclerosis in the arteries (both large and medium sized), which in turn, is responsible for supplying oxygen and nutrients to the muscles of heart. CVDs is a group of diseases or interrelated diseases which include hypertension, atherosclerosis, heart failure (HF), ischemic heart disease and peripheral vascular disease. The partial or total occlusion of the arterial lumen causes atherosclerotic lesions. The cause for angina pectoris (chest pain which is caused by exercise), myocardial infarction (death of the tissues of muscles of the heart) and ischemic death (insufficient supply of blood) are due to the development of cracks and fissures in the lesions, which in turn, leads to thrombosis.

Cardiovascular disorders, heart strokes, cancers, these are the most common causes of death in both males and females. Many more people are affected by the heart diseases or heart related problems.

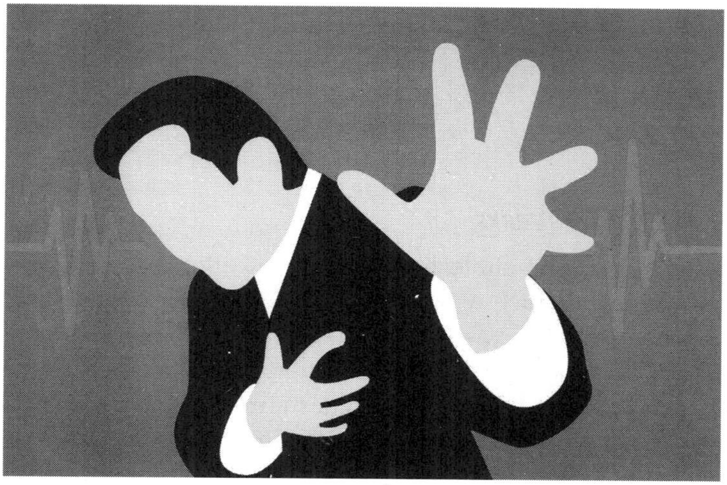

3.2 ATHEROSCLEROSIS

It is the most common reason for many cardiovascular diseases around the world. Atherosclerosis is a type of disorder in which the deposition of fatty plaques are present and accumulated within the arteries. Due to which the walls of the arteries become thicker that leads to slow levels of the blood flow in it. The medium sized arteries which include the coronary, carotid, cerebral arteries and the arteries which supply the blood to the lower limbs like the iliac and the femoral arteries are mainly affected with atherosclerosis.

3.2.1 Stages of Development in Atherosclerotic Lesions

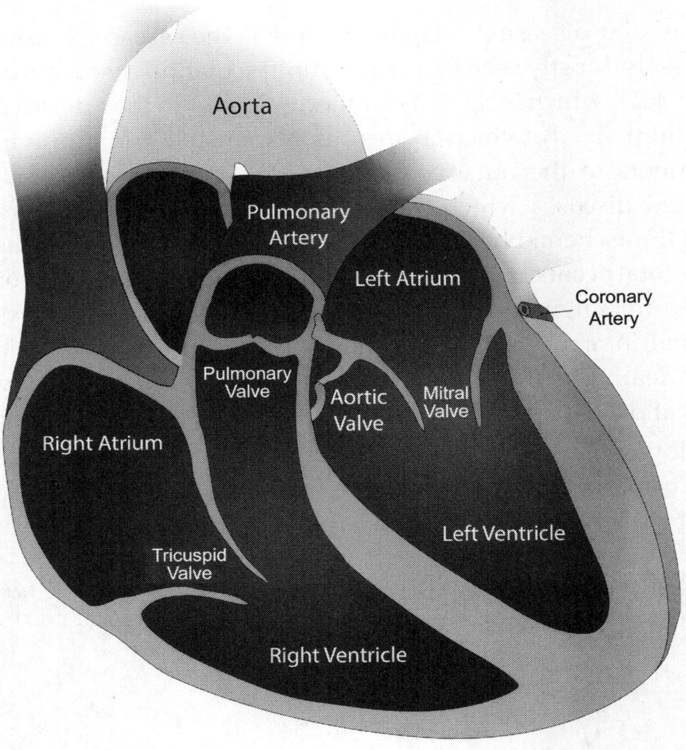

3.2.1.1 Stage I: Fatty streaks

Development of fat and cholesterol leads to swelling of the newly formed connective tissue because of which certain inner membrane which runs longitudinally along the vessels get thickened. Initially, it does not show any symptom. At this stage there are only fatty streaks which do not hinder any activity or function, as there is chronic injury in the arterial endothelium in response to that the macrophages and smooth muscle cells of the artery forms a bend. It is not necessary that all fatty streaks will develop into complicated lesions. Commonly seen in people below 30 years of age.

3.2.1.2 Stage II: Plaque

The layers of plaque combine to destroy the innermost lining which involves the inner medial layer. It can be of two types:

Soft or atheromatous: The lesions which contain more amounts of lipid.

Hard or fibrous plaque: The lesions which contain more amount of fibrous tissue.

This stage contains soft or atheromatous plaque that may get ruptured. High amount of lipid comes from the plasma LDL which enters the injured endothelial wall. At this stage the lesions are unstable.

3.2.1.3 Stage III: Complicated Lesions

There is development of ulcers and some amount of fat gets dissolved in the blood stream due to loss of endothelium. Fibrin gets deposited and thrombosis develops–presence of free blood and calcification. This stage has complicated ruptured lesions and are non-occlusive thrombus. At this stage the lesions are in acute phase.

3.2.1.4 Stage IV

This stage may lead to serious problems like angina or myocardial infarction and in some cases sudden death can also occur.

3.2.1.5 Stage V

At this stage the blood supply is cut off from the lesions.

3.3 ANGINA PECTORIS

It is a type of pain in chest which is caused because of reduced blood flow to the heart. It is a symptom of coronary artery disease and the main reason for angina pectoris is atherosclerosis The term has been taken from a Greek word *at here* which means gruel, because the lesion has a yellow deposition. Its onset starts from the childhood and it usually affects the inner membrane of the elastic and muscular arteries where the lipids like cholesterol, its esters, triglycerides, ceroid, in macrophages and smooth muscle cells there is deposition of calcium, iron, red blood cells and fibrous tissue. The deposition of various substances causes fatty streaks, which during initial stage of childhood is not of much concern as it has only minimal thickening in the inner walls and therefore there is not much obstruction in the flow of the blood but as the adolescence approaches the problem and effect become severe. In the adults of young age, there is deposition of lipids in or around some places, the smooth muscle and fibrous tissue covers the core of lipid and necrotic debris. These symptoms produce fibrous plaques (severe form of lesion) which hinder the flow of blood by projecting into the lumen.

3.4 HYPERLIPIDEMIA/ HYPERLIPOPROTEINEMIA

Traditionally, lipid disorders have been classified in a descriptive typing system, but currently these have been given a functional classification.

Traditional descriptive typing system was proposed by Fredrickson and others.

Classification of traditional descriptive of hyperlipidemia are:

Type I : Chylomicrons elevated, rare condition

Type IIa : LDL elevated, common condition

Type IIb : LDL and VLDL elevated, common condition

Type III : LDL elevated, uncommon condition

Type IV : VLDL elevated, common condition

Type V : LDL and chylomicrons elevated, uncommon condition.

Current functional classification: This approach classifies lipid disorders in four major groups based on the underlying functional problems:

(a) Defects in apolipoprotein synthesis (apolipoprotein is the protein fraction of lipoprotein molecule)

(b) Enzyme deficiencies

(c) LDL, receptors deficiency

(d) Other inherited hyperlipidemias.

(e) These disorders are described in detail and show their corresponding type as given in the descriptive classification. It may be noted that some of the disorders which could not be explained in the earlier traditional classification have now been taken care of in the functional classification.

3.5 CONGESTIVE HEART FAILURE

In the congestive heart failure the heart gets impaired which can be seen with the development of dyspnea (breathing difficulty) due to exertion or weakness or chest pain. The dilation of the heart occurs in severe failure. Impairment is so severe that the circulation to the tissues via kidney could not take place properly which results in the blockage of sodium and water in the tissue spaces. Oedema fluid (the arteries or tissues of the body gets filled with an excess of watery fluid) starts collecting first in the extreme end and as the failure increases it starts collecting in the cavities of abdomen and chest. In chronic CHD, congestive heart failure may develop over a period of time. The heart muscle–myocardium–gets progressively weakened and is not able to maintain normal cardiac output and thus normal circulation. This results in fluids imbalance, which causes oedema especially pulmonary oedema, leading to problems in breathing as well as greater strain on the already weakened heart.

Cardiac oedema: The fluid imbalance resulting in cardiac is caused by three different mechanisms.

Imbalance in capillary fluid shift mechanism: The normal capillary fluid shift mechanism is responsible for maintaining the flow of the fluids of the body. The mechanism fails to operate properly in congestive heart failure. The failing heart is not able to pump out the blood fast, resulting in blood accumulation in the vascular system of the right side of the heart, thus affecting normal circulation. This affects the normal flow of fluids between the tissue space and the blood vessels and instead of the fluid being returned to the circulation, it starts accumulating in the tissue spaces causing oedema.

Hormonal influences: Two hormonal mechanisms, aldosterone and anti-diuretic hormone (ADH) that control water balance in the body also contribute to the cardiac oedema in congestive heart failure. Aldosterone mechanism also called the renin - angiotensin - aldosterone mechanisms, is a sodium and water conserving mechanism. The failing heart is not able to maintain normal cardiac output and thus the blood flow through kidney nephrons is also reduced. This triggers the renin - angiotensin mechanism, which in turn, stimulates the adrenals to secrete aldosterone. Aldosterone hormone causes the tubules of kidney to reabsorb more sodium and water and this results in still more fluid being held in the tissues. The cardiac stress and resulting reduced renal blood flow causes the release of water from the nephrons of the kidney and thus fluid accumulation in the tissues.

Increased free-cell potassium: Reduced blood circulation depresses the cell metabolism resulting in the cell protein breakdown and release of potassium in the cell. Increased amount of intra-cellular free potassium increases the osmotic pressure. In order to balance this increase as well as to prevent cell dehydration, there follows an increase of sodium in the extra- cellular fluid. Excess of sodium eventually causes still more retention.

3.6 MYOCARDIAL INFARCTION (HEART ATTACK) AND HEART STROKE

Myocardial infarction is the starting phase in childhood with the deposition of excess fat present in the blood or the minerals such as calcium, iron or clotting caused by the red blood cells, triglycerides and the fibrous tissues in the macrophages and smooth muscle cells. Myocardial infarction (death of the tissues muscles of the heart) and ischemic death (insufficient supply of blood) are due to the development of the cracks and fissures in the lesions, which in turn, leads to thrombosis.

3.7 CEREBROVASCULAR DISEASE

The word cerebrovascular is made up of two parts – "cerebro" which refers to the large part of the brain, and "vascular" which means arteries and veins. Together, the word cerebrovascular refers to blood flow in the brain. The term cerebrovascular disease includes all disorders in which an area of the brain is temporarily or permanently affected by ischemia or bleeding and one or more of the cerebral blood vessels are involved in the pathological process. Cerebrovascular disease includes stroke, carotid stenosis, vertebral stenosis and intracranial stenosis, aneurysms, and vascular malformations.

Restrictions in blood flow may occur from vessel narrowing (stenosis), clot formation (thrombosis), blockage (embolism) or blood vessel rupture (haemorrhage). Lack of sufficient blood flow (ischemia) affects brain tissues and may cause a stroke.

Because the brain relies on only two sets of major arteries for its blood supply, it is very important that these arteries are healthy. Often, the underlying cause of an ischemic stroke is blocked carotid arteries with a fatty buildup, called plaque. During a haemorrhagic stroke, an artery in or on the surface of the brain ruptures or leaks, causing bleeding and damage in or around the brain.

3.8 PERIPHERAL VASCULAR DISEASE

Peripheral vascular disease (PVD) is a blood circulation disorder that causes the blood vessels outside the heart and brain to narrow, block, or spasm. This can happen in the arteries or veins. PVD typically causes pain and fatigue, often in your legs, and especially during exercise. The pain usually improves with rest. It can also affect the vessels that supply blood and oxygen to your:

- arms,
- stomach, intestines, and
- kidneys.

In PVD, blood vessels become narrowed and blood flow decreases. This can be due to arteriosclerosis, or "hardening of the arteries," or it can be caused by blood vessel spasms. In arteriosclerosis, plaques build up in a vessel and limit the flow of blood and oxygen to your organs and limbs. As plaque growth progresses, clots may develop and completely block the artery. This can lead to organ damage and loss of fingers, toes, or limbs, if left untreated.

Peripheral arterial disease (PAD) develops only in the arteries, which carry oxygen-rich blood away from the heart. According to the CDC, approximately 12 to 20 per cent of people over age 60 develop PAD, about 8.5 million people in the United States. PAD is the most common form of PVD, so the terms are often used to mean the same condition.

PVD is also known as:

- arteriosclerosis obliterans,
- arterial insufficiency of the legs,
- claudication, and
- intermittent claudication.

3.9 AETIOLOGY OF CARDIOVASCULAR DISORDERS

The factors like nutritional and non-nutritional which have been found as the cause of atherosclerosis have different effects in the process of disease.

(a) **Sex:** The men has higher risk of developing coronary heart disease, the death rate is almost three times when it is compared with women. Women are at lower risk with respect to men but once the women reach menopause then the ratio of death rate of men : women becomes narrower.

(b) **Age:** The risk for developing arthrosclerosis or death rate due to arthrosclerosis increases with increase in age and it almost doubles in every 5 years once the person approaches the age above 24 years.

(c) **Heredity:** A person who is born in a family which already has a running history of cardiovascular disease is more likely to develop heart diseases and at an early age. Men are almost 1.5 to 2 times more prone to heart diseases because of running family history of coronary heart disease with respect to men whose family does not have any history of cardiovascular diseases but in case of women the risk of developing heart diseases is less even with a family history.

(d) **Smoking:** Cigarette is one of the leading causes of coronary heart disease. It is mainly made up of nicotine and carbon monoxide both of which are dangerous as they directly affect the heart and blood vessels. Nicotine affects the heartbeat, it puts an intense pressure on the heart muscles to pump blood leading to increase in the heart beat which therefore results in higher demand for oxygen. Carbon monoxide affects the oxygen supply to the heart muscles by blood cells and ultimately stops it. It also affects the consistency of the blood making it thick, which in turn, results into the formation of clots.

(e) **Physical inactivity:** The involvement in physical activity lowers the risk factor for cardiovascular diseases because when a person is engaged in any direct or in direct physical activity the concentration of high density lipoprotein (HDL) cholesterol level increases which has a protective function. Inactivity will lead to several heart diseases.

(f) **Psychosocial factors:** The risk of heart disease increases with the increase in the sense of competitiveness, excessive drive and time urgency and all these factors together constitute a pattern of behaviour termed as Type A behaviour.

(g) **Obesity:** It is primarily one of the major causes of heart diseases. The body mass index (BMI) is directly proportional to the chances of development of coronary heart disease. There are several ways in which the risk of development of coronary heart disease can be predicted such as increased level of cholesterol in the body which is again proportional to body mass index and the distribution of weight, i.e., upper body to lower body ratio; it is also related to how the body tolerates the level of glucose and lipid serum.

(h) **Hypertension:** The risk factor for cardiovascular disease can be lowered with the proper and controlled treatment of high blood pressure. The pressures on the arterial wall worsens the condition of atherosclerosis by fibromuscular thickening.

(i) **Diabetes mellitus:** Another condition which affects the atherosclerotic process is diabetes mellitus and its treatment does not guarantee that it will lower the risk of coronary heart disease. It accelerates the process of atherosclerosis as the count of lipids in the blood increases.

(j) **Hyperhomocysteinemia:** It is mainly a causal factor for early onset of atherosclerosis in the children who have deficiency of cystathionine B synthase which is an enzyme for homocysteine which are catabolically involved in the reaction.

(k) **Thrombogenic or haemostatic factor:** It is related with the plasma fibrinogen and the level of fibrinogen is affected with smoking, high levels of triglycerides, genetic factor and sedentary lifestyle. It plays a major role in the development of heart disease like myocardial infraction and coronary heart disease.

(l) **Inflammatory markers such as C-reactive protein:** It is one of the several causes of the diseases of heart like stroke, peripheral vascular disease and angina. The dietary factors are major contributors in development of heart problems because the foreign material deposited in the heart enters through diet only.

3.9.1 Prevention

Most subjects with elevated blood lipid levels have no overt symptoms and may be diagnosed during routine medical examination. Individuals with two or more risk factors listed under multiple risk factors are highly susceptible to coronary heart diseases. To avoid the risk of developing clinical manifestations of coronary heart diseases, interventions in the form of diet and behaviour modification are essential for these persons. Moderation in all the things is the advice given to them that is regular daily exercise, cessation of smoking, a prudent diet and avoidance of alcohol as far as possible.

3.10 DIETARY MANAGEMENT OF THE DISEASE

The aim of treatment in congestive heart failure is to secure maximum rest for the heart and to remove oedema. Basis of treatment are:

- Complete rest.
- Administration of diuretics and cardiac stimulants.
- Administration of a diet low in sodium and energy.

Energy: To maintain the proper body weight as per once height, age and sex the person suffering from any heart disease (who are mostly overweight or obese) should be provided with diet low in calories.

Fat: The recommended amount of fat in the diet less than 30 per cent of total intake of energy and for people with hypercholesterolemia should consume only 20 per cent of total energy from fat as the patient has to lose weight and one should also check the quality of fat.

Cholesterol: A diet which is low in cholesterol should be provided to the patient who is suffering from hypercholesterolemia with a daily intake of 200 mg/day and for normal person it is 300 mg/day.

Dietary fibre: Several studies have suggested that increased dietary intake of fibre may lower blood pressure. Vegetarians whose diets are usually high in fibre generally have blood pressure but a number of other differences in vegetarian and non-vegetarian diets may also account for this variation. High fibre diets are associated with lower postprandial insulin levels, greater faecal water and electrolyte excretion and altered absorption rates for fat. These may be some of the mechanisms through which dietary fibre may influence the blood pressure and, thus, it has a beneficial effect here.

Sodium: 250-500 mg per day as suggested by the ICMR. Moderate salt restrictions should be included for the treatment of the hypertension.

Potassium and calcium: These two are very important in the relation to hypertension. Adequate amount of potassium should be taken because it is an essential part of the treatment. The products which are high in potassium are milk, fruits and vegetables. These things should be included in the diet.

Saturated fatty acids (SFAs): Normally, SFAs have the tendancy to increase or elevate the blood cholesterol in all the lipoprotein fractions during the time of substitution of carbohydrates or other fatty acids. A dose response relationship is there between SFA and LDL-C. Lauric, myristic and palmitic acids are the most hypercholesterolemic or atherogenic. The most potent is the myristic and it is followed by palmitic acid though it's an SFA. In blood lipoprotein stearic acid has no effect and hence it is considered neutral which is similar to carbohydrates. The most prevalent hypercholesterolemic SFA is palmitic acid, that include 60% of the total SFA consumed. Most of the palmitate is present in animal foods but it also comes from plant sources. Myristic acid is mainly present in coconut, palm kernel oils and butterfat. In palm kernel and coconut oil lauric acid is mainly present which is a medium chain triglycerides. Saturated fatty acids are also considered hypercholesterolemic. In men with the progression of coronary artery disease dietary fatty acid has also been introduced. Palmitic and palmitoleic acids are also responsible for the progression of the disease, but not when the disease is controlled. The sources of fatty acid are milk, cheese, butter, lamb, bakery goods, fast foods and snack items that provide an additional source in many of the diets.

During the trial of secondary prevention, replacement of saturated fatty acid with monounsaturated fatty acid and alpha-linolenic acid with increasing amount of fruits and veggies can be beneficial or can prevent fatal and nonfatal CVD problems. And this way fatty acid affects the progression of the disease through lipids and other mechanisms, mainly thrombosis.

Polyunsaturated fatty acids

Omega-6 Polyunsaturatedfatty acids

If linoleic acid is introduced in place of carbohydrates then the dietary omega-6 polyunsaturated fatty acid, LDL cholesterol is decreased and HDL cholesterol is increased. When PUFA in low fat diet is introduced in place of SFAs, LDL and HDL cholesterol levels are lowered. Overall replacing SFA is twice as effective in decreasing serum cholesterol level in increasing PUFA. PUFA decreases the very low density lipoprotein, apo B, and synthesis of HDL. Omega-6 PUFA are mainly present in foods and their major sources are vegetable oils, salad dressings and margarine produced with oils. If linoleic acid is not consumed in large amounts then it increases oxidation of LDL, an increase in linoleic acid is not recommended more than current consumption.

Omega-3 polyunsaturated fatty acids

The main omega-3 fatty acids are eicosapentaenoic acid (EPA) and docosahexaenoic acid (DHA). These are mainly present in fish oils, fish oil capsules, and fishes from ocean. Most of the studies proved that total cholesterol is not affected by omega-3 fatty acids, they increase the LDL cholesterol level and decrease the level of triglycerides. Patient with hypertriglyceridemia have the trend to increase LDL cholesterol. VLDL and apo B-100 synthesis and also by reducing postprandial lipaemia can be inhibited or reduced by lowering triglycerides omega-3 fatty acids.

Omega-3 fatty acids' effects on triglycerides levels are dose dependent, i.e, the greater effect is produced by high doses. With hyperlipoproteinemia triglycerides level is also elevated. Many other steps are affected in atherogenesis by omega 3 fatty acid and they are the precursors of prostaglandins which involves the clotting of blood. So high intake can extend the bleeding time. It is now experimented that consuming fish and fish oils rich in EPA and DHA reduce cholesterol,LDL, and triglyceride levels with sudden reduction in cardiac arrest. Consumption of little amount of fatty fish, meal per week results 50% decrease in the risk of cardiac arrest. Dietary supplementation should be 1 gm of omega-3 PUFA decrease the risk of CVD daily. So omega-3 PUFA is known for its cardioprotective effect in the prevention of primary and secondary steps.

Trans fatty acids: In the hydrogenation process sterio-isomers of naturally occuring cis-linoleic acid are produced and their uses are widely spread in the food industry to harden unsaturated oils and to make the margarine soft. 50% of trans fatty acids mainly comes from animal sources like beef, butter and milk fats and remaining 50% comes from vegetable oils. Trans isomer of oleic acid and elaidic acid raises the blood cholesterol in comparison to PUFA. Moreover, it has less capacity to raise cholesterol level in comparison to lauric or myristic acid. The estimated average intake of trans fatty acid is 7% to 8% of total fat intake.

Fibre: Fibres which are soluble like pectins, gums, mucilages, algal polysaccharides and some of the hemicelluloses in oats, fruits, legumes and psyllium have the capacity to lower serum cholesterol and LDL cholesterol.

Coffee: By the studies it came to focus that result of having coffee and its effect on serum lipid is mixed. Regularly consuming strong coffee can lead to slight increase in total cholesterol, HDL cholesterol. In comparison to filtered coffee, boiled coffee increases the plasma lipids. People who drink coffee have the high chance of consuming saturated fat and cholesterol, they smoke more cigarettes, and even they exercise less than than coffee drinkers.

3.11 HYPERTENSION

It is a risk factor for CHD, stroke and congestive heart failure. Due to hypertension development of disease caused by vascular injury and stresses to the myocardium. About 50% of first mayocardial infarction patients and 66% of stroke patients have high blood pressure, i.e., 160/90 mm Hg. Along with other risk factors hypertension is also present such as hypercholestrolemia and obesity. So treating hypertension can play a major role in reducing the risk of stroke, CHD, and CHF.

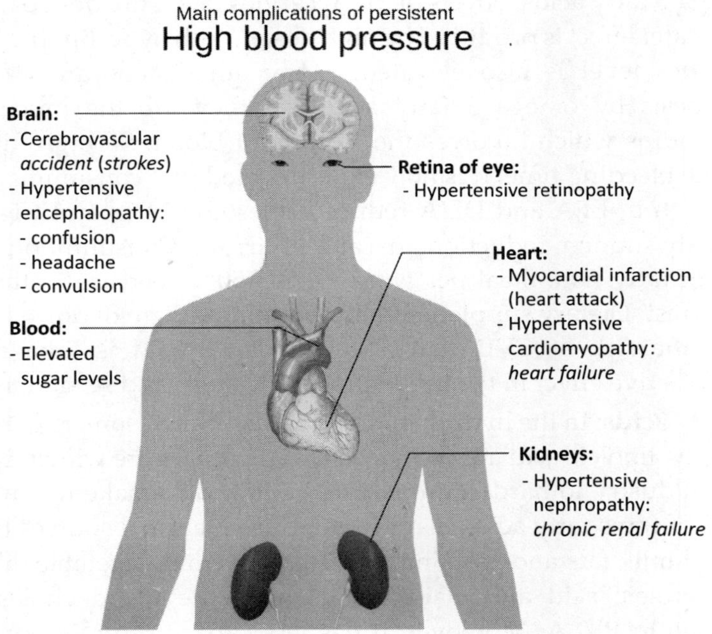

Primary hypertension is not known and can ever be identified in more than 95% cases. It is more frequently seen in Black and Japanese people–occurring between the ages of 25–55 years.

Secondary hypertension is directed towards diagnosis and treatment of the underlying cause. Hypertension is a chronic disease, it's a long condition that may lead to the development of the coronary heart disease and stroke. In the mild to moderate hypertension may achieved by the diet restriction, controlling weight, cessation of smoking, alcohol restriction, regular sustained physical activity and its moderation in the life.

Left ventricular hypertrophy (LVH): In response to high blood pressure and if workload increases then left ventricle increases. LVH is a risk factor in all age, gender and ethnic groups. Some trials are conducted to know the progression of LVH will be improved by clinical course or not.

3.11.1 Symptoms

- Headache
- Dizziness
- Impaired vision
- Failing memory
- Shortness of breath
- Pain
- Gastrointestinal disturbances

3.11.2 Aetiology of Hypertension

Primary hypertension can result from multiple factors, including:

- Volume of plasma.
- Blood volume and pressure maintained by medicines affect endocrine system.
- Environmental factors, such as stress and lack of exercise.

Secondary hypertension has specific causes and is a complication of another health problem. Chronic kidney disease (CKD) is a common cause of high blood pressure, as the kidneys no longer filter out fluid. This excess fluid leads to hypertension.

Conditions that can lead to hypertension include:

- diabetes, due to kidney problems and nerve damage,
- kidney disease,
- pheochromocytoma, a rare cancer of an adrenal gland,
- cushing syndrome that corticosteroid drugs can cause,
- congenital adrenal hyperplasia, a disorder of the cortisol secreting adrenal glands,
- hyperthyroidism, or an overactive thyroid gland,
- hyperparathyroidism, which affects calcium and phosphorous levels,
- pregnancy,
- sleep apnea, and
- obesity.

3.11.3 Risk Factors

A number of factors increase the risk of hypertension.

- **Age:** Hypertension is more common in people who are more than 60 years of age. Blood pressure can increase steadily with age as the arteries stiffen and become narrow due to plaque buildup.

- **Ethnicity:** Some ethnic groups are more prone to hypertension than others. African Americans have a higher risk than other ethnic groups, for example: Size and weight: Being overweight or obese is a primary risk factor.
- **Alcohol and tobacco use:** Regularly consuming large quantities of alcohol or tobacco can increase blood pressure.
- **Sex:** According to a 2018 review, males have a higher risk of developing hypertension than females. However, this is only until after women reach menopause.
- **Existing health conditions:** Cardiovascular disease, diabetes, chronic kidney disease, and high cholesterol levels can lead to hypertension, especially as people age.

Other risk factors include:

- Sedentary lifestyle
- Salt rich, high fat diet
- Low potassium intake

Poorly managed stress and a family history of high blood pressure can also contribute to the risk of developing hypertension.

3.11.4 Prevention

Dietary approaches to stop hypertension (DASH), studies the efficacy of dietary change in preventing hypertension or lowering blood pressure in persons with high normal pressure.

3.11.5 Nutritional Management

The nutritional management is as follows.

Energy: A weight loss in the obese hypertensive is often accompanied with a fall in the blood pressure, also the majority of the hypertensive patients are overweight thus a hypocaloric diet is suggested. The ratio of the carbohydrate, proteins and the fat in the overall diet for patients who are hypertensive is an important consideration. All these nutrients contribute towards energy content of the diet.

Protein: It should contribute about fifteen to twenty per cent energy in a low energy diet. The excess amount of the animal protein should be avoided. Include vegetables, whole pulses, and legumes more in the diet. They are low in fat and sodium and are high in the dietary fibre.

Fats: Low fat diets are essential as they are low in energy or low energy diets. The quantity of the fat should be reduced to a certain level.

Carbohydrates: About sixty to sixty five percent should be taken from the carbohydrate foods. High complex carbohydrates should be included. Example: starch and dietary fibres.

Sodium: Sodium chloride was linked to body fluid volume, in the mid-nineteenth century. There are some isolated population groups such as of culturally homogenous people, lean people, isolated people, physically active people, people who gain weight with the age, and consuming high potassium diet and those who are consuming low sodium diet. They have been described as populations with low blood pressure. But there is no evidence of the effect of sodium chloride on the blood pressure of the people or population.

Potassium: There are many ways through which the dietary potassium can influence the blood pressure. These are as follows:

- The effect of the sodium balance that is potassium supplementation causes increased excretion of the sodium by the kidneys.
- Supplementation of potassium may decrease in the blood pressure by the response to the circulating norepinephrine.
- Arteriolar smooth muscle activity and vascular tissue may directly modify and provide relax to the excitability through the potassium.

There is evidence that dietary potassium supplementation lowers the blood pressure but it should not be widely prescribed. It has the risk of hyperkalemia in the hypertensive subject with the renal insufficiency and or diabetes.

Intake of potassium per day is 90 mmol (that is 90 mEq daily).

Calcium and magnesium: High dietary intake of calcium which has been associated with the lowering blood pressure in the men. 1000-2000 mg daily is the recommended intake of the dietary calcium to meet the RDA.

A number of studies suggest that the lower dietary magnesium levels may be associated with the higher blood pressure. And large number of doses of magnesium salts may lower the blood pressure. Calcium and magnesium both are involved in several physiological mechanisms that influence blood pressure. However, it is not known whether dietary modifications in the calcium and magnesium within the physiological range can affect these mechanisms.

Alcohols: A strong association exist between moderate to heavy alcohol consumption and hypertension. This may be due to an indirect rather than to a direct effect of alcohol. Frequent alcohol consumption is correlated with high energy intake and obesity. It may be an indication of increased psychological stress and thus indirectly influences the blood pressure.

Caffeine: Caffeine is not considered a nutrient. It does form a common part of the diet. The small amount of caffeine present in a cup of coffee that can produce a short term increase in the both SBP and DBP.

Dash diet: As dash diet is popularly known for preventing various diseases such as cancers, heart diseases, strokes, diabetes, etc., so proper attention should be given for including dash diet in our regular diet to attain various health benefits. Generally the term dash diet includes vegetables, low fat dairy product and fruits and moderate amount of poultry, fish, whole grains and nuts. If one follows a dash diet regularly, chances of blood pressure come to normal level within just 1-2 weeks. Moreover the consumption of salt is restricted to 2.3 gm a day and finally cut down to 1.5 gm a day.

- Addition of one vegetable or fruit after every meal.
- Consider having meal free of meats
- Substitute salt with herbs and functional spices
- Use nuts instead of junk and fats greasy food
- Avoid using refined/white flour
- Perform an exercise for about 15-20 minutes a day

3.12 RELATIONSHIP BETWEEN OMEGA THREE POLYUNSATURATED FATTY ACIDS AND OMEGA SIX POLYUNSATURATED FATTY ACIDS

Essential fatty compounds are those that are not produced or generated in the body of humans and hence, are needed to be consumed from outside through diet. The omega three polyunsaturated series acids and omega six range fatty acids are structurally not same depending on the location of initial double bond when we count from the methyl group end of the molecule of fatty acid.

3.12.1 Omega Six Fatty Acids

Structurally omega six fatty acids have the double bond at sixth carbon from methyl end group. Three fatty acids come under the category of omega six range fatty acids.

1. **Linoleic acid:** It is an eighteen-carbon chain with two double bonds. Oils extracted from vegetables such as oil extracted from safflower, corn, oil extracted from sunflower, soybean, sesame, rapeseed, cottonseed have abundance of linoleic acid in them.
2. **Gamma linoleic acid (GLA):** It is a carbon chain of eighteen carbons which has three double bonds.

3. **Arachidonic acid (AA):** It is a 20-carbon chain with 4 double bonds. Due to 4 double bonds it is highly flexible and strong. It can be produced from linoleic acid but cannot be synthesized in human body. It is present mainly in animal based foods. It has been found out that, the more is the amount of fat in the meat the more it contains arachidonic acid.

3.12.2 Omega Three Fatty Acids

Both Plant and animal sources constitute the oil provided with the omega three fatty acids. In animal sources tuna fish, salmon, sardines, herring, mackerel, spirulina and fish oil are the richest sources of omega three fatty acids. The damage to the omega three fatty acids is very easy and also they are liable for oxidation in a quick and easy manner. Hence, they need to be stored in airtight packages.

The major sources of omega three fatty acids are flax, seeds of pumpkin, whole pulses, nut walnuts, cow pea, black gram, kidney beans, green leafy vegetables, wheat, spinach, bajra, brussels sprouts, rapeseed oil, linseed oil and soybean oil.

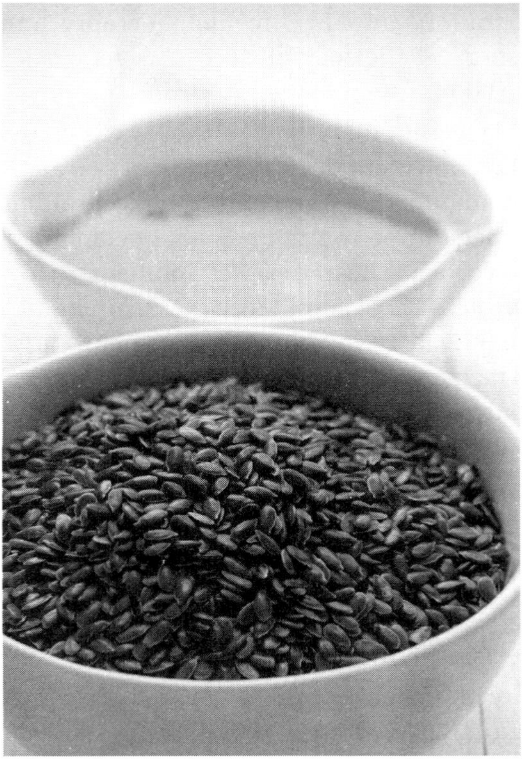

The classification of major three omega three fatty acids are given below.

1. **Alpha linolenic acid (ALA):** It is an eighteen-carbon chain having three double bonds. Alpha linolenic acid is very beneficial in reducing the blood pressure and keeping the blood cholesterol levels low and also prevents various heart related disorders. Deficiency of alpha linolenic acid may result in retardation of growth and cognitive disorders.
2. **Eicosapentaenoic acid (EPA):** It is a twenty-carbon chain with five double bonds. Eicosapentaenoic acid has anti-inflammatory properties and is very helpful in blood clotting, immune function, triglyceride levels, and platelet accumulation. It competes with omega six fatty acids and generates more helpful and crucial eicosanoids.
3. **Docosahexaenoic acid (DHA)**: It is a twenty-two-carbon chain with six double bonds. It is a crucial part of phospholipids present in the cell membrane of retina and myelin sheath in brain. Docosahexaenoic acid is very influential in the functioning of membranes. It is found in the grey matter of the brain and affects or controls concentration ability, cognition, thinking, feeling, memory and various other brain functions. Deficiency of docosahexaenoic acid may result in various nervous system related disorders.

Both omega six compounds and omega three compounds work in coordination and complement the functioning of one another. If these two are taken in right amounts then the aim of good health can be achieved. Omega six and omega three compounds act in combination and provide protection against coronary heart diseases and helps in lowering the blood low density lipoprotein cholesterol levels. Consuming omega six alone in excess amount may lead to inflammatory and chronic diseases such as atherosclerosis. The oils used in cooking are main sources of omega fatty acids. People consuming more fried and processed food are actually consuming large quantities of omega six acids which further causes harm to the human body. That is why omega six fatty acids must be consumed in right amount and incorporation with omega three acids. In experimental studies it is clearly stated that the ideal ratio between omega six vital acid series and omega three polyunsaturated compounds should be 5 to 1 to 10. The efforts should be made to include more and more incorporation of omega three fatty acids in the diet.

The availability of omega six fatty acids is at a rise and this is the main reason that omega three are consumed less in human body. The ratio for omega six and omega three in diet is being increased day by day. Various studies have shown that omega six and omega three vital PU acids lead to the gaining of fat through various mechanisms such as formation of adipose tissues, browning of adipose tissues, homeostasis of lipids, brain gut adipose tissue axis and systemic inflammation. Various studies have proved that when there is increase of omega 6 fatty acids in RBC membranes there is automated increase of compounds in the phospholipids hence, the risk of fat gain and obesity also increases. This mechanism is reversed when there is increase in omega three fatty acids, there is automatic decrease in risk of obesity. The balance of omega six series acids and omega three series compounds is very crucial for good health and preventing and managing the obesity.

To reach to a conclusion the more omega six leads to disorders while the increased ratio of omega three fatty acids decreases incidence of metabolic disorders. Therefore a right combination of omega six and omega three fatty acids are important for maintaining balance. The chances for developing cardiovascular disorders are more in people consuming omega six series acids. And the consumption of omega three range acids was observed to repress the formation of such diseases. The ratio of omega six and omega three essential acid chain should be low to prevent diseases and to maintain good health status. But the level of ratio required still depends upon the disease or existing medical condition. Some disease may require a little bit of high ratio to get healed and some diseases may require very small ratio for complete effective healing.

CASE STUDIES

1. TO PLAN A DAY'S DIET FOR A MAN, 32 YEARS OLD SUFFERING FROM A GRADE I OBESITY AND HYPERLIPIDEMIA

Personal Information

Age: 30 years

Sex: male

Physiological condition: Grade 1 obesity and hyperlipidemia

RDA: 1700 kcal/day

CHO: 55% of total energy requirement = 233-260 gm/day

Protein: 15% of the total energy requirement = 63 gm/day

Fat: 12% of the total energy requirement = 22 gm/day

Principal Diet

Low calorie, high protein, low carbohydrate, low fat and high fibre.

Comprehensive Exchange List

Food group	Exchange number	Protein	Carbohydrate	Fat	Energy
Milk	1.5	12	24	3	270
Meat	1	7		10	140
Pulses	4	28	68		400
Cereals	7.7	15.4	115.5		539
Veg A	4		14		80
Veg B					
Fruits	3		30		120
Fats	2			10	90
Sugar					

Distribution from the Table

Food group	No. of exchange list	Bed tea	Breakfast	AM snack	Lunch	PM snack	Dinner	Post dinner snack
Milk	1.5		1		0.5			
Meat	1				1			
Pulses	4		2		2			
Cereals	7.7		3		2.7		1	
Veg A	4		1		1		2	
Veg B								
Fruits	3		1			1		1
Fat	2		0.5		1		0.5	
Sugar								

Meal	Quantity	Food item	Energy (kcal)	CHO (g)	Proteins (g)	Fats (g)
Bed tea	1 glass	Apple cider	-	-	-	-
Breakfast	1 glass	Skim milk	90	12	8	3.2
	1 bowl	Wheat noodles	300	45	6	-
	1 small bowl	Blue berries	60	13	-	-
	1 small bowl	Chick pea sprouts	160	30	14	--
Mid-morning	1 medium	Grape fruit	60	12	-	-
	1 glass	Luke warm water	-	-	-	-
Lunch	3 serving	Brown rice	240	47	6	-
	2 small bowl	Mixed vegetables curry (carrot + collard greens + artichokes)	4	1.3	-	-
	1 medium	Egg white + Carrot + Cucumber salad	80	-	8	3

	2 nos	Pears	40	13	-	-
Evening tea	1 small bowl	Roasted chickpea	160	32	15	-
	1 glass	Green tea	-	-	-	-
Dinner	2 medium	Whole wheat chapattis	160	30	4	-
	1 large bowl	Fish soup with garlic flavour	4	-	2	-
	1 small bowl	Mixed vegetables	-	-	-	-
Post-dinner	1 cup	Grilled tofu	180	30	14	-

2. TO PLAN A DAY'S DIET FOR A FEMALE, WHO SUFFERED FROM A STROKE AND IS 51 YEARS OLD

Let us assume that the patient is 155 cm tall and weighs 60 kg

- Calories : 1500 kcal
- Protein : 55-65 gm
- Carbohydrate: 200 gm
- Fat: 33 gm

	Servings	Energy	Protein	Carbohydrates	Fats
Milk	2½	232.5	20	36.4	-
Meat	1	80	7	-	-
Pulses	2½	250	17.5	42.5	-
Cereals	7	490	14	105	-
Vegetable A	6	120	6	21	-
Vegetable B	-	-	-	-	-
Fruit	1	45	-	10	-
Fat	5	225	-	-	25
Sugar	3	60	-	15	-
Total		1502.5 kcal	64.5 gm	222.9 gm	25 gm

	Early morning	Break-fast	Mid morning	Lunch	Evening tea	Dinner	Post dinner
Milk		1 ¼		¼	½	½	
Meat		1					
Lean meat							
Pulses				1	½	1	
Cereals		2		2		2	1
Vegetable A		1		2	1	2	
Vegetable B							
Fruit			2				
Fat	5						
Sugar		1			1		1

Meal	Menu
Early morning	• Soaked methi dana- I tsp (empty stomach) • Cinnamon tea/ green tea/black tea – 1 cup • Almonds-3, walnuts- 2
Breakfast	• Skimmed milk- 200 mL • Missi roti/whole wheat bread/brown bread/multigrain bread- 1 • Hung curd with vegetables- 10 gm • Egg white/paneer- 40 gm
Mid-morning	• Fruit- 150 gm • Pudina water/lemon water/vegetable juice/vegetable soup – 1 cup
Lunch	• Brown rice - 40 gm or 2 chapatti (wheat flour+ chana flour) • Seasonal vegetables 1 katori • Dal- 30 gm/ lean chicken • Curd/raita 100 gms • Salad – 100-150 gm with sprouts – 10 gm
Tea	• Lassi/soup/soy milk – 1 cup • Sprouted dal chaat/roasted chana/wheat puff- 20 gm/2 marrie biscuits
Dinner	• Brown rice -40 gm or 2 chapatti (wheat flour + chana flour) • Seasonal vegetables 1 katori • Dal- 30 gm/lean chicken • Curd/raita 100 gm • Salad – 100-150 gm with sprouts – 10 gm
Bedtime	• Cinnamon tea or green tea- 1 cup • Oats/ragi biscuit- 2

General Instruction

- Skimmed milk
- Whole grain cereal
- Vitamin A rich foods, e.g., papaya, carrots, red capsicum, broccoli, fish, egg, milk.
- Vitamin C rich foods, e.g., guava, black-kishmish, papaya, broccoli
- Calcium rich foods, e.g., milk, cottage cheese, yogurt, fish, tofu, channa
- Folic acid rich foods, e.g., cabbage, cauliflower, oats, peas, beans, lettuce.
- Reduce excess weight.
- Reduce total fat in diet; increase the fibre intake, particularly the soluble fibre and soy based products.
- Reduce sugar and salt intake.
- Intake of plenty of fluids.

- Be physically active. Avoid intake of alcohol and avoid smoking.
- Foods that help in increasing HDL:
  1. Fenugreek seeds
  2. Flax seeds
  3. Garlic, ginger
  4. Green tea, cinnamon tea
  5. Almonds and walnuts
  6. Fish oil
  7. Olive oil
  8. Whole grain cereals
  9. Soya beans
  10. Red and purple fruits and vegetables which contain antioxidants anthocyanin
- Fruits such as:
  1. Blueberries, plums, grapes, apple, strawberries and jamun should be included.
- Vegetables such as:
  1. Cabbage, brinjal, red raddish and red onions should be included.

3. TO PLAN A DAY'S DIET FOR A MALE, 69 YEARS OLD WITH VLDL- 180 AND HIGH LDL.

- **Calories:** 2075 kcal
- **Protein:** 73-75 gm
- **Carbohydrates:** 311.2 gm
- **Fats:** 46 gm

	Servings	Energy	Protein	Carbohydrates	Fats
Milk	2½	232.5	20	36.4	-
Meat	1	80	7	-	6
Pulses	2½	250	17.5	42.5	-
Cereals	10	700	20	150	-
Vegetable A	9	180	9	31.5	-
Vegetable B	1	40	2	7	-
Fruit	2	90	-	20	-
Fat	9	405	-	-	45
Sugar	5	100	-	15	-
Total		2067 kcal	75.5 gm	302.4 gm	51 gm

	Early morning	Break-fast	Mid morning	Lunch	Evening tea	Dinner	Post dinner
Milk		1		½	½	½	
Meat							
Lean meat		1					
Pulses				1	½	1	
Cereals		2½		2½		2½	2
Vegetable A			2	2	2	3	
Vegetable B			1				
Fruit		1	1				
Fat	7						
Sugar							

Meal	Menu
Early morning	• Soaked methi dana- I tsp (empty stomach) • Cinnamon tea/green tea/black tea – 1 cup • Almonds-5, walnuts-2
Breakfast	• Skimmed milk- 200 mL • Oats/dalia/muesli- 30 gm multigrain bread- 1 • Any fruit -1 • Egg white/paneer- 40 gm
Mid-morning	• Fruit-150 gm • Vegetable juice –1 cup
Lunch	• Brown rice-40 gm or 2 chapatti (using sattu) • Seasonal vegetables 1 katori • Dal-30 gm/lean chicken • Curd/raita 100 gms • Salad – 100-150 gm with sprouts – 10 gm
Tea	• Lassi/soup/soy milk – 1 cup • Sprouted dal chaat/roasted chana/wheat puff- 20 gm/2 Marrie biscuits
Dinner	• Brown rice -40 gm or 2 chapatti (using sattu) • Seasonal vegetables 1 katori • Dal- 30 gm/ lean chicken • Curd/raita 100 gm • Salad – 100-150 gm with sprouts – 10 gm
Bedtime	• Cinnamon tea or green tea- 1 cup • Oats/ragi biscuit-2

General Instruction

- Skimmed milk
- Whole grain cereal

- Vitamin A rich foods, e.g., papaya, carrots, red capsicum, broccoli, fish, egg, milk.
- Vitamin C rich foods, e.g., guava, black-kishmish, papaya, broccoli
- Calcium rich foods, e.g., milk, cottage cheese, yogurt, fish, tofu, channa
- Folic acid rich foods, e.g., cabbage, cauliflower, oats, peas, beans, lettuce.
- Reduce excess weight.
- Reduce total fat in diet; increase the fibre intake, particularly the soluble fibre and soy based products.
- Reduce sugar and salt intake.
- Intake of plenty of fluids.
- Be physically active. Avoid intake of alcohol and avoid smoking.
- Foods that help in increasing HDL:
    1. Fenugreek seeds
    2. Flaxseeds
    3. Garlic, ginger
    4. Green tea, cinnamon tea
    5. Almonds and walnuts
    6. Fish oil
    7. Olive oil
    8. Whole grain cereals
    9. Soya beans
    10. Red and purple fruits and vegetables which contains antioxidants anthocyanin
- Fruits such as:
    1. Blueberries, plums, grapes, apple, strawberries and jamun should be included.
- Vegetables such as:
    1. Cabbage, brinjal, red raddish and red onions should be included.

4. TO PLAN A DAYS DIET FOR A PATIENT 38 YRS OLD FEMALE SUFFERING FROM SYSTEMATIC LUPUS ERYTHROMATOSUS.

Nutritional Requirement

Energy: 1950 acc. to RDA

Protein: 20% of total energy = 97 g

CHO: 60% of total energy = 292 g

Fat: 20% of total energy = 43 g

Menu

Meal timing	Menu
Early morning	Skimmed milk-200 mL Soaked almond -10 g Dates-20 g
Breakfast	Veg sandwich • Bread slices-60 g • Cabbage-100 • Onion-30 g • Cheese -60 g • Tomato-30 g • Garlic-5 g • Egg white-40 g • Oil-5 g
Mid-morning	Orange-100 g Kiwi-50 g Apple -50 g
Lunch	Veg pulao- 1 katori • Rice-100 g • Onion-30 g • Peas-50 g • Broccoli-50 g • Spinach-50 • Curry leaves-50 g • Oil-5 g Baked fish-50 g Salad • Lettuce-100 • Kale-30 g • Lemon-10 g
Evening	Upma-1 katori • Oats-40 g • Black olives-10 g • Onion-30 g • Tomato-30 g • Beans-30 g • Oil-5 g
Dinner	Roti -2 nos. Chole curry-1 katori • Cow pea-50 g • Onion-30 g • Tomato-30 g • Oil-5 g
Bedtime	Skimmed milk-200 mL

Nutritive Value

Ingredients	Amount	Energy	Protein	CHO	FAT
Milk	200 mL	58	5	9.2	-
Almond	10 g	6.9	1.8	1.05	5.8
Dates	20 g	56.4	0.5	15	0.08
Egg	40 g	69.2	5.32	-	5.32
Cabbage	100 g	27	1.8	4.6	0.1
Onion	30 g	15	0.36	3.33	0.03
Cheese	60 g	208.8	14.46	3.78	11.06
Bread slices	60 g	146.4	5.28	29.4	0.84
Tomato	30 g	12	0.54	2.16	0.12
Garlic	5 g	7.25	0.18	1.49	0.005
Oil	5 g	45	-	-	5
Orange	100 g	9	0.2	1.9	0.1
Kiwi	50 g	21	0.4	5	0.2
Apple	50 g	29.5	0.1	6.7	0.25
Onion	30 g	15	0.36	3.33	0.03
Rice	100 g	349	8.9	77.4	0.6
Fish	50	60	10	-	1.9
Peas	50 g	46.5	3.6	7.95	0.05
Broccoli	50 g	15.5	1.25	3	0.2
Spinach	50 g	13	1	6.45	0.35
Curry leaves	50 g	54	3.05	9.35	0.5
Lettuce	100 g	29	3.6	3.2	0.2
Kale	30 g	10.5	0.876	1.326	0.426
Lemon	10	5.7	0.1	9.9	0.05
Oil	5 g	45	-	-	5
Oats	40 g	154	4.6	27.6	1.8
Black olives	40 g	14.5	0.08	0.63	1
Onion	30 g	15	0.36	3.33	0.03
Tomato	30 g	12	0.54	2.26	0.12
Beans	30 g	47.4	2.22	8.94	0.03
Oil	5 g	45	-	-	5
Cow pea	30 g	12.9	7.53	17.7	0.21
Wheat flour	100 g	341	12.1	69.4	1.7
Oil	5 g	45	-	-	5
Milk	200 mL	58	5	9.2	-
Total		2000 kcal	100.9 g	335 g	49.9

Energy: 2000 kcal Protein : 100.9 g CHO : 335 g Fat : 49.9 g

QUESTIONS

1. What is atherosclerosis? Describe its causes, symptoms management and prevention.
2. Differentiate between peripheral vascular disease and cerebrovascular disease.
3. Write short notes on the following-
   (i) Angina pectoris
   (ii) Hyperlipidemia
   (iii) Myocardial infarction
   (iv) Heart stroke
4. Discuss about management of at least four cardiovascular disorders.
5. Define hypertension and discuss about its aetiology, symptoms, risk factors associated along with dietary management.
6. Write about the importance of omega 3 and omega 6 fatty acids in light of cardiovascular disorders.
7. What is DASH diet? Write about its relevance in management of hypertension.
8. What is the difference between angina pectoris and myocardial infarction?
9. Plan a day's diet for a 55 years old male patient of atherosclerosis with acute kidney failure. Weight = 65 kg, Height = 162 cm.
10. Plan a day's diet for a female of age 45-year suffering from hyperlipidemia. Weight = 60 kg, Height = 164 cm

4

Diabetes Mellitus

4.1 INTRODUCTION

Diabetes, or more specifically diabetes mellitus, is a category/group of metabolic disorders which are characteristic of high sugar levels in the blood, for a continuing period of time. The symptoms of the same include frequent thirst, increase in quantity and frequency of urination and increase in hunger. Untreated diabetes is prone to cause multiple complications. Some immediate and short term, or acute complications may include hyperglycaemic state caused due to hyperosmosis, diabetic ketoacidosis, etc., however, complications that continue for longer terms of time are much more serious and may include stroke, cardiovascular disease, foot ulcers, CKD, eye damage, etc. Such is the nexus of diabetes mellitus that it may even result in death.

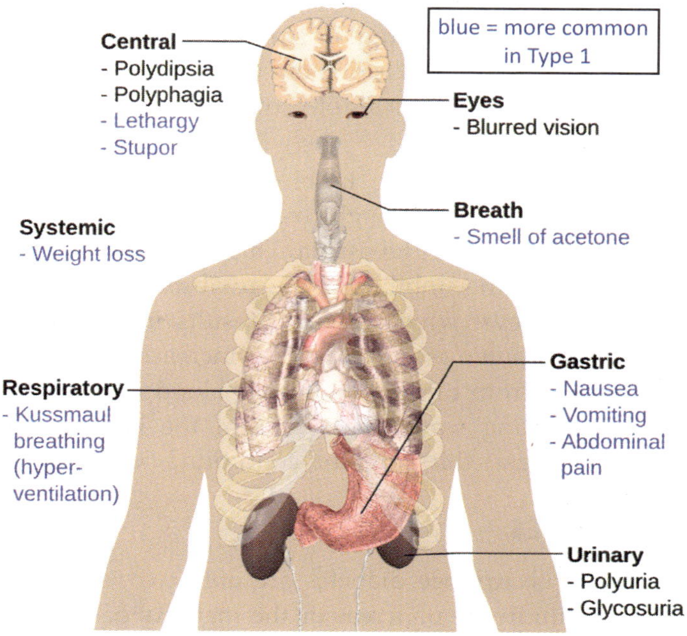

Main symptoms of diabetes

Insulin is the principle hormone that accounts for the uptake of glucose, or blood sugar from blood into cells, tissues, etc. It happens specifically in the liver, adipose tissues and muscle, with the exception of smooth muscle, wherein the same is carried out by IGF-1. Hence, whenever there is a deficiency of insulin or when the insulin receptors become insensitive to it, it generally acts as a pilot for diabetes mellitus.

The balance of glucose in the body is maintained largely by insulin. Insulin has the potential to prevent utilization of glycogen and also gluconeogenesis, mainly by stimulating the transport of glucose into the cells of fat and muscle. It also triggers the storage of glucose in the body in the form of glycogen.

Beta cells release insulin into the body. These cells are found in the islets of Langerhans in the pancreas. Insulin is released as a responsive measure when the blood sugar levels rise, conventionally upon the consumption of a meal. Two-thirds of all cells in the body need insulin to utilize glucose from the bloodstream, which acts as a fuel for the cellular functions. When the glucose levels are low, it is observed that there is a decrease in the secretion of insulin and breakdown of glycogen into glucose. The hormone glucagon is mainly responsible to carry out this process, known as glycogenolysis. The action of glucagon is seen to be as opposed to that of insulin.

In case of inadequacy in the availability of the insulin hormone or its ill-usability or defectiveness, the glucose is absorbed improperly in the body in the cells where it is required. Its storage in the form of glycogen in the liver and muscles is also not carried out properly. The end result is the rise in blood glucose, poor synthesis of proteins and also other metabolic abnormalities like acidosis.

Upon the prolonged increase in blood glucose, the kidneys find themselves unable to re-absorb the glucose and this leads to the excretion of glucose in urine, known as glucosuria. This causes an increment in the osmotic pressure of urine, inhibiting the re-absorption of water done normally by the kidneys, which in turn, results in an increase in the production of urine, known as polyuria. This increases the fluid loss from the body. To recover from this fluid loss, the blood volume is recovered osmotically by deducing water from cells of the body, which causes dehydration and increases thirst and this condition is known as polydipsia.

4.2 TYPES OF DIABETES

The reasons of the occurrence diabetes are only two, either insufficient production of insulin in the pancreas or the inability of the body cells to utilize it. Diabetes mellitus may be sub-divided into three types.

4.2.1 Type I or Insulin Dependent Diabetes Mellitus (IDDM)

It results due to the failure of the pancreas on the front of secretion of insulin. This is generally attributed to the loss of beta cells. This is also known as juvenile diabetes. The exact cause of IDDM remains unknown.

Type 1 diabetes mellitus is characteristically signified when the cells that produce insulin, i.e., the beta cells of the pancreatic islets are lost. This leads to the deficiency of insulin. Further classification of type I diabetes is made into idiopathic or immune mediated. The most commonly seen type I diabetes is of the immune mediated type. In this, an autoimmune attack mediated by the T-cells destroys the beta cells, leading to the loss of insulin. This type (immune mediated) accounts for nearly 10% of all cases in North America and Europe combined. Although this type of diabetes may affect all ages, it was initially termed 'juvenile diabetes', owing to majority of the diagnosed patients being children.

Unstable, labile or brittle diabetes is the name given to conditions that are characterized by the sudden changes in glucose levels which may also recur without apparent reason, generally in insulin dependent diabetes. However, this name has been found to be biologically illogical and thus isn't used anymore. However, similar symptoms still accompany type I diabetes, with fluctuations in the levels of blood sugar, which may be too high or too low. Ketosis also occurs frequently and seriously low sugar levels in the blood are often observed.

4.2.2 Etiology of Type I Diabetes Mellitus

Causes of type I diabetes rely partly on genetics, helped by multiple genes, inclusive of the genotype HLA, which is particularly known to increase the risk of diabetes. However, genetics alone cannot be held responsible for the onset on diabetes. The provision of the right environmental factors is very important for the expression of diabetic genes. These factors may include viruses and/or diet. Several viruses have been accredited with this act, none of which are evidently convicted of causing diabetes in humans as yet. Although it is unclear, the development of type I diabetes may also be aided by gliadin, a type of protein present in gluten.

4.2.3 Type II or Non-Insulin Dependent Diabetes Mellitus (NIDDM)

It begins with the resistance of insulin in the body. Herein, the body cells fail to utilize the insulin and thus the glucose of the blood. Insulin deficiency may also occur with the progression of the disease. This is also called adult onset diabetes. Insufficient exercise and high body weight combined contribute to the incurrence of NIDDM.

Insulin resistance is what characterizes the onset of type II diabetes mellitus, combined with lowered secretion of insulin. This may be caused by a relatively lower secretion of insulin in quantity. Insulin receptors are believed to be involved in this defective utilization of the hormone in the body tissues; even though the exact defects are unknown. The classification of those types of diabetes mellitus whose defects are known is done separately. The most common type of diabetes mellitus has been found to be type II DM.

The initial or early stages of type II diabetes mellitus are marked by the predominating abnormality of loss of sensitivity of the body towards insulin. Medications and a variety of other measures might help at this stage to reverse the impeccably high levels of blood sugar. These medications generally either improve the sensitivity of the body towards insulin or carry out a reduction in the production of glucose from the liver.

The occurrence of type II diabetes is accredited largely to lifestyle factors and also to genetics. Numerous lifestyle factors such as obesity (which is defined as the acquisition of a body mass index over 30), sedentary lifestyle that lacks activity, poor diet, urbanization and stress. The relation of excess body fat to diabetes has deeply been studied, with 30% occurrence in Chinese and Japanese cases, 60-80% in African and European cases and a whole 100% in Indian and Pacific Islander cases. People that do not fall into the category of obese may also possess a high waist to hip ratio.

4.2.4 Etiology of Type II Diabetes Mellitus

The risk of development of type II DM is also affected by dietary practices. The association of the consumption of sweetened or carbonated beverages in excess with an increased risk of occurrence of the condition has been made out. Fats also influence the risk of occurrence of type II diabetes mellitus. Saturated and trans fats are known to increase the risk of this type of diabetes, whereas PUFAs and MUFAs are known to decrease the risk. The consumption of large portions of white rice and other starches for long periods also aids the occurrence of type II diabetes mellitus. 7% of total cases of type II are believed to have their causes in the lack of physical activity of the patients. The heredity also plays an important role in development of this type of diabetes mellitus. Obesity also contributes to development of diabetes mellitus. The adipose tissue acts as a barrier in uptake insulin by the cells so the more the weight the strong the barrier for uptake of insulin. Any injury to pancreas is also a major factor in its development.

4.2.5 Gestational Diabetes

This condition is known to occur when diabetes prevails in pregnant women who have no history of the condition.

The treatment and also the prevention of the condition discussed here includes the maintenance of a healthy diet, a regular exercise regime, maintenance of a normal body weight and boycotting tobacco use. Also, emphasis must be laid upon the maintenance of a healthy blood pressure and also on foot care for the patients of this disease. The management of IDDM must be done by the administration of insulin injections. NIDDM, or type II diabetes mellitus treatment includes medication with or without the use of insulin. Insulin, coupled with some oral medicines, is known to lower the levels of glucose in blood. Surgery for weight loss is also considered effective in patients with NIDDM. Gestational diabetes generally disappears after childbirth.

Gestational diabetes mellitus, shortened as GDM, is similar to type II DM in various means, as it involves a combination of impaired responsiveness to insulin and also its relatively lower production. Its occurrence is known to be in 2-10% of pregnancies and it may either improve or completely vanish post childbirth. However, it may give birth to type II DM, as is seen in 5-10% of all cases of gestational diabetes mellitus. Although completely treatable, GDM patients need careful and special medical supervision throughout the course of the pregnancy. Monitoring of blood glucose, dietary changes and in some cases, insulin may be required to manage GDM.

However, transient it may be, GDM is known to cause damage to the mother as well as to the foetus. Multiple problems may be caused to the foetus due to GDM, some of which may include congenital heart abnormalities, abnormalities of the CNS, macrosomia (or high birth weight) and malformations of the skeletal/cranial muscles. Inhibition of production of foetal surfactant in foetus is seen due to increase in levels of insulin in the blood of the foetus, which may cause infant respiratory distress syndrome. The destruction of red blood cells may also cause a rise in the levels of bilirubin. Vascular impairment causes poor perfusion of the placenta, which, in turn, may result in prenatal deaths. Decreased placental function may be an indication for the induction of labour. C-section or caesarean section may need to be performed in case of remarkable distress on the foetus, or when the risk of injury is high, which is generally linked to macrosomia. An example of such an injury is dystocia of the shoulder, which is the retraction of the baby's anterior shoulder above the pubic bone of the mother after the head comes out during childbirth.

4.2.6 Maturity Onset Diabetes of the Young (MODY)

This is a rare form of autosomal dominant diabetes, which is inherited. The cause of this form of diabetes is known to be the mutation of one of several single genes. The occurrence of this type of diabetes is much lower than the pre-discussed forms of diabetes. The reference of the name of this disease is to the early hypotheses that relate to its nature. Due to its cause being a defective gene, the presentation of the disease varies largely in ages; whereas its severity varies, based on the particular gene defect that causes that particular case of MODY, which points to the fact that there exist 13 different sub-types of this type of the disease. Controlling of MODY may be done often without the use of insulin.

4.2.7 Other Types

Prediabetes: it is the name given to the condition wherein the blood glucose levels of a person are higher than the normal ranges, but not yet high enough for their classification into the category of type II diabetes mellitus. Patients of type II DM may have spent years in this stage without knowledge of the same.

LADA (latent autoimmune diabetes of adults): This is the condition wherein the development of type I diabetes mellitus takes place in adults instead of in children or in juvenile ages. The diagnosis of adults with this type of diabetes is often conducted wrongly into the class of type II DM, primarily due to the age and not the cause of the condition.

A very uncommon form of diabetes may also be caused by the irresponsiveness of the receptors of the body tissues even when the levels of insulin are adequate, as opposed to that of type II DM. Mitochondrial or autosomal genetic mutations may also lead to the defection of beta cells and their functioning. In some cases, even the determination of the abnormal action of insulin may be done by genetics. Pancreatic damage resulting from diseases like chronic pancreatitis and cystic fibrosis may also lead to diabetes. Diseases that are known to increase the secretion of the hormones that are antagonistic to the production of insulin may also cause diabetes. However, this type of diabetes is generally known to disappear once the disease causative of it is cured and the excess of the antagonistic hormone is removed. Numerous drugs are also known to impair the secretion of insulin. Certain toxins are also found to damage the beta cells of the pancreas which are responsible for the secretion of insulin. Another rare type of diabetes is **MRDM, or malnutrition related diabetes mellitus**. It is associated with the persistence of malnutrition for a long period of time. The characterization of this type of diabetes may be done by insulin resistance, insulinopaenia, hyperglycaemia and the failure of beta cells of the pancreas. Patients of MRDM are generally thin, young and severely hyperglycaemic, i.e. they maintain a high blood sugar level. As opposed to type I diabetes, these patients do not show ketonuria and there is requirement of high doses of insulin for the control of this condition.

There are also other forms of diabetes mellitus, of which one is congenital diabetes. This specific type of diabetes finds its cause in the genetic defects that relate to the secretion of insulin, diabetes related to cystic fibrosis, diabetes induced by uncontrolled usage of high doses of steroids like glucocorticoids and also some forms of monogenic diabetes (forms of diabetes caused by mutation of a single gene).

Another suggestion is for the renaming of "Alzheimer's disease" as "Type 3 diabetes", owing mainly to the underlying process, which causes the brain to resist insulin.

4.3 OTHER FACTORS THAT CAUSE DIABETES MELLITUS

Given below is a comprehensive list of other factors that cause diabetes:

- Defects owing to genetics affecting the functioning of beta cells
  - ◊ MODY
  - ◊ DNA mutations of the mitochondria
- Genetic defects that affect the processing of insulin or its activity
  - ◊ Defect in the conversion of proinsulin
  - ◊ Gene mutations of insulin
  - ◊ Mutations of receptor of insulin
- Defects of pancreas (exocrine)
  - ◊ Pancreatectomy
  - ◊ Cystic fibrosis
  - ◊ Fibrocalculouspancreatopathy
  - ◊ Chronic pancreatitis
  - ◊ Pancreatic neoplasia
  - ◊ Haemochromatosis
  - ◊ Excess of growth hormone
  - ◊ Hyperthyroidism
  - ◊ Endocrinopathies
  - ◊ Pheochromocytoma
  - ◊ Cushing's syndrome
  - ◊ Glucagonoma

- Drugs
  - ◊ Thyroid hormone
  - ◊ Statins
  - ◊ β-adrenergic agonists
  - ◊ Glucocorticoids
- Infections
  - ◊ Coxsackievirus B
  - ◊ Cytomegalovirus infection

A study conducted in the year 2018 suggested that the three basic types of diabetes be abandoned due to them being too simplistic. The study further classified the disease into five sub-groups. Type I diabetes and autoimmune late onset diabetes were made into one group. Type II diabetes covers four sub-groups. This is aimed at improving the way diabetes is treated, as management and treatment can now be more specifically tailored and targeted.

4.4 SIGNS AND SYMPTOMS

The conventional symptoms of diabetes are enlisted as follows:

- Polyuria: frequent and increased urination
- Polydipsia: frequent and unquenchable thirst
- Polyphagia: frequent and increased thirst
- Nocturia: random and increased passage of urination during the night

Symptoms may develop rapidly over several weeks or months, or even years; especially in type I diabetes or insulin dependent diabetes mellitus. In type II diabetes mellitus, the development of the symptoms is slower and might also be subtle and/or absent.

There are other signs and symptoms that may be present at the time of diabetes' occurrence in the body, although they aren't specific to diabetes alone. Added to the pre-discussed symptoms, these may be as follows:

- Blurring of vision
- Fatigue
- Headache
- Delayed wound healing
- Itchy skin
- Change in vision and shape of eye lens, due to glucose absorption, although this only occurs in case of long-term diabetes without treatment.

- Prolonged vision loss may lead to a condition called diabetic retinopathy.
- Diabetic dermadromes are skin rashes that occur in diabetes.

4.5 EMERGENCIES OR SUDDEN COMPLICATIONS OF DIABETES MELLITUS

Hypoglycaemia, or low blood sugar, is a common emergency that occurs in both type I and type II diabetes. Most of these cases are mild and may or may not be considered emergencies that require medical attention. The effects of the same may be mild to severe, with the mild ones being uneasiness, sweating, increased appetite and trembling; ranging towards more serious ones like changes in behaviour, confusion, seizures, unconsciousness, fits, aggressiveness, permanent brain damage (although rare), and even death. Moderately low blood sugar is commonly confused with drunkenness. Characteristics of low blood sugar include sweating, rapid and heaved breathing, pale skin; however, these symptoms may not be too definitive. Mild, or even moderate cases may be self treated with methods like drinking high sugar beverages or eating foods high in sugars. Severe cases may require medical attention and are generally restored with the usage of IV glucose.

Diabetic ketoacidosis is also a condition that may occur in people with type I diabetes, which is characterized by nausea, abdominal pain, or vomiting. Common symptoms are the smell of acetone on breath or deep breathing. Decreased consciousness levels may also be recorded in severe cases.

Another very severe possibility is hyperosmolar state of hyperglycaemia or hyperosmolar hyperglycaemic state (HHS). Although rare, this condition may occur in patients of type II diabetes due to dehydration.

4.6 METABOLISM OF CARBOHYDRATES, PROTEINS AND FATS IN DIABETES MELLITUS

4.6.1 Carbohydrates Metabolism

The major function of insulin is to increase glucose utilization in the skeletal muscles and adipose tissues. Insulin maintains glucose homeostasis in the body and helps in its absorption and utilization. The concept of insulin resistance was proposed as early as 1936 and is defined as the decreased sensitivity or decreases response to the glucose uptake or disposal or the hindrance in the hepatic glucose production. When carbohydrates are ingested they are broken into simpler carbs and all the carbohydrates are digested and form glucose. This glucose is primary source of energy and enters the blood. As blood sugar rises, insulin is secreted from the pancreas to transport the glucose to provide energy or to be stored as glycogen. As cells of the body become deficient of glucose the glucagon hormone is secreted from pancreas which, in turn, releases stored blood sugar.

The complex carbohydrates are converted to simple carbohydrates after digestion and then it is simplified to glucose which is then being transported to the liver for further metabolism. Insulin is responsible to transport glucose to cells for further use as well. The rest glucose which is not used by the body, i.e., in the fed state of body the Glycolysis takes place and then glucose is stored as glycogen in liver and muscles. In starvation state or when body requires energy the glucagon hormone is secreted and the stored glycogen undergoes glycogenolysis and the glycogen is converted to glucose. This glucose is then transported to cells for further usage and providing energy.

Various biochemical procedures for the metabolic development, break down and transformation of sugar to the living creatures. Despite the fact that a range of sugars is used, complex starches are processed into a number of basic monomers, namely glucose, fructose and galactose, for digestion. Glucose is the essential structure that is suitable for cells in tissues.

The objective of processing and assimilation of starches is to separate them into little particles of sugar known as glucose. Glucose is an essential fuel that drives the digestion and capacity of each cell in the body. For instance, the mind and red platelets rely upon glucose for vitality since they don't utilize fat or protein under typical conditions. The ingestion, assimilation and digestion of sugars are in this manner basic for every single substantial capacity.

The activities of biting and gulping food invigorate the stomach to discharge stomach corrosive, which keeps on separating the sugars, despite the fact that the corrosive itself has no particular proteins to process starches. When the mostly processed starches touch base of the small digestive system, more chemicals are discharged to additionally separate the sugars into glucose particles. Gastric purging happens quicker with straightforward starches contrasted with complex carbs, as indicated by "utilitarian food carbohydrates." Simple sugars are made out of it is possible that one sugar atom or two sugar particles connected together. Complex starches likewise regularly contain fibre; models incorporate beans, lentils and entire grains. The rate of starch assimilation and ingestion impacts sugar digestion. As per "useful food carbohydrates," a fast breakdown of sugars prompts an over-burden of glucose in the circulation system. The pancreas reacts by siphoning out insulin to rapidly bring down glucose. In the event that quickly required by organs and tissues in the body, the glucose atoms are conveyed there. Something else, the abundant glucose atoms are removed in the liver and muscles like glycogen, and the glycogen capacities as a reserve of promptly accessible glucose. The flood of insulin additionally prompts the change of overabundance glucose atoms to muscle to fat ratio. Complex starches are processed and digested at slower rate; they are more averse to make a fast ascent in glucose and the trademark insulin spike is found in simple sugars. Complex starches in this way furnish the body with an unfaltering supply of glucose and they are less likely to be put as fat versus muscle.

4.6.2 Protein Metabolism

The methods by which the body makes proteins with protein breaking up procedures for creating energy that is used by the body. In the circulation system at that point, the nutrient proteins are broken down to amino acids, and finally used in the structure of the body cells to make new proteins. Amino acids can be transformed into keto acids and urea when the body needs. Urea is released with sweat and urine.

Dietary proteins are separated by different chemicals and corrosive hydrochloric agents in the gastrointestinal tract into individual amino acids. These amino acids can be reused in the body to produce glucose, fat and other amino acids and are also separated into alpha-keto acids. A compound called peptidases may separate the proteins or they may separate due to denaturation

The process by which proteins are separated into amino acids is the catabolism of protein. This is also called proteolysis and further breakdown of amino acids can lead to it.

Proteases (otherwise known as peptidases) were initially designed only to mitigate enzymatic responses and actually help catabolize proteins with cleavage and produce new proteins previously absent. Proteases also aid in the management of metabolism. In pathways that do not work (for example, gluconeogensis, when the fixation of blood glucose is strong), they are one way to separate carbon atoms. However, much vitality can be expected, this moderates and stays away from unnecessary cycles. Difficult cycles occur when both catabatic and anabolic paths have basically been followed by a similar response rate. As the intermediates are expended, there are no net gains for the body. Through purposeless cycles, vitality is lost. Proteins prevent this cycle by changing the rate of a path or by separating a key compound can stop one path.

The digestion of protein results in formation of amino acids which are then transported to liver through portal vein. The liver then starts protein synthesis or the cycle of gluconeogenesis starts based on the needs of the body. In the patient suffering from diabetes mellitus muscle wasting is seen and also sometimes the person experiences weight loss as well. It has been shown that in subjects without and with mild type 2 diabetes, ~50–70% of a 50-g protein meal is accounted for over an 8-hour period by deamination in the liver and intestine and synthesis to urea. Now the amino acids which are left are sent to give carbon skeleton for glucose synthesis in liver. The essential amino acids freely flowing in the body are utilized by the muscles as fuel. These amino acids are responsible to increase insulin and glucagon secretion. The insulin deficiency enhances the oxidation of branched chain amino acids in muscle and uptake of alanine (the principle glycogenic amino acid) by the liver, resulting in increased gluconeogenesis and augmented protein catabolism. Therefore an imbalance in the metabolism of the body is observed in the diabetes mellitus. Insulin also inhibits the degradation of body proteins and lowers the circulating concentration of many amino acids. Now when insulin is deficient in the body the glucose is not uptaken so the amino acids are utilized to provide energy which results in the protein impaired functions.

4.6.3 Fat Metabolism

Lipid digestion is the blending or degradation of lipids in cells, including the breakdown or the ability of vitality fats and, for example, the combination of auxiliary and utilitarian lipids, those involved in cell layer development. An unsaturated fat is essentially a carbon chain linked to hydrogen in a carboxylic collection. They vary in length and in the number and area of double-bonds between carbon and carbon. These fats are obtained from food or are blended in the liver. The way to combine these fats is lipogenesis. Triglycerides and cholesterol are the dominant parts of lipids found in the human body from ingestion. Unsaturated fats and layer lipids are other kinds of lipids found in the body. Lipid digestion is often viewed as an assimilation and intake of dietary fat; however, two sources of fat can be used by the living beings for vitality: consumed fats and discharged fat.

The lipid digestion regularly begins with hydrolysis, with various compounds of the stomach. Further, lipid digestion occurs in plants but here and there, in contrast to livestock, the procedures contrast. The second step following hydrolysis is the assimilation of unsaturated fats into the intestinal epithelial cells. Unsaturated fats are grouped in the epithelial cells and transported to the rest of the body.

Assimilation is the first step in the process of lipid digestion, and is the way to separate triglycerides by lipase chemicals into littler monoglyceride units. Fat uptake begins in the mouth through lingual lipase compound assimilation. Cholesterol ingested by lipases is not separated and remains unblocked until the small digestive tract enter the epithelium cells. At this point, lipids proceed to the stomach where the absorption of compounds begins by gastric lipase and mechanical assimilation (peristalsis).

At a couple distinctive strides in this procedure, carbon dioxide is created. Additionally, at a few distinct advances, hydrogen particles are expelled from the particles and those hydrogen molecules are then consequently permitted to respond with oxygen to shape water. So during the time spent the oxidation of fats, the oxygen really comes into the procedure very late.

Next, we should think about every one of the parts of the general procedure thusly: hydrolysis of fats, glycerol to acetyl CoA, unsaturated fat winding (to acetyl CoA), citrus extract cycle, and electron transport framework (oxygen at last gets the electrons).

Fats metabolism is by oxidizing methods and it is completed in the muscles. The fats require glucose to complete their oxidation. Fats are first oxidized in the liver to ketone bodies plus a two-carbon compound (acetic acid). And then the ketones are utilized by periphery of the body. The fats are converted to ketone bodies carbohydrate oxidation in the periphery. If insulin is given in IDDM then the carbohydrates are oxidized and the coupled ketone body-carbohydrate oxidation, viz.:

$$\text{Ketones} + \text{Carbohydrate} + O_2 = CO_2 + H_2O.$$

But insulin is not present in the body in DM so incomplete oxidation of fatty acids is very common and this results in formation of ketone bodies.

4.6.4 Complications

There are some severe complications that are related to diabetes mellitus. They include retinopathy, nephropathy and neuropathy.

The risk of long term complications is increased by all forms of diabetes. The development of the same occurs in 10-20 years. However, the symptom of these complications may be the first for the patients that have received no diagnosis or treatment for diabetes before that time. Majority of the long-term complications occurring due to diabetes mellitus are known to occur due to damage in blood vessels. The risk of CVD increases to double due to diabetes and 75% diabetic deaths find the reason as coronary artery disease. Other diseases falling into the category of macrovascular diseases are stroke and peripheral artery disease. The kidneys, eyes and nerves are damaged due to damage in the smaller blood vessels in diabetes. Gradual vision loss and eventual blindness is caused by damage to the blood vessels in the retina of the eyes, known as diabetic retinopathy. The diabetic patient is also more prone to other eye problems like glaucoma and cataracts. An annual eye check-up is recommended for diabetic patients. Diabetic nephropathy is the name given to kidney damage owing to diabetes, which is characterized by scarring of kidney tissue, protein loss of urine and gradually leads to chronic kidney disease. Untreated cases may also need dialysis or even transplant. The most common complication of diabetes may be regarded as diabetic neuropathy, which is the damage to the nerves or the body due to diabetes. Symptoms are recognized as tingling, pain, numbness and altered sensation of pain; which in turn, may lead to skin damage. Diabetes also affects the feet characteristically, causing severe problems like diabetic foot ulcers, which are not only difficult to treat but may also require amputation. Weakness and painful atrophy in the muscles is also caused by proximal diabetic neuropathy.

Diabetes is also linked to cognitive defects. People with diabetes are found to have a higher rate of cognitive decline, almost by 1.2 to 1.5 times.

4.7 ASSESSMENT OF DIABETES MELLITUS

Diabetes mellitus evaluation: Easily available blood tests are conducted on patients, The fasting blood glucose should be less than 100 mg per dL. The post-prandial blood sugar levels should be less than 140 mg per dL.

4.8 INSULIN AND TYPES OF INSULIN

4.8.1 Pancreas and Its Function

Insulin is the hormone that is produced by pancreas. Insulin is a hormone that helps in controlling the blood glucose level in the human body and making it possible so that every cell can get the glucose to perform the specific function. Pancreas comes under digestive system and helps in the digestion of the foods by secreting digestive juice. The presence of pancreas is just behind the stomach. It is 12-14 cm long, being a part of the gastric system it helps in digestion by secreting juices into the duodenum with the help of the pancreatic ducts. Bicarbonate is present in this juice which helps in neutralizing the acids that comes from the stomach and gastric enzymes and also it helps in the breaking of the carbohydrates, protein and fats of the foods entering the duodenum from the stomach.

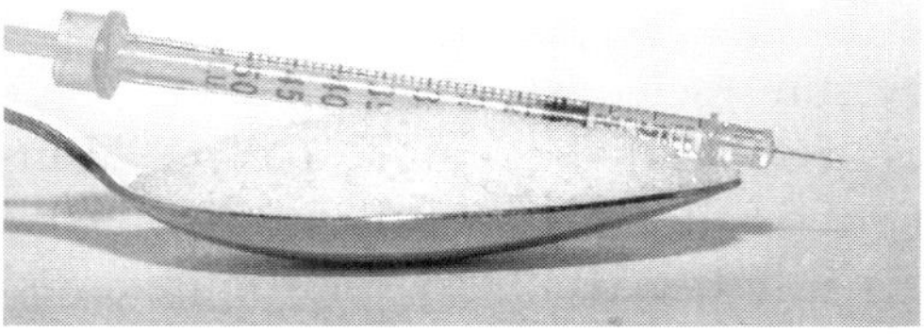

4.8.1.1 Glucose Regulation

Pancreas not only helps in digestion but also helps in the regulation of blood glucose level of blood or controls the blood glucose level and the metabolism inside the body. The role of the pancreas is divided on the basis of endocrine role and exocrine role in which the former is related to the secretion of insulin and the next is helps in regulation of blood sugar level and the metabolism inside the body. Cells in the pancreas help regulating the blood sugar level. The cells which perform this function surround this pancreas. Glucagon is secreted by the alpha cells which gets stimulated when the level of the glucose is less in the body then the glucagon helps by raising the level, and just the same work is done by the insulin which is secreted by the beta cells of the pancreas that is when the level of the glucose rises then the insulin is secreted by the pancreas to decrease or reduce the level of the glucose.

4.8.2 Characteristics of Insulin

Insulin has 3 qualities:

- Beginning is the period of time before insulin achieves the circulatory system and starts bringing down blood glucose.
- Peaktime is the time amid which insulin is at greatest quality as far as bringing down blood glucose.
- Time or duration to what extent insulin keeps on bringing down the blood glucose.

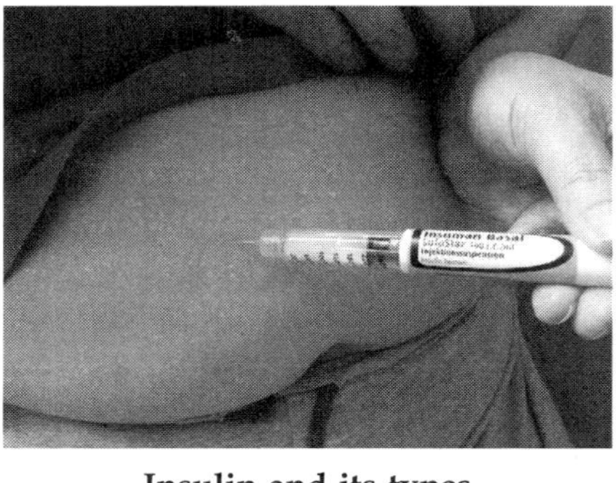

Insulin and its types

4.8.3 Formation of the Insulin

In the 19th century some scientists from Canada saw response from the patient suffering from type 1 diabetes mellitus. In 1955 insulin was the first protein to be sequenced fully. Insulin is formed by the two chains A and B where A contains 51 amino acids and b chain contains 21 amino which are linked by the two disulphide bonds. The Golgi body of the beta cells of pancreas imports the precursor of insulin, that is, proinsulin which is then processed and packaged into granulated forms. The proinsulin is a single chain amino acid peptide bond which is divided into or cleaved into insulin and c-peptide and they both are secreted in equal quantity by the beta cells when there is stimulation from the glucose and other insulin secretagogues. The c-peptide has no other function in the body but can help in estimate measurement of insulin production by the beta cells.

4.8.4 Sources of Insulin

During early days the persons with deficiency of insulin were injected insulin derived from the pigs and the cows but it was seen that the people started having allergy from this animal insulin and hence the process was stopped. Thereafter by using the recombinant DNA technology the use of the animal's insulin was also reduced. The insulin of the beef, pork and pork is not used anymore.

In the recombinant DNA technology the gene of the precursor proinsulin gene is inserted in the *Saccharomyces cerevisiae* or *E. coli* which acts as a production organism, after insulin is produced it is isolated and purified. This recombinant technology has helped in the development and the production of analogs to human insulin. With analogs the molecule of the insulin is changed somewhat to change the pharmacokinetic properties of the insulin hormone.

4.8.5 Immunogenicity

The insulin that is being sold in the markets are contamination free. The formation of insulin before was found more contaminated which contained cell peptides, proinsulin and glucagon, etc. The constituents that are used in the preparation of insulin and the little amount of inside human body insulin they both together form the antibodies in the humans. Now the exogenous human insulin are all free form the contamination and the resistance of insulin is rare to be seen in any individual.

The responses that the human body shows are of two types: first is local or systemic IgE-mediated reaction, second is immediate type. After the insulin is injected in the human body there are two conditions which can occur, first is lipodystrophy which results in the loss of the fat at the area where insulin is injected and occur in only the insulin that is purified and the second is lipohypertrophy. This is the next condition in which if the person is injected with the insulin in the same area many times the effect of the insulin decreases in the body. In lipohypertrophy there is reduced absorption of insulin and it will be good if the patient does this.

4.8.6 Concentration

In some countries like US the concentration of insulin is 100 units/mL. Therefore, insulin syringes are designed according to the concentration of the insulin. The insulin that is used by the patient frequently is more concentrated. The concentration of the insulin depends or varies according to the regions so the person travelling should always look after this and also should match the insulin with the syringes as the syringes depend on the concentration of insulin.

4.8.7 Absorption

When insulin is administered through the subcutaneous route it is directly absorbed into the blood where a very little support is provided by the lymphatic system. The time or the rate of absorption of the insulin depends on the activity of the insulin in the body. The activity of the insulin also depends on the place of the syringe injected because basically after insulin is injected into the body the insulin is absorbed in the blood and from the blood it is passed into the sites. As in the case of regular insulin it is seen that the rate of absorption insulin is two times faster in the abdomen than in the other subcutaneous sites. This means that person should avoid using random places for injecting the insulin. For instance, if the person has injected the insulin in the thigh in the afternoon then he should use the same area constantly for the injection. And after so many cases it is found that the abdomen is the preferred site for the insulin to be injected.

4.8.8 Elimination

The degradation of insulin is mainly done by kidney and the liver where the pancreas secreted insulin in the portal vein is degraded by the liver which is up to 50-60% and 35-45% by kidney. But it is seen that the amount of insulin that is exogenous in nature its profile of degradation is different as it is not directly imported in the portal vein.

4.8.9 Types of Insulin

4.8.9.1 Short (Prandial or Bolus) Acting Regular Insulin

Regular insulin is prescribed to give before the meal so that the level of the postprandial rise in sugar does not increases. There is formation of hexamers in the subcutaneous layers by insulin which reduce the rate of absorption of insulin in the body. This insulin is then divided into absorbable form. That is why the activity of the insulin is noticed after 30-60 minutes and therefore should be injected before meal by 30 minutes approximately to dull the postprandial rise in blood sugar level.

4.8.9.2 Rapid Acting (Prandial or Bolus) Insulin Analog

Rapid acting insulin analogs are different from the human insulin in amino acid structure because of which the formation of hexamers from the rapid acting insulin is decreased after the syringe is injected in the subcutaneous space. And this results in the sudden absorption of the insulin in the blood and the activity of the insulin starts in shorter duration. The pre- and post-prandial hypoglycaemia level of rapid acting insulin is less than regular insulin. Rapid insulin is injected 15-20 minutes before meal and the results in maximum reduction in post-prandial glucose is seen in relation with the regular insulin which is injected 30 minutes before the meal.

4.8.9.3 Inhaled Insulin

In this there is delivery of insulin of powered form in the lower air parts using inhaling devices. As it is absorbed pulmonary the absorption rate is higher than the regular insulin injected in subcutaneous layers.

4.8.9.4 Intermediate Acting Insulins

The effects of NPH (neutral protamine hagedorn) can be prolonged by the addition of the protein protamine during production. It is intermediate acting insulin whose action time is two hours and will work for 6-14 hours and the duration is 10-16 hours. NPH inulin is available in many types of mixture with regular insulin.

4.8.9.5 Long Acting(basal) Insulin Analogs

This insulin gives basic insulin coverage. It inhibits the process of hepatic gluconeogenesis so that the level of glucose does not increase after the meal in the insulin deficient patient. In type 1 diabetes the patient who is taking basal insulin is prevented from ketogenesis.

4.8.9.6 Mixed Insulins Along with Short or Rapid Acting Insulins

Proinsulin or NPH can be mixed with the rapid acting insulin analogs together with regular or rapid acting insulin analogs in fixed combinations. They are given either before heavy breakfast or dinner meal as once daily or it can be given twice daily before breakfast and dinner. There can be high risk of hypoglycaemia with these preparations of insulins if comparing with basal and pre-meal bolus insulins advices.

4.8.10 Storage of Insulin

When insulin is produced in the industries the insulin are marked with the date of manufacturing and expiry and are asked to keep it in the refrigerator. Insulin should not be kept in direct sunrays or at room temperature. If the insulin is kept in the direct sunrays then the effectiveness of the insulin is reduced. Some insulins are colourless and clean but become cloudy like basal insulin analogs, rapid acting insulin analogs and regular insulin.

4.8.11 Adverse Effect of Insulin

- **Weight gain:** This is the most common effect seen in the person having insulin doses. This is due to the hypoglycaemic changes due to which a person consumes more calories to counter the hunger and the low level of blood glucose level in the body. The one drawback of insulin is that it causes the uptake of the fatty acids into the adipose tissues.
- **Hypoglycaemia:** This is the worst effect of insulin therapy in the patient suffering from type 1 and type 2 diabetes which make it impossible to reach the glycaemic target. The factors that can be responsible for the hypoglycaemia are older age, longer duration of diabetes, renal insufficiency, hypoglycaemia unawareness, precedinghypoglycaemia and lower Hb1Ac. All persons should be aware who is having insulin therapy and therefore they should know how to treat low glucose levels.
- **Mitogenic properties:** Some of the observational studies have shown that there is a relation between cancer and the person taking insulin therapy.

4.9 HYPOGLYCAEMIC DRUGS

4.9.1 Pathophysiology

4.9.1.1 Medications

A delayed progression of diabetes has been seen in predisposed patients by the prophylactic use of rosiglitazone, valsartan or metformin. However, regardless of weight loss, lifestyle changes and interventions have been known to be more effective than these drugs.

Various other drugs are used to modify the risk of type II diabetes mellitus, even when they're prescribed to cure other conditions that are completely unrelated to type II diabetes mellitus. For rheumatoid arthritis, patients prescribed hydroxychloroquine show a 77% decline in the incidence of diabetes. The exact mechanisms and reasons for the same are unknown. Glycaemic control shows improvement upon administration of dopamine receptor agonists. They also reduce the resistance of insulin and help in weight loss.

4.9.1.2 Management

Diabetes mellitus is a chronic disease with no known cure except for some very select and specific incidences. The concentration of the management is primarily upon keeping the blood sugar level close to normal without it dropping below the lower points. The accomplishment of this can be done with a combination of a healthy diet, physical activity, loss of weight and medication like insulin for type I diabetes and oral and/or insulin medications in type II diabetes.

Active participation and gaining knowledge about the disease is important during the treatment as complications are reduced along with their severity in patients with blood sugar levels in check. The treatment aims at reaching an HbA_{1C} level of 6.5% but not lower. It may even be set higher than this. Emphasis is also laid upon other health issues that might increase the negative effects of diabetes. These effects include smoking, high cholesterol levels, hypertension, obesity and inactiveness on the physical front. There is specialized footwear being used extensively in order to reduce the risk of foot ulcers in diabetic feet. However, there is no clear evidence that points towards the efficiency of this method.

4.9.2 Oral Hypoglycaemic Drugs

The use of oral hypoglycaemic drugs is done only in the treatment of type II diabetes mellitus, which is a condition wherein there is resistance to the insulin that has been secreted. There is a lack of insulin in type I diabetes mellitus and hence treatment requires administration of insulin. Now, hypoglycaemic drugs are classified into four subtypes:

- Metformin
- Alpha-glucosidase inhibitors
- Thiazolidinediones
- Sulphonylureas

However, the approval of these drugs is only for the patients diagnosed with type II diabetes mellitus. Optimal utilization of these medicines is seen in those patients whose bodies do not respond well to weight reduction, exercise and/or dietary changes. However, approval of these drugs for the treatment of pregnant ladies diagnosed with diabetes, is given.

Sulphonylureas: These drugs are most widely used to treat type II diabetes mellitus. Sulphonylureas' function is to stimulate the secretion of insulin hormone, the end result of which is the increase in the response of the beta cells in the islets of langerhans in the pancreas. This responsiveness is increased to both types of secretagogues, i.e., glucose and non-glucose; which in turn, ultimately causes a higher release of insulin at all concentrations of blood glucose. There are also supportive effects of sulphonylureas, like increment in the sensitivity of the tissues to insulin. However, these supportive extra pancreatic effects of sulphonylureas are of low clinical importance.

Pharmacokinetics: The difference between sulphonylureas and pharmacokinetics is mainly in the potency and duration of the two. Some examples of the second generation drugs of sulphonylureas are glimepride, glyburide and glipizide. Their potency is high enough for them to be administered in low dosages.

The drugs with a longer half-life; like glimepride, glyburide and chlorpropamide, may be given once in a day. However, the benefits of these are countered by the significantly increased threat of hypoglycaemia.

This makes it important to shed light on the side effects of these drugs. The tolerance of sulphonylureas is generally good in the human body. The most common side effect is hypoglycaemia. Patients discharged from hospital are most susceptible to it in the initial days of recovery.

Following are the situations which aid the occurrence of hypoglycaemia:

- Right after exercise or skipping of meal.
- Upon administration of higher drug doses.
- Usage of drugs that take longer to act, like chlorpropamide and glyburide.
- Patients undergoing undernourishment or abusing alcohol.
- Patients that have impaired function of the cardiovascular system or renal function, and also patients with gastrointestinal diseases.
- Immediately after discharge from the hospital.

Other infrequent and non-significant side effects are nausea, abnormal liver function test reports and skin reactions. Also, if the dietary management is improper along with imbalanced physical activity, weight gain may occur. There are two very unique effects of chlorpropamide: it may cause hyponatraemia, which is the phenomenon of low sodium in blood, mainly due to the increase in activities of diuretic hormones; and an unpleasant flushing reaction to consumption of alcohol, immediately after ingestion.

The clinical use of sulphonylureas is made in order to lower the levels of blood glucose by around 20%. These are most effective in patients who maintain a normal or slightly higher than normal body weight. On the contrary, administration of insulin is done in those patients who are losing weight, are underweight or show ketosis even upon adequacy in calorie intake.

The choice of the drug within the sulphonylureas depends mainly upon the availability and affordability, since the efficiency of all of them is similar. However, the drug type may need to be changed in case of recurrence of hypoglycaemia in patients taking longer duration drugs, such as glyburide and chlorpropamide; to which short acting drugs are given, especially in elderly patients.

Another drug that has been recently brought into use for treatment of diabetes is **repaglinide**. It is a short acting drug that helps in lowering the levels of blood glucose. It has been approved by the Food and Drug Administration Department of the US for the treatment of type II diabetes mellitus, either alone or in combination with metformin. The differences between repaglinide and sulphonylureas are primarily structural, although with a similar action in the body of increment in the secretion of insulin.

The clinical efficiency of repaglinide is also similar to that of sulphonylureas. Recommendation for initial use is a dose of 0.5 mg right before meals for those patients who have never used hypoglycaemic drugs in the past. The highest dose that must be administered before a meal is 4 mg and doses must be skipped in case meals are skipped. Again, the most common side effect is hypoglycaemia.

Another significant drug is **natiglinide** or **starlix**. It is a very short acting drug that helps to lower the levels of blood sugar. Again, the mode of action is the increment in levels of secretion of insulin. However, this drug is pending approval from FDAD. The biggest advantage of this is the short length and brisk working of the first phase of release of insulin. It is this phase in diabetic patients that is found to be abnormal in early stages of the condition of diabetes and is often found in patients who have an impaired tolerance to glucose before diabetes. The usual dose of starlix is estimated at 120 mg before each meal.

The use of **metformin** has been done for the management of diabetes for over 30 years in Europe. It has also found its way into the US since March 1995. As opposed to the other drugs mentioned above, it is, however, only effective in the presence of insulin. Rather than acting as a stimulant to secrete insulin, it only helps in increasing the action of insulin in the body. The exact mechanism behind the increment of the action of insulin in the body due to metformin is unknown, even though it is known to affect multiple tissues. One of its prime effects is that it suppresses the output of glucose from the liver. Due to its actions of aiding weight loss and stabilization of body weight, metformin's clinical use is mostly done upon patients who are obese or overweight. This provides a stark contrast to the action of sulphonylureas, which promote weight gain and a provide a generalized sense of an increase in appetite. As also achieved by the administration of sulphonylureas, metformin lowers the fasting blood sugar by about 20%. However, contrasting and similar their effects may be, either of the drugs (metformin and sulphonylurea) work best in combination with each other.

In addition to the aid to weight losss, metformin has the following advantages over sulphonylureas:

- It doesn't cause hypoglycaemia.
- It is known to have activity that lowers lipid, giving prominent reductions in the concentrations of serum triglyceride and free fatty acid. It also shows a minute reduction in the levels of serum LDL and an elevation in the levels of HDL.

However, metformin also comes with its disadvantages, which can be noted as below:

- Increased risk for lactic acidosis.
- Prominent side effects on the gastrointestinal front (described below).

Metformin intake must be done with meals and should initially be started on a low intake if one must look at avoidance of gastrointestinal side effects. A maximum of 2550 mg/day may be reached, in forms of 850 mg 3 times a day (TID).

The most common side effects of metformin are generally gastrointestinal. It may cause nausea, mild anorexia, diarrhoea, and discomfort in the abdomen and a general metallic taste in the mouth. However, these side effects are generally short lived and transient and can be curbed by either reduction in the dosage or intermittent discontinuation of the drug.

Another rare issue is lactic acidosis. This may be fatal in half of all cases in which it occurs. However, the risk of this in metformin is much lower than in the drugs that were previously used in the US but are now banned (biguanide and phenformin), primarily only due to this complication. Alarming lactic acid accumulation is seen in the following prone-to conditions:

- Instability in the haemodynamics
- Liver disease or abuse of alcohol
- Heart failure
- State of hypoxia
- Ages more than 80 years
- Acute illnesses
- Renal insufficiency

4.9.3 Drug Interactions

There is a notably important potential drug interaction that may occur between cimetidine and metformin. This results in an increase in the blood levels of metformin.The aforementioned drug interaction may cause hypoglycaemia, especially in patients who are taking sulphonylureas and/ or insulin along with. It also increases the risk of lactic acidosis in patients who have an impaired function of the kidneys. These risks may increase as cimetidine is now available for free purchases over the counter. This problem is less likely to occur with other H2 blockers.

There is also a recommendation for the discontinuation of metformin post-radiological procedures that administer iodinated material into the blood for 48 hours after the procedure. It is recommended to do so in order to prevent the increase in plasma concentrations of metformin in case of development of acute renal failure in the patient owing to the iodine contrast material.

The efficacy of thiazolidineiones has been tested in a study conducted upon 284 patients diagnosed with type II diabetes. They were treated with rezulin. There was a significant but non-dramatic fall in the mean fasting levels of blood glucose over a period of 12 weeks. However, treatments done with placebo showed only a fall in the blood glucose levels of 4 mg/ dL. The value of HbA_{1C} in the group treated with troglitazone reduced from 8.6% to 8.1%.

4.9.4 Alpha Glucosidase Inhibitors

These include miglitol and acarbose and are available for sale in multiple countries, including the United States. They work by the inhibition of the upper GI enzymes which convert dietary starches and other complex carbohydrates into simpler ones for their utilization in the body. This slows down the absorption of glucose post the consumption of meals.

There are side effects of this type of drugs, mainly in the form of diarrhoea and flatulence. These are generally mild and do not require discontinuation of the drug.

4.10 MANAGEMENT OF DIABETES MELLITUS

4.10.1 Diets for Diabetes Mellitus

For type I diabetes, no method of prevention has been found yet. However, for type II diabetes, which causes for 85-90% of all diabetes cases worldwide, prevention can be done by maintaining a healthy body weight, regular physical activity, and intake of healthy diet. Higher than 90 minutes a day's physical activity is known to decrease the incidence of diabetes straight by 28%. The dietary changes which aid the prevention or delaying of type II diabetes mellitus include high intake of whole grains and fibre, and also the consumption of good fats, like PUFAs, found in nuts, fish and vegetable oil. Certain things must be avoided, like sugary beverages and red meat along with other sources that provide high amounts of saturated fats. Smoking of tobacco has been linked multiple times with the incidence of diabetes, hence curbing smoking is another effective measure to fight the onset of diabetes.

It is seen that the link between diabetes and the factors that may prevent it (like body weight, unhealthy diet, tobacco and lack of physical activity) is the same throughout the world. A link has been made out between diabetes and matters of international and global importance, such as population explosion, urbanization, aging, globalization and a general unhealthy environment.

Type II diabetes mellitus may be prevented by changes in lifestyle and by administration f proper medication. Pre-diabetes has been classified as a group that is at high risk in accordance to the increased glycaemic levels which doesn't meet the criteria for diabetes, by the American Diabetes Association. Without preventive measures, patients falling into the category of pre-diabetes advance to the diabetes stage (type II) with a rate of 5-10%. Prevention of diabetes may be achieved by a combination of weight loss and increase in a physical activity. This reduces the risk of diabetes by 50-60%.

It has been made evident with the help of multiple clinical studies that sensitivity is increased by resistant starch, in a manner independent of the glycaemic response that our body gives to the food intake. This reduces the risk of diabetes. The FDA in the US (Food and Drug Administration) has claimed that this type of starch can reduce the incidence of type II diabetes, along with scientific evidence that limits support for this claim.

With more significant and substantial evidence, foods with lower glycaemic index and rich in fibre are known to help in the prevention of diabetes.

Significance of the dietary fat types has been made out by various sources. Unsaturated fats have been found to have a positive effect, as proposed on theoretical grounds as well as by observations made in animal studies. Harmful effects of hydrogenated fats have been seen universally upon the cardiovascular system.

Connections have been made out by numerous studies between certain aspects of type II diabetes mellitus and the ingestion of particular foods or drugs. In mothers, breastfeeding may be linked to the prevention of type II diabetes mellitus.

The consumption of coffee has also been linked to the prevention of type II diabetes mellitus by various studies, although it remains unclear if there's any change in the risk of diabetes due to the consumption of coffee, as yet. This holds true for all kinds of coffee, whether potboiled or not, caffeinated or decaffeinated or with or without sugar.

4.10.2 Lifestyle

Many interventions that promote a healthy lifestyle show a positive effect in the prevention of diabetes. Diet and physical activity combined supported by counselling with programmes to reduce weight, maintain a healthy blood pressure, and improve levels of cholesterol are known to decrease risk of diabetes mellitus.

Prevention of type II diabetes mellitus may be aided by increment in physical activities, especially when the physical activity is conducted soon after the intake of a meal rich in carbohydrates, as it increases blood sugars. It has been recommended by the American Diabetes Associaction (ADA) that a healthy weight be maintained, along with at least 2½ hours of weekly exercise and a modest intake of fat (30% of energy intake) and fibres from whole grains.

Different diets are being recommended for diabetes, the main aim of the diet intervention and the nutritional therapy is to provide proper nutrition along with suppressing the clinical manifestations of the disease. Other objectives of the diet therapy in diabetes are to:

- improve the quality of life of the patient along with his life span;
- help body perform all basic metabolic functions properly on its own; and
- provide relief from the symptoms.

To achieve all these objectives, the best way is to have a healthy lifestyle along with proper and timely food and medications.

Energy requirements: It varies with age, BMI, gender, lifestyle and the type of diabetes a person is suffering from. Complications of the disease also play a major role in the determination of his energy requirements. If the person is of normal body weight and height, then normal calorie diet is given, keeping in mind his physical activities. If the person is malnourished, then a calorie increase of 500 kcal per day is required to reach the target of normal body weight and help body perform proper functions. If the person is required, then a reduction of 300 and 500 kcal per day for woman and man is done, respectively. With normal BMI, the calorie requirements for sedentary man and woman are 2320 and 1920 kcal/day respectively.

Carbohydrates: 1 gm of carbohydrate provides 4 kcal. Total energy derived from carbs should not be more than 50-60% of the total energy requirement. Complex carbs are given more along with good amount of dietary fibre. Simple carbohydrates are reduced. Complex and simple carbs should be in the ratio of 4:1. Dietary fibre is given, so as to reduce the calorie intake in case of overweight patients. Daily carbohydrate intake of the patient should be between 250 and 325 g.

Proteins: Just like carbs, protein also provides 4 kcal of energy for every 1 gm. Daily protein requirement of the patient is 1 g/kg body weight, and is increased in case of malnourishment. Protein should provide 25% of the total energy. Proteins should be of high biological value. All the essential amino acids should be provided in the diet.

Fats: 1 gm of fat provides 9 kcal of energy. Fats should not provide more than 25% of the total energy required. Per day requirement of fat should not be more than 60 gm per day. Of the total fats given per day, 50% should be monounsaturated fatty acids, 25% each saturated and polyunsaturated fats. Ratio of MUFA and PUFA should be 2:1.

Dietary fibre: Daily requirement of fibre is between 25 and 30 gm. Fibre helps in achieving early satiety, thus decreasing the food intake. It also provides bulk to the stools. Both soluble and insoluble fibres should be given. Fibre intake can be increased up to 60 gm per day.

Vitamins and minerals: A close check on the vitamin and mineral levels should be kept, and proper supplementation is to be done in case of low levels.

Foods to be included: Whole cereals, pulses, egg, milk, buttermilk, paneer, curd, fish, meat, fruits, vegetables, nuts and olive oil.

Foods to be excluded: Refined cereals, packed, processed food, alcohol, sugar, cake, jams, jellies, biscuits, pickles, fried, fatty food, khoya, ice-cream, butter and cream.

Several diets are being prescribed, 1 diet each of 1200, 1600 and 1800 kcal are given below along with calorie count and carbohydrate, protein, fat and fibre calculations.

4.10.3 1200 kcal Diet for Obese Diabetic

Required amount	Calculated amount
Total calories: 1200 kcals	**Total calories:** 1194.2 kcal
Carbohydrates: 189 g (63%)	**Carbohydrates:** 191.38 g
Protein: 60 g (20%)	**Protein:** 55.02 g
Fat: 29.3 g (22%)	**Fat:** 22.49 g
Fibre: 15 g	**Fibre:** 14.65 g

4.10.3.1 Menu

Meal	Food
Early morning	Amla (2) + Apple (1 small)
Breakfast	Skimmed milk (1 glass) + Uttapam (2)
Mid-day	Watermelon (250 g)
Lunch	Buttermilk (1 glass) + Chapatti (2) + Dal (1 bowl) + Salad (Tomato, cucumber)
Evening snack	Roasted Channa + Nuts (Almonds, Pistachios)
Dinner	Veggie Stew (beans, carrot, cauliflower and tomato)
Post-dinner	Skimmed milk (1 glass)

4.10.3.2 Diet Chart

Meal	Food	Calories (kcal)	Carbohydrates (g)	Protein (g)	Fats (g)	Fibre (g)
Early morning	Amla (30 g)	17.4	4.11	0.15	0.03	1.02
	Apple (60 g)	35.4	8.04	0.12	0.3	0.06
Breakfast	Skimmed milk (250 mL)	72.5	11.5	6.25	0.25	-
	Sooji (60 g)	208.8	44.88	6.24	0.48	0.12
	Onion (20 g)	10	2.22	0.36	0.02	0.12
	Tomato (20 g)	4	0.72	0.18	0.04	0.16
	Oil (3 g)	27	-	-	3	-
Mid-morning	Water melon (250 g)	42.5	8.25	0.5	0.05	0.5
Lunch	Buttermilk (250 mL)	100	12	8.25	2.25	-
	Cucumber (40 g)	5.2	1	0.16	0.4	0.16
	Tomato (40 g)	8	1.44	0.36	0.8	0.32
	Missi chapatti (2*20 g)	136.4	27.76	4.84	0.68	0.76
	Bengal gram (30 g)	104.1	17.88	7.2	0.42	0.27
	Tomato (30 g)	6	1.08	0.27	0.06	0.24
	Onion (30 g)	15	3.33	0.54	0.03	0.18
	Oil (1.5 g)	13.5	-	-	1.5	-
Evening	Roasted channa	109.2	18.3	5.7	1.8	5.1
	Almonds	65.5	1.05	2.08	5.89	0.17
	Pistachios	62.6	1.62	1.98	5.35	0.21
Dinner	Stew- carrot (50 g)	24	5.3	0.45	0.1	0.6
	Beans (20 g)	31.6	5.96	1.48	0.2	0.38
	Cauliflower (50 g)	15	2	1.3	0.2	0.6
	Tomato (50 g)	8	1.44	0.36	0.08	3.2
Post-dinner	Skimmed milk (250 mL)	72.5	11.5	6.25	0.25	-
Total	-	1194.2	191.38	55.02	22.49	14.65

4.10.3.3 Food Exchange Value

Food group	Weight
Cereals	30 g
Legumes and pulses	30 g
Milk and products	240 mL/100 g
Meat and products	70-80 g
Vegetable A	120-150 g
Vegetable B	70-80 g
Fruits	80-100 g
Oil	1 teaspoon/5 g
Nuts and seeds	10 g
Sugars	10 g

4.10.3.4 Food Exchange Table

Food group	Servings	Calories (kcal)	Carbohydrates (g)	Proteins (g)	Fats (g)	Fibre (g)
Cereals	4	345.2	72.64	11.08	1.16	0.88
Legumes and pulses	2	213.3	36.18	12.9	2.22	5.37
Milk products	3	245	35	20.75	2.75	-
Meat products	-	-	-	-	-	-
Vegetable A	-	-	-	-	-	-
Vegetable B	3	95.6	18.81	4.13	0.55	1.88
Fruits	4	121.3	25.08	1.94	1.09	2.84
Oil	1	40.5	-	-	4.5	-
Nuts and seeds	2	128.6	2.67	4.06	11.24	0.29
Sugars	-	-	-	-	-	-
Total	-	1194.2	191.38	55.02	22.49	14.65

4.10.4 1600 kcal Diet for Diabetes Mellitus

Required amount	Calculated amount
Total calories: 1600 kcals	**Total calories:** 1595.95 kcals
Carbohydrates: 220 g (55%)	**Carbohydrates:** 218 g
Protein: 80 g (20%)	**Protein:** 72 g
Fat: 44.5 g (25%)	**Fat:** 44.5 g
Fibre: 13.36 g	**Fibre:** 14.49 g

4.10.4.1 Menu

Meal	Food
Early morning	Pomegranate (1) + Raisins (10 g)
Breakfast	Skimmed milk (1 glass) + Stuffed roti (2)
Mid-day	Orange (80 g)
Lunch	Curd (100 g) + Brown Rice (60 g) + Dal (1 bowl) + Salad (Tomato, cucumber)
Evening snack	Veggie Poha + Nuts (Almonds, walnuts) + Buttermilk (1 glass)
Dinner	Bottlegourd raita (1 bowl) + Salad (Cucumber, carrot, lettuce, tomato and beetroot)+ Missi Roti
Post-dinner	Skimmed milk (1 glass)

4.10.4.2 Diet Chart

Meal	Food	Calories (kcal)	Carbohydrates (g)	Protein (g)	Fats (g)	Fibre (g)
Early morning	Pomegranate (80 g)	52	11.6	1.28	0.08	4.08
	Raisins (10 g)	30.8	0.4	0.18	0.03	0.11
Breakfast	Skimmed milk (250 mL)	72.5	11.5	6.25	0.25	-
	Stuffed roti (2*30 g)	204.6	41.64	7.26	1.02	1.14
	Potato (20 g)	19.4	4.52	0.32	0.02	0.08
	Paneer (20 g)	53	0.24	3.66	4.16	-
	Onion (20 g)	11.8	2.52	0.36	0.02	0.12
Mid-morning	Orange (80 g)	48	10.9	0.7	0.2	0.3
Lunch	Curd (100 g)	60	3	3.1	4	-
	Brown rice (60 g)	66.6	13.8	1.56	0.54	1.08
	Blackgram (45 g)	156.15	26.82	10.8	0.63	0.4
	Onion (50 g)	29.5	6.3	0.45	0.05	0.3
	Tomato (50 g)	10	1.8	0.9	0.1	0.4
	Oil (3 mL)	27	-	-	3	-
	Salad- Tomato (100 g)	20	3.6	0.9	0.2	0.8
	Cucumber (100 g)	15	2.5	0.4	0.1	0.4
Evening	Poha (30 g)	103.8	23.19	1.98	0.36	0.21
	Tomato (30 g)	6	1.08	0.27	0.06	0.24
	Onion (30 g)	17.7	3.78	0.54	0.03	0.18
	Peanuts (20 g)	113.4	5.22	5.06	8.02	0.62
	Almonds (10 g)	65.5	1.05	2.08	5.89	0.17
	Walnuts (10 g)	68.7	0.11	1.56	6.45	0.26
	Oil (3 mL)	27	-	-	3	-
	Buttermilk (250 mL)	100	12	8.2	2.25	-

Dinner	Salad- carrot (50 g)	24	5.3	0.45	0.1	0.6
	Cucumber (50 g)	13	2.5	0.4	0.1	0.4
	Tomato (50 g)	10	1.8	0.45	0.1	0.4
	Beetroot (50 g)	21.5	4.4	0.85	0.05	0.45
	Missi Roti	21	2.5	2.1	0.3	0.5
	Curd (100 g)	60	3	3.1	4	-
	Bottle gourd (50 g)	6	1.25	0.1	0.05	1.25
Post-dinner	Skimmed milk (250 mL)	72.5	11.5	6.25	0.25	-
Total	-	1606.45	219.82	71.51	45.41	14.49

4.10.4.3 Food Exchange Value

Food group	Weight
Cereals	30 g
Legumes and pulses	30 g
Milk products	240 mL/100 g
Meat products	70-80 g
Vegetable A	120-150 g
Vegetable B	70-80 g
Fruits	80-100 g
Oil	1 teaspoon/5 g
Nuts and seeds	10 g
Sugars	10 g

4.10.4.4 Food Exchange Table

Food group	Servings	Calories (kcal)	Carbohydrates (g)	Proteins (g)	Fats (g)	Fibre (g)
Cereals	5	375	78.63	10.8	1.92	2.43
Legumes and Pulses	1.5	156.15	26.82	10.8	0.63	0.4
Milk products	5	418	41.24	30.56	14.91	-
Meat products	-	-	-	-	-	-
Vegetable A	1	21	2.5	2.1	0.3	0.25
Vegetable B	5	157.9	33.07	3.87	0.52	3.78
Fruits	5	176.8	31.18	6.03	0.57	6.33
Oil	1.2	54	-	-	6	-
Nuts and seeds	5	247.6	6.38	8.7	20.36	1.05
Sugars	-	-	-	-	-	-
Total	-	1606.45	219.82	72.86	45.21	14.24

4.10.5 1800 kcal Diet for Diabetes Mellitus

Required amount	Calculated amount
Total calories: 1800 kcals	**Total calories:** 1789.1 kcal
Carbohydrates: 238.5 g (53%)	**Carbohydrates:** 238.94 g
Protein: 99 g (22%)	**Protein:** 100.59 g
Fat: 50 g (25%)	**Fat:** 46.5 g
Fibre: 12 g	**Fibre:** 11.09 g

4.10.5.1 Menu

Meal	Constituents
Early morning	Skimmed milk (1 glass)+ 1 apple (80 g)
Morning	Omelet (2 eggs, onion, tomato)
Mid-morning	Makhana chaat
Lunch	Rajmah (30 g) + Brown rice (60 g) + Buttermilk (250 mL)
Evening snack	Upma (60 g) + curd (100 g)
Dinner	Soybean, Spinach, Chapatti rolls

4.10.5.2 Diet Chart

Time	Meal	Calories (kcal)	Carbohydrates (g)	Proteins (g)	Fats (g)	Fibre (g)
Early morning	Skimmed milk (250 mL)	72.5	11.5	6.25	0.25	-
	Apple (60 g)	35.4	8.04	0.12	0.3	0.06
Breakfast	Omelet (2 eggs)	173	-	13.3	13.3	-
	Onion (50 g)	29.5	6.3	0.9	0.05	0.4
	Tomato (50 g)	10	1.7	0.25	0.05	0.3
	Oil (3 mL)	27	-	-	3	-
Mid-morning	Makhana Chaat					
	Makhana (30 g)	104.1	23.07	2.91	0.03	2.28
	Curd (100 g)	98	3.4	11	4.3	-
	Onion (50 g)	29.5	6.3	0.9	0.05	0.3
	Coriander chutney (10 g)	4.4	0.63	0.33	0.06	0.12
Lunch	Rajmah (30 g)	207.6	36.36	13.74	0.78	1.44
	Onion (30 g)	17.7	3.78	0.54	0.03	0.18
	Tomato (30 g)	20	3.4	0.15	0.1	0.24
	Oil (2 mL)	18	-	-	2	-
	Brown rice (60 g)	66.6	13.8	1.56	0.54	1.08
	Buttermilk (250 mL)	100	12	8.2	2.25	-
Evening snack	Upma					
	Sooji (60 g)	208.8	44.88	6.24	0.48	0.12
	Onion (50 g)	25	5.55	0.6	0.05	0.3
	Tomato (50 g)	10	1.7	0.25	0.05	0.4
	Oil (2 mL)	18	-	-	2	-
	Curd (100 g)	98	3.4	11	4.3	-

Dinner	Soybean Spinach Chapati Rolls					
	Soybean (30 g)	129.6	6.27	12.96	5.85	1.11
	Spinach (100 g)	26	2.9	2.0	0.7	0.6
	Onion (100 g)	59	12.6	1.8	0.1	0.6
	Tomato (100 g)	20	3.4	0.5	0.1	0.8
	Oil (5 mL)	45	-	-	5	-
	Chapatti (2*20 g)	136.4	27.76	4.84	0.68	0.76
Total		1789.1	238.94	100.59	46.5	11.09
%			53	22	25	44.36

4.10.5.3 Food Exchange Value

Food group	Weight
Cereals	30 g
Legumes and pulses	30 g
Milk products	240 mL/100 g
Meat products	70-80 g
Vegetable A	120-150 g
Vegetable B	70-80 g
Fruits	80-100 g
Oil	1 teaspoon/5 g
Nuts and seeds	10 g
Sugars	10 g

4.10.5.4 Food Exchange Table

Food Group	Servings	Calories (kcal)	Carbohydrates (g)	Proteins (g)	Fats (g)	Fibre (g)
Cereals	6	411.8	86.44	12.64	1.7	1.96
Legumes and pulses	2	337.2	42.63	26.7	6.63	2.55
Milk products	4	368.5	30.3	36.45	11.1	-
Meat products	1	173	-	13.3	13.3	-
Vegetable A	1	30.4	3.53	2.33	0.76	0.72
Vegetable B	4	165.2	35.28	5.04	0.28	2.18
Fruits	3	95.4	18.24	1.27	0.6	1.9
Oil	2.5	108	-	-	12	-
Nuts and seeds	3	104.1	23.07	2.91	0.03	2.28
Sugars	-	-	-	-	-	-
Total	-	1789.1	238.94	100.59	45.5	11.09

4.11 GLYCAEMIC INDEX AND GLYCAEMIC LOAD

4.11.1 Glycaemic Index (GI)

The GI is helpful for evaluating the relative velocity with which the body separates sugar. It considers just the accessible starch (complete sugar less fibre) in a nourishment. Glycaemic file does not foresee a person's glycaemic reaction to nourishment, however can be utilized as an instrument to survey the insulin reaction weight of a food, arrived at the midpoint of over an examined populace. Singular reactions change incredibly.

The glycaemic file is typically connected to the amount of the diet and the measure of sugar in the nourishment that is really expanded. A related measure, the glycaemic load (GL), factors this in by duplicating the glycaemic file of the nourishment being referred to by the sugar substance of the genuine serving.

A reasonable confinement of the glycaemic list is that it doesn't quantify insulin generation because of ascends in glucose. Thus, two nourishments could have the equivalent glycaemic file, yet produce distinctive measures of insulin. Moreover, two eatables could have the equivalent glycaemic load, however motivates diverse insulin reactions. Moreover, both the glycaemic file and glycaemic load estimations are characterized by the starch substance of diet. For instance, when eating steak, which has no sugar content yet gives a high protein consumption, up to half of that protein can be changed to glucose when there is practically no starch, but since it contains no starch itself, steak can't have a glycaemic record. For some nourishment examinations, the "insulin record" might be increasingly valuable.

4.11.1.1 Measurement

The glycaemic list of foods is characterized as the gradual zone under the two-hour blood glucose reaction bend AUC (glucose area under the curve) following a 12-hour quick and ingestion of a nourishment with a specific amount of accessible sugar (not more than 50 g). The AUC of the test nourishment is isolated by the AUC of the standard (either glucose or white bread, giving two distinct definitions) and duplicated by 100. The normal GI estimation is determined from information gathered in 10 human subjects. Both the standard and test food must contain an equivalent measure of accessible starch. The outcome gives a relative positioning for each tried nourishment.

Food with starches that separate rapidly amid absorption and discharge glucose quickly into the circulatory system will, in general, have a high GI.

Nourishments with sugars that separate all the more gradually, discharging glucose all the more step by step into the circulation system, will in general have a low GI. A lower glycaemic list proposes slower rates of processing and assimilation of the nourishment's sugars and can likewise demonstrate more noteworthy extraction from the liver and fringe of the results of starch absorption. The current approved strategies use glucose as the reference nourishment, giving it a glycaemic record estimation of 100 by definition. This has the benefits of being widespread and creating greatest GI estimations of around 100. White bread can likewise be utilized as a source of prospective food, giving an alternate arrangement of GI increments (in the event that white bread = 100, at that point glucose ≈ 140). For individuals whose staple starch source is white bread, this has the benefit of passing on legitimately whether supplanting of the dietary staple with an alternate nourishment would result in quicker or slower blood glucose reaction. An inconvenience with this framework is that the reference diet isn't very much characterized, in light of the fact that there is no all inclusive standard for the sugar substance of white bread.

Glycaemic record diagrams regularly give just a single raise for every nourishment, except varieties are conceivable due to

- Ripeness: Riper organic products contain more sugars, expanding GI like banana.
- Cooking techniques: The more cooked, or overcooked, a nourishment, the more its cell structure is broken, with a propensity for it to process rapidly and raise GI more. Fat, fibre, and acids, (for example, lemon juice or vinegar) bring down the glycaemic file.
- Processing – Flour has a higher GI than the entire grain from which it is ground as pounding breaks the grain's defensive layers) and the their strength. Potatoes are an outstanding precedent, extending from moderate to high GI even in a similar assortment.

All the more vitally, the glycaemic reaction is unique in relation to one individual to another, and furthermore in a similar individual from everyday, contingent upon blood glucose levels, insulin opposition, and different components. Our age, how dynamic we are, and how quick we digest nourishment likewise influence how our body responds to carbs. In the event that we have a diabetes difficulty called gastroparesis which postpones our stomach from purging, our body will retain nourishment significantly more gradually. The glycaemic list just demonstrates the effect on glucose level two hours subsequent to eating the food. Individuals with diabetes have raised dimensions for four hours or longer subsequent to eating certain nourishments.

A low GI nourishment will cause blood glucose levels to build all the more gradually and relentlessly, which prompts lower postprandial (after feast) blood glucose readings. A high-GI diet causes a progressively fast ascent in blood glucose level and is reasonable for vitality recuperation after exercise or for an individual encountering hypoglycaemia. Cut down the general glycaemic list of a dinner by consolidating a high glycaemic record diet with nourishments that have lower ones.

Bread is a standout amongst the most generally expended staple nourishments around the world. White-wheat bread, generally devoured in France, is produced using profoundly refined flour, which prompts a low supplement thickness. Because of an exceedingly permeable structure and gelatinized starch, it is effectively separated amid assimilation, prompting a fast increment of glucose discharged into the circulation system. Low glycaemic reactions are viewed as great to well-being, particularly against a foundation of diabetes. Writing reports demonstrate that choice of crude material is a fundamental factor in diminishing the glycaemic list (GI) of white bread. There are two methods for diminishing the rate of starch corruption: it is possible that (i) abating gastric exhausting rate as well as glucose diffusion– retention through the intestinal mucosa, which can be accomplished by consolidating solvent fibre or natural corrosive in bread, or (ii) constraining starch availability to α-amylase by utilizing high-amylose oat assortments and additionally fusing unblemished oat grains. Concentrates on grain items demonstrate that conservation of the food structure amid processing is by all accounts a more imperative GI-lessening factor than the level of starch crystallinity or the nearness of solvent fibre. Consequently, we should hope to create bread with an increasingly smaller nourishment structure or higher thickness, which is the situation in raised wholewheat bread or bread with flawless oat grains. The preparing procedure ought to likewise be improved to accomplish this objective, by utilizing, for instance, a diminished working time or less yeast than expected.

Foods grown from the ground, in general, have a low glycaemic record. The glycaemic record can be connected just to food's where the test depends on subjects expending a measure of nourishment containing 50 gm of accessible sugar, however numerous foods grown from the ground (not potatoes, sweet potatoes, corn) contain under 50 gm of accessible starch per ordinary serving. Carrots were initially and inaccurately revealed as having a high GI. Mixed drinks have been accounted for to have low GI qualities, yet brew was at first answered to have a moderate GI because of the nearness of maltose. This has been disproved by industry experts, who state that all maltose sugar is devoured in the fermenting procedure and that bundled brew has practically zero maltose present. Ongoing investigations have demonstrated that the utilization of a mixed beverage preceding a feast lessens the GI of the dinner by around 15%. Moderate liquor utilization over 12 hours preceding a test does not influence the GI.

For certain individuals, a low GI diet may give required heading to enable them to settle on better decisions for a solid eating regimen plan. The analysts who keep up the GI database alert, nonetheless, that the "glycaemic file ought not be utilized in confinement" and that other wholesome elements — calories, fat, fibre, nutrients and different supplements — ought to be considered.

Surveys of preliminaries estimating the effect of low GI file counts calories on cholesterol have appeared predictable proof that such weight control plans may help lower all out cholesterol, just as low thickness lipoproteins (the "awful" cholesterol) — particularly when a low GI diet is joined with an expansion in dietary fibre. Low-to-direct GI nourishments, for example, natural products, vegetables and entire grains are commonly great wellsprings of fibre.

One hypothesis about the impact of a low GI diet is craving control. The reasoning is that high GI diet causes a fast increment in blood glucose, a quick insulin reaction and an ensuing fast come back to feeling hungry. Low GI nourishments would, thus, postpone sentiments of yearning. Clinical examinations of this hypothesis have delivered blended outcomes. Additionally, if a low GI diet smothers hunger, the long haul impact ought to be that such an eating regimen would result over the long haul in individuals eating less and better deal with their weight. The long haul clinical research does not, be that as it may, show this impact.

4.11.1.2 Limitation

4.11.1.2.1 Contrasted with Amount of Sugar

Contingent upon amounts, the quantity of grams of starch in a nourishment can affect glucose levels more than the glycaemic list does. Devouring less dietary vitality, getting in shape and starch checking can be better for bringing down the glucose level. Starches sway glucose levels most significantly with a similar carb content are, by and large, practically identical in their consequences for glucose. Diet with a low glycaemic file can have a high sugar substance or the other way around; this can be represented with the glycaemic load (GL) where GL= GI% × grams of starch per serving (Louie JCY, et al., 2015]. Devouring starches with a low glycaemic record and ascertaining starch admission would create the most steady glucose levels.

GI estimations don't mirror the presumable amount we would eat of a specific food. For instance, watermelon has a GI estimation of 80, which would place it in the class of food to maintain a strategic distance from. However, watermelon has generally couple of absorbable sugars in a regular serving. At the end of the day, we need to eat a tonne of watermelon to fundamentally raise your blood glucose level.

To address this issue, scientists have built up the possibility of glycaemic load (GL), a numerical estimation that shows the adjustment in blood glucose levels when you eat a run of the mill serving of the food. For instance, a 4.2 ounce (120 gram, or 3/4 glass) serving of watermelon has a GL estimation of 5, which would recognize it as a solid nourishment decision. For examination, a 2.8 ounce (80 gm, or 2/3 container) serving of crude carrots has a GL estimation of 2.

Sydney University's table of GI estimation likewise incorporates GL values. The qualities are commonly gathered in the accompanying way:

- Low GL: 1 to 10
- Medium GL: 11 to 19
- High GL: at least 20

4.11.1.2.2 Contrasted with Insulin File

While the glycaemic file of nourishments is utilized as a manual for the ascent in blood glucose that ought to pursue supper containing those nourishments, real increments in blood glucose show extensive fluctuation from individual to individual, even after utilization of vague dinners. This is to some degree on the grounds that glycaemic record does not consider different factors other than glycaemic reaction, for example, insulin reaction, which is estimated by the insulin file and can be increasingly suitable in speaking with the impacts from some food substances other than starches. Specifically, since it depends on the zone under the bend of the glucose reaction after some time from ingesting a subject nourishment, the state of the bend makes little difference to the relating GI estimation. The glucose reaction can ascend to an abnormal state and fall rapidly, or rise less high however stay there for a more drawn out time, and has a similar territory under the bend.

4.11.1.2.3 Diabetes Mellitus

For subjects with sort 1 diabetes who don't have an insulin reaction, the rate of appearance of glucose after ingestion speaks to the assimilation of the food itself. This glycaemic reaction has been displayed, where the model parameters for the diet empower expectation of the persistent impact of the nourishment after some time on glucose estimations, and not simply a definitive impact that the GI speaks to.

In spite of the fact that the glycaemic record gives a few bits of knowledge into the relative diabetic hazard in explicit nutritional categories, it contains some illogical appraisals. These incorporate proposals that bread for the most part has a higher glycaemic positioning than sugar and that a few potatoes are more glycaemic than glucose.

A GI estimation reveals nothing about other healthful data. For instance, entire milk has a GI estimation of 31 and a GL estimation of 4 for a 1 container (250 millilitre) serving.

4.11.2 Glycaemic Load

The glycaemic record shouldn't be the main thing we think about when settling on decisions about what to eat. The reality a nourishment has a low glycaemic list doesn't mean it's super-solid, or that we ought to eat a great deal of it. Calories, nutrients, and minerals are as yet imperative. For instance, potato chips have a lower glycaemic record than oats and is about equivalent to green peas.

Segment sizes matter, as well. The greater amount of whatever sort of carbs we eat, the more they'll influence our glucose. That is the thing that the glycaemic load lets us know. It's a number we may see alongside the glycaemic record in records. Consider it the glycaemic list for a particular measure of that nourishment.

The glycaemic load of nourishment is a number that gauges how much the diet will raise an individual's blood glucose level subsequent to eating it. One unit of glycaemic load approximates the impact of expending one gram of glucose. Glycaemic load represents how much sugar is in the nourishment and how much every gram of starch in the food raises blood glucose levels. Glycaemic load depends on the glycaemic list, and is determined by duplicating the grams of accessible sugar in the food by the nourishment's glycaemic file, and afterwards partitioning by 100.

4.11.2.1 Estimation

Glycaemic load (GL) evaluates the effect of starch utilization utilizing the glycaemic file while considering the measure of sugars that are expended in a serving. GL is a GI weighted proportion of starch content. For example, watermelon has a high GI, yet a regular serving of watermelon does not contain numerous starches, so the glycaemic heap of eating it is low. Though glycaemic file is characterized for each sort of nourishment, glycaemic burden can be determined for any size serving of a food, a whole supper, or a whole day's dinners.

Glycaemic heap of a 100 gm serving of nutrition can be determined as its starch content estimated in grams (gm), increased by the nourishment's GI, and isolated by 100.

The glycaemic heap of a nourishment positions the impact of a particular serving size of that food on the glucose levels. The GL utilizes white bread as a pattern standard, where every unit of GL mirrors the glycaemic impact of 1 gm of sugar from white bread. In the event that we take a typical natural product, for example, an apple, the GL is resolved as:

GI of a standard apple = 40

Starch substance of a standard apple = 15

GL = (GI × Carbohydrate content)/100 = (40 × 15)/100 = 6

In the event that we take two foods with a similar GI estimation, however Food A contains 5% sugars and Food B contains 80% starches, Food B has a lot higher GL and ought to be eaten in lesser extents. All in all terms, nourishments with high sugar levels and low fibre substance have high GI and GL values, though those with high fibre substances have lower GLs.

For instance, watermelon has a GI of 72. A 100 gm serving of watermelon has 5 gm of accessible sugars (it contains a great deal of water), making the figuring 5 × 72/100=3.6, so the GL is 4. A food with a GI of 90 and 8 gm of accessible sugars has a GL of 7.2 (8 × 90/100 = 7.2), while a nourishment with a GI of only 6 and with 120 g of starch likewise has a GL of 7.2 (120 × 6/100 = 7.2).

4.11.2.2 Components Influencing Glycaemic Load

There are different elements that influence the GL of a food. A large number of these are like those that additionally impact the GI of a food item. These include: the sorts of sugar and starches in the nourishment, the manner in which it is readied, its fat, fibre and sugar content, and the serving size. The rate of ingestion and processing of food items additionally impact the GI and GL. Glycaemic load represents both the amount and the nature of our carbs. For one serving of a food, a GL more noteworthy than 20 is viewed as high, a GL of 11– 19 is viewed as medium, and a GL of 10 or less is viewed as low. Nourishments that have a low GL in a common serving size quite often have a low GI. Diets with a middle or high GL in an average serving size range from an extremely low to high GI. The accompanying qualities are connected to characterize the GL every day:

- Low GL – under 80
- High GL – more than 120

High GL nourishments incorporate white rice and refined nibble food products, for example, chips and improved beverages. By consuming foods that have a low GL, there is a general slower and lower ascend in glucose levels.

4.11.2.3 Applications

4.11.2.3.1 Digestion and Glycaemic Load

The GL is more mind boggling than the GI. Starches differ as far as amount and quality in various foods. Give us a chance to contrast the GI estimations of nourishments and distinctive starch densities.

4.11.2.4 Usefulness

The value of the GL has been illustrated, especially in connection to diabetic patients. If you experience the ill effects of diabetes, GL is an increasingly precise and intelligent indicator of glucose levels. By clinging to an eating regimen with a low GL, diabetics can decrease their normal glucose levels and lessen the dangers of creating entanglements, for example, eye, kidney and nerve harm.

Glycaemic burden can include a specific measure of estimation which may not be commonsense for everybody, notwithstanding, those with time to get the computations right may observe glycaemic burden to be a useful additional apparatus in picking which nourishments and which portions are appropriate for keeping up great blood glucose levels.

Surveying the glycaemic heap of nourishments can be especially helpful in the event that we have a particular dinner regularly or on the off chance that we are considering attempting another supper yet don't know how it might affect our blood glucose levels.

Note that diverse individuals with diabetes will have distinctive resistances to the starch in foods. Some people might almost certainly endure dinners with a medium glycaemic load, while others may find that they can just endure low glycaemic load estimations. In the event that we approach blood glucose testing supplies, we may wish to test which glycaemic load increments enable you to keep our sugar levels in the suggested rule blood glucose levels. A decent method to survey the impact of a specific supper is to test our blood glucose before eating, 2 hours subsequent to eating and again 4 hours in the wake of eating.

For an eating regimen with a lower glycaemic load, eat:

- more entire grains, nuts, vegetables, natural products, vegetables without starch, and different foods with a low glycaemic list;
- fewer nourishments with a high glycaemic file, similar to potatoes, white rice, and white bread;
- less of sugary nourishments, including treats, cakes, and sweet beverages;

Food	GI (glucose = 100)	Serving size	Carbohydrate* per serving (g)	GL per serving
Russet potato, baked	111	1 medium	30	33
Potato, white, boiled (average)	82	1 medium	30	25
Puffed rice cakes	82	3 cakes	21	17
Cornflakes	79	1 cup	26	20
Jelly beans	78	1 oz	28	22
Doughnut	76	1 medium	23	17
Watermelon	76	1 cup	11	8
Soda crackers	74	4 crackers	17	12
Bread, white-wheat flour	71	1 large slice	14	10
Pancake	67	6″ diameter	58	39
Rice, white, boiled	66	1 cup	53	35
Table sugar (sucrose)	63	2 tsp	10	6
Dates, dried	62	2 oz	40	25
Spaghetti, white, boiled (20 min)	58	1 cup	44	25
Honey, pure	58	1 Tbsp	17	10
Pineapple, raw	58	½ cup	19	11
Banana, raw	55	1 cup	24	13
Maple syrup, Canadian	54	1 Tbsp	14	7
Parsnips, peeled, boiled	52	½ cup	10	5
Rice, brown, boiled	50	1 cup	42	20
Spaghetti, white, boiled (average)	46	1 cup	44	20
Whole-grain pumpernickel bread	46	1 large slice	12	5
All-Bran™ cereal	45	1 cup	21	10
Spaghetti, whole-meal, boiled	32	1 cup	37	14
Orange, raw	42	1 medium	11	5
Apple, raw	39	1 medium	15	6
Pear, raw	38	1 medium	11	4
Skim milk	33	8 fl oz	13	4
Carrots, boiled	33	½ cup	4	1
Lentils, dried, boiled	29	1 cup	24	7
Kidney beans, dried, boiled	28	1 cup	29	8
Pearled barley, boiled	28	1 cup	38	11
Cashews	25	1 oz	9	2
Peanuts	18	1 oz	6	1

*Amount of available carbohydrates in a food serving that excludes indigestible carbohydrates, i.e., dietary fibre.

- replace starches with protein;
- eat low GI starch nourishments rather than high GI sugar food; and
- try and have no less than 3 low GL nourishments for the duration of the day, with every feast.

We can in any case eat food with a high glycaemic record. Simply appreciate them in little segments, and balance them with nutritious, low-glycaemic file food.

4.11.3 Low GI/GL Diet versus High GI/GL Diet

Amid the post-prandial period, blood glucose and insulin rose higher after the high GI supper than after the low GI feast. Also, because of the overabundance insulin emission, blood glucose dipped under fasting conditions three to five hours after high-GI dinner consumption. Cerebral blood stream was essentially higher four hours after ingestion of the high GI feast (contrasted with a low GI dinner) in a particular locale of the striatum (right core accumbens) related with food consumption reward and longing for. On the off chance that the information recommended that devouring low as opposed to high GI diet may help limit gorging and secure against weight gain, this has not yet been affirmed in long haul randomized controlled preliminaries.

Way of life alteration programmes don't as of now incorporate the decrease of calories from starch as an option in contrast to standard medicine of low-fat weight control plans, nor do they propose utilization of GI/GL as a manual for more beneficial dietary decisions.

4.12 CONCLUSION

Diabetes, or more specifically diabetes mellitus, is a category/group of metabolic disorders which are characteristic of high sugar levels in the blood for long. The symptoms include frequent thirst, increase in quantity and frequency of urination and increase in hunger. The reasons of the occurrence diabetes are only two, either insufficient production of insulin in the pancreas or the inability of the body cells to utilize it. There are mainly 3 types of diabetes:

- **Type I diabetes** results due to the failure of the pancreas on the front of secretion of insulin. This is generally attributed to the loss of beta cells. This is also known as juvenile diabetes.
- **Type II diabetes** begins with the resistance of insulin in the body. Herein, the body cells fail to utilize the insulin and thus the glucose of the blood.

- **Gestational diabetes** occurs in pregnant women and generally vanishes after childbirth. May give rise to type II diabetes.

Insulin is the principal hormone that accounts for the uptake of glucose, or blood sugar from blood into cells, tissues, etc. It happens specifically in the liver, adipose tissues and muscle, with the exception of smooth muscle, wherein the same is carried out by IGF-1. Hence, whenever there's a deficiency of insulin or when the insulin receptors become insensitive to it, it generally acts as a pilot for diabetes mellitus.

The use of oral hypoglycaemic drugs is done only in the treatment of type II diabetes mellitus, which is a condition wherein there is resistance to the insulin that has been secreted.

Following are the drugs used mainly for management and treatment of diabetes mellitus:

- Metformin
- Alpha-glucosidase inhibitors
- Thiazolidinediones
- Sulphonylureas

Conclusively, diabetes, although a severe metabolic disorder that requires attention of the highest order, can be managed and treated. The aim of treatment is to lower the blood glucose and HbA_{1C} levels. This is done with a combination of dietary changes, medications and physical activity.

CASE STUDIES

Juvenile Diabetic

To plan a day's diet for a girl, 7 years old suffering from diabetes (height = 145 cm and weight = 29 kg)

Personal Information

Age: 7 years old

Sex: female

Physical activity: moderate

Physiological condition: diabetes

RDA: 1200-1250 kcal/day

CHO: 55% of total energy requirement = 165 gm/day

Protein: 10-12% of the total energy requirement = 30-35 gm/day

Fat: 15-17% of the total energy requirement = 20-22 gm/day

Principal Diet

Low calorie, high protein, low carbohydrate, low fat and high fibre

Comprehensive Exchange List

Food group	Exchange number	Protein	Carbohydrate	Fat	Energy
Milk	1	8	12	8	170
Meat					
Pulses	1,5	10	25		150
Cereals	6	12	90		420
Veg A	6		21		120
Veg B	1		6		40
Fruits	5		25		200
Fats	5			15	45
Sugar					

Distribution from the Table

Food group	No. of exchange list	Bed tea	Breakfast	After meal snack	Lunch	Post meal snack	Dinner	Post-dinner snack
Milk	1		1					
Meat								
Pulses	1.5		0.5		1			
Cereals	6		3		3			
Veg A	6		2		2	1	1	
Veg B	1			1				
Fruits	5		1	1	1	1	1	1
Fat	5		2		2		1	
Sugar								

Meal	Quantity	Food item	Energy (kcal)	CHO (g)	Proteins (g)	Fats (g)
Bed-tea	1 glass	Lemon water	-	-	-	-
Breakfast	1 glass	Milk	150	12	8	3.2
	1 bowl	Cornflakes	320	150	10	-
	1 medium	Apple	60	15	11	-
	1	Paneer sandwich	90	20	-	-

Mid-morning	1 cup	Coconut water	-	-	-	-
	1 tablespoon	Flaxseed	69	6	2	4.5
Lunch	3 serving	Boiled rice	160	45	6	-
	2 small bowl	Mixed vegetables curry	50	9	3.5	-
	1 large bowl	Salad	20	4	1	-
	1 small bowl	Curd	155	8.7	8	10.3
Evening tea	1 small bowl	Baked tuna	110	-	14	6
	Green tea	-	-	-	-	-
Dinner	2 medium	Chapattis	160	30	4	-
	1 cup	Dal	101	10	8	3.2
	1 large bowl	Salad	20	3.5	1	-
	1 small bowl	Mixed vegetables	25	3.5	1	-
Post-dinner	1 cup	Chicken soup	5.7	-	1.2	3.2

QUESTIONS

1. What is diabetes mellitus? Describe causes, symptoms and risk factors associated with it
2. How does diabetes mellitus affects the metabolism of carbohydrates, proteins and fats?
3. What are the types of assessment techniques that are used for detecting of diabetes melltitus?
4. Differentiate between type I and type II diabetes mellitus in terms of etiology, symptoms and management.
5. Differentiate between glycaemic index and glycaemic load.
6. What are hypoglycaemic drugs? Write about their role in treatment of diabetes.
7. Discuss about the dietary management of diabetes mellitus with reference with:
   (i) 1400 kcal
   (ii) 1600 kcal
   (iii) 1800 kcal
8. Write a brief note on insulin. Discuss about its types, formation, role in diabetes mellitus, absorption and elimination.

9. Write a short note on:
   (i) Immunoginicity
   (ii) Adverse effects of insulin
10. Write about low glycaemic index foods and their role in the management of diabetes mellitus.
11. Plan a day's diet for a male patient of 65 years suffering from type II diabetes mellitus and hypertension.

5

Gastrointestinal Disorders and Gastrointestinal Surgeries

A. DIETARY MANAGEMENT IN GASTROINTESTINAL DISORDERS

5.1 PEPTIC AND DUODENAL ULCER

5.1.1 Peptic Ulcer

This disease mainly occurs in the stomach. The mucosal lining of the alimentary tract comes in close association with the acid, that is, gastric acidic juice. It can cause ulceration in the tissue. Peptic ulcer disease is curable and also avoidable. For *Helicobacter pylori* infection in the stomach anti-inflammatory non-steroidal drugs are given. The person who is infected from *Helicobacter pylori* has 10 to 20 per cent chances of peptic ulcer.

Peptic ulcers are classified as under–

Gastric ulcers are produced on the inner lining of the stomach.

Duodenal ulcers are found on the inner lining of the upper portion of small intestine (duodenum).

Oesophageal ulcers: They develop in the inner lining of the oesophagus.

Ulcers are formed when acids in stomach break down the lining of gastrointestinal tract. General reasons are bacteria, i.e., *Helicobacter pylori* and anti-inflammatory pain relievers including aspirin, cigaratte smoking, Crohn disease. Doctors call this type of peptic ulcer oesophageal ulcer.

Patients wake up at night with upper abdominal pain. The pain develops with eating, the pain might worsen with excess eating. It is also called burning or dull ache. Some other symptoms are also seen like belching, vomiting, bleeding, and poor appetite. Bleeding occurs in 15% of cases. The mucous membrane in the inner lining of stomach, oesophagus, small intestine becomes more sensitive to the action of *Helicobacter pylori*.

Helicobacter infection diagnosed in the 60 to 100% in the peptic ulcer while 90 to 100 % in the duodenal ulcer. The symptoms of the peptic ulcer are:

- Nausea
- Heart burn
- Intolerance of foods like fatty food
- Stomach pain
- Satiety
- Belching
- Bloating
- Vomiting trouble in breathing
- Feeling of faint

Most common symptom being burning sensation in stomach with pain. Pain worsens on empty stomach because of excessive acid production; pain lasts from few minutes to many hours. Foods which are basic in nature or act as buffer are found to be useful in neutralizing the acid, thus giving a temporary relief. Antacids also help in reliving the symptoms temporarily. Pain generally increases during night or between the meals. About three quarter patients are asymptomatic. Vomiting or hematemesis, dark coloured, black and tarry stools, breathlessness, nausea, anorexia, fatigue, unexplained weight loss, pale skin colour are the rare symptoms which are observed in different patients.

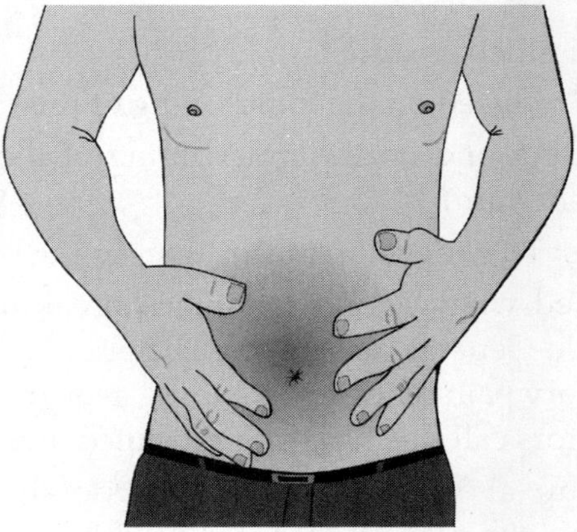

Stomach pain is the most common symptom. The acids present in the stomach at the time of peptic ulcer disease make the pain worse. For relaxation one can eat certain foods that neutralize the acid in the stomach or create buffer, or by taking medicines.

5.1.1.1 Pathophysiology

Back in time when *H. pylori* weren't discovered, scientists found three major physiological disturbances in the gastrointestinal tract of the patients suffering from duodenal ulcers. Abnormalities observed were impaired acid inhibition releasing from the antral mucosa, elevated basal along with stimulated acid secretion by stomach's body and elevated acid in the duodenum of the small intestine. After the discovery of *H. pylori*, these abnormalities were justified with the bacterial infection like the elevated secretion of gastrin by the antral mucosa in the patients suffering from duodenal ulcers. Genetic or environmental factors also contribute to these abnormalities. Inhibition of the bacterial growth was seen with the critical nature of gastric load in precipitating and washing out of the bile. Gastric metaplasia is promoted in cases of progressive damage to the duodenum. Gastric metaplasia promotes the growth of the bacteria and thus causing more inflammation. Repetitive and increased inability of the duodenal bulb to neutralize the acid coming from stomach makes the condition favourable for the development of ulcer by altering the structure and function of the duodenal bulb. Treating *H. pylori* infection helps in restoring the duodenum's normal pH making a marked decrease in the duodenal acid load. Decreased acid load in the duodenum helps against inflammation which finally helps in the cure of chronic ulcer disease.

5.1.1.2 Diagnosis

Different tests are done to explore the site, type and severity of the ulcer formed. Some tests are listed below.

Gastroscopy: Commonly known as endoscopy. This test confirms the presence of the wounds or ulcers in different sites. This is done by passing an endoscope or a thin flexible telescope down the oesophagus, and looking for any inflammation or ulcerations.

Test to detect *H. pylori*: It is generally done in the case of duodenal ulcer. The bacterium can be detected in stool test, breath test, blood test and even in the biopsy sample taken during endoscopy. If test comes positive, then the cause of ulcer is bacteria and patient is put on antibiotics along with other anti-ulcerative medicines.

5.1.1.3 Causes of Peptic Ulcer

Peptic ulcer occurs when the acid causes ulceration in the wall of the small intestine or the inner surface wall of the stomach. The acid in the stomach and in the intestine may sore which is very painful and which can bleed too.

Peptic ulcers are formed when acids in the gastrointestinal tract breaks down the inner lining of the stomach, oesophagus, and small intestine. This acid forms a sore that is open and very painful. Sometimes this sore bleeds. In humans digestive tract is layered with mucous membrane that generally protects the inner lining from wear and tear and also from acids. But, if the acid production is more and the mucus production is less than acid, then there is chance of ulcer formation on major side. The clinical observations are limited and non-specific. Patients having this have sudden onset of severe, sharp abdominal pain.

The common causes of peptic ulcer are:

5.1.1.3.1 *Helicobacter Pylori*

Helicobacter pylori are the bacteria which survive in the small intestine. They survive in the mucus layer of the membrane which protects and covers the tissue layer of the stomach. The *H. pylori* causes no problem in the stomach but when their number increases in the stomach, they react with the acid present in the stomach and cause ulcer in the wall of the stomach and intestine. The *H. pylori* spread through the contaminated food and water.

5.1.1.3.2 Use of Painkillers on Regular Basis

Non-steroidal anti-inflammatory drugs: Before understanding how NSAIDs' cause peptic ulcer, first we have to understand NSAIDs' work. Non-steroidal anti-inflammatory drugs reduce pain, swelling, inflammation and fever. Every human being has two types of enzymes that produce two types of cells, that give inflammation and fever. The role of NSAIDs' is to reduce the amount of enzymes that body produces. However, one of the two enzymes protect the inner lining from wear and tear. If the amount of these enzymes is reduced by this, NSAIDs that increase the chances of developing peptic ulcer.

These medicines are aspirin, naproxen, etc. Sometimes anti-coagulants, steroids, selective serotonin inhibitor also cause irritation on the lining of the stomach and have great chances to cause peptic ulcer.

5.1.1.3.3 Smoke and Drink Alcohol

It the people who are infected with *H. pylori* continue to smoke then they cause ulceration in the stomach. Some of them are consuming alcohol after the infection, so the alcohol erodes the lining of mucus in the stomach and increases the amount of acid present in the stomach.

5.1.1.3.4 Spicy foods

During the infection there is restriction on eating spicy and junk foods. If anyone consumes, it can cause inflammation in the stomach and cause ulcer.

Tumours from ZES: Zollinger Ellison syndrome is a rare type of disorder and occurs when two or more tumours form in pancreas or duodenum.

These tumours release large amounts of gastrin. Gastrin stimulates the stomach to produce large amounts of acids. This extra acid causes peptic ulcers in the stomach and duodenum.

5.1.1.4 Risk Factors

There are several factors which put an individual on the stake of getting duodenal ulcers. Some are explained below.

- **Heredity:** Genetics and heredity play a key role in determining the physical makeup of an individual. It also tells about the risk of getting certain diseases and defects from the ancient family of an individual. If duodenal ulcer is present in close family of the individual, then the chances of getting them increases manifolds.
- **Lifestyle:** Another important factor which can either favour the hereditary complications or can even suppress their effects is lifestyle. Lifestyle plays a key role in avoiding the disease. A decent daily routine can delay the appearance of the disease despite being hereditary.
- **Smoking tobacco:** Smoking tobacco and cigarettes increases the risk of getting duodenal ulcers.
- **Age:** People of age 70 and above are more prone to the disease.
- Physical trauma
- **Medications:** NSAIDs (non-steroidal anti-inflammatory drugs) are the leading medicines which cause duodenal ulcers. Other medicines include anti-coagulants, steroids and selective serotonin reuptake inhibitors (SSRIs).

From recent studies it has been found that alcohol consumption or regular consumption of spicy food is not a contributing factor of the disease, but they tend to worsen the pain and hinder the process of wound healing. The role of stress as a risk factor in the ulcer formation is not specific yet. Some researchers think stress of a direct risk factor while for others it is an indirect one. From a study, it was found that psychological stress is directly linked with duodenal ulcer formation, but it was also found that the stress is indirectly linked to ulcers as the subjects were under either NSAIDs prescription or were into smoking.

5.1.1.5 Complications of the Peptic Ulcers

If peptic ulcer is not managed properly, it can cause many serious problems which may become life threatening. The complications of peptic ulcers are:

- Anaemia
- Intestinal bleeding

- Perforation in the stomach and intestine
- Inflammation in the lining of abdominal cavity
- Shock
- Obstruction of intestine

Treatment of the peptic ulcer is therapy as well as proper eating habit that is, diet. Treating involves inhibitors of acid and the second one is most common antacid.

The solution of magnesium hydroxide and aluminum hydroxide is a common antacid which is present in the market. The drugs which are used as inhibitors of acid are H2 receptor blocker and proton pump inhibitor such as omeprazole.

Several other complications occur in peptic ulcer, and are listed below:

Internal bleeding: In case of ulceration at the site of blood vessel, vessels are at a risk of eruption and thus bleeding. It is one of the most common and drastic complication of ulcer. 15-20 per cent cases of the total experiences internal bleeding. Risk factors include overconsumption of non-steroidal anti-inflammatory (NSAID) drugs over a long period of time. People who are 60 years of above are at a greater risk. Based on the type and site of the blood vessel inflamed, long-term and short-term bleeding can be observed. Long-term bleeding leads to the development of anaemia (drop in the number of RBCs, oxygen carrying blood cells). In some cases symptoms of anaemia include bleeding that can be rapid and severe, and may lead to vomiting blood, tar-like or dark coloured stools. In case of moderate bleeding, proton pump inhibitor injections are found to be useful. It has been found that lowering acid around the bruised sites helps in faster blood clotting and thus ceasing the bleeding. In case of severe bleeding, blood transfusion is found to be useful. Blood vessels can be repaired using surgery. Endoscopy is used to check for the bruising and chances of recurrence of the disease. If the patient is at the risk of recurrence, further medications and PPI's are given as a part of eradication therapy.

Perforations: It implies to the fact that ulcer has digested the lining of the stomach. Probability of getting perforations is very low, about 2- 10 per cent. Perforations are severe and deadly, as it may lead to peritonitis, a condition in which peritoneum lining of the abdomen is infected with the bacteria. Peritonitis is a medical emergency because peritoneum is sterile and doesn't have any defense mechanism of its own to protect itself. The infection from the peritoneum can travel to different organs via blood, leading to multiple organ failure and finally death. Sudden onset of abdominal pain which eventually worsens with time is among the most common symptom of peritonitis. This condition requires urgent hospitalization, where the patient is given antibiotics and surgery to close up the wounds of stomach lining.

Gastric obstruction: In some cases it has been found that peptic ulcer can cause swelling thus leading to the obstruction in passage of food in the further parts of the digestive tract. This obstruction is termed gastric obstruction. Though it is rare, and is seen in 5 to 8 per cent of the total cases. Symptoms include vomiting containing major parts of bolus (mass of undigested food), bloating, anorexia, belching, excessive and unexplained weight loss. Endoscopy is used as a tool to diagnose the site, type and severity of the obstruction. In case of obstruction due to inflammation, histamine 2 receptor antagonists or proton pump inhibitors are given to reduce the inflammation. In case of obstruction due to scar tissue formation, surgical procedures are required for treatment. In severe cases, the scarred tissue is surgically removed out of the stomach and the remaining part is ligated thereafter. But in case of less or moderately complicated cases, side of obstruction is widened using a balloon, which is passed through an endoscope and then is inflated at the site of obstruction.

Duodenal ulcers: A condition in which formation of scar tissue or ulcer takes place in the starting region of small intestine particularly named duodenum is duodenal ulceration. *Helicobacter pylori* are the infection causing bacteria in ulcers. Other contributing factors to the ulcer formation are cigarette smoking and anti-inflammatory medicines. Pain caused in ulcers is not linked with the size and severity of the scar tissue formed. Food after leaving stomach enters directly into the duodenal part of the small intestine, thus making duodenum an active site for ulceration. Ulceration can take place both in the stomach as well as in the duodenum. Both stomach and duodenal ulcers are categorized under peptic ulcers. Ulcers heal with a medication course of about 4-8 weeks. Along with it, 1 week course of antibiotics is given along with medicines which suppress the production of acid in the stomach. This is done to remove any bacteria in the gut, which might cause reinfection. Anti-inflammatory medicines are very useful against duodenal ulcers.

5.1.1.6 Management of Peptic Ulcer through Drugs

Carifate, omeprazole, ranitidine and sucralfate are the most common drugs prescribed in duodenal ulcers.

Carifate: Its action is very similar to sucralfate, as it acts on the active ulcers by adhering to the bruised site and making a protective shield against the acid, bile and enzymes. It is not absorbed in the body, and is a very potent anti-ulcerative drug. It doesn't guarantees non-recurrence of the ulcers at new sites.

Sucralfate: It is used in the treatment of an active ulcer, and is given for a short duration of time, up to 8 weeks. Main site of action of the drug is stomach mucosal lining, and is absorbed in less amounts in the body. It protects the stomach lining from acid produced, enzymes and bile by adhering to the site of ulceration. This medicine can help in healing of the current ulcers, but doesn't help against further wound formation. It is consumed orally, and its IV administration can be fatal. Stop consuming the medicine if you are allergic to it or have diabetes, kidney disorder, or on dialysis or have trouble swallowing tablets. It is not to be consumed by children of age below 18 years. Consult your physician before taking this medicine if you are pregnant or lactating.

Antibiotics: For *Helicobacter pylori* infecting ulcers you have to take antibiotics along with proton pump inhibitors. It helps in healing peptic and duodenal ulcers. Mostly used antibiotics are amoxicillin, clarithromycin, metronidazole, and tetracycline. They are given through doctor's prescription and this drugs are available in capsules and tablets.

Proton pump inhibitors (PPIs): PPIs have direct role in inhibiting the acid production by interfering with the proton pumps of the gastric parietal cell which is responsible for acid production and thus healing the ulcer. The effects of PPIs are stronger than that of histamine 2 receptor antagonists. They are omeprozole and the pharmacy only medicine lansoprazole, rabeprazole, esomeprazole, pantoprazole and aripiprazole. They are available in different forms like tablets, capsules and injections.

Omeprazole: It is a type of proton pump inhibitor (PPI). It works against ulcers by depressing the quantity of acid formed in the stomach. It is helpful in treating conditions in which excess acid is produced, like gastroesophageal diseases. It is also helpful in treating oesophagitis (inflammation of the oesophagus due to acid, infection or some drugs). Administration along with antibiotics helps in treating gastric ulcers caused as a result of bacterial infection. It is also used against heart burn. Course period of this medicine is of 14 days in a row. It acts slowly and doesn't provide immediate relief against heart burn. It may worsen the existing lupus (an inflammatory disease caused when immune system starts attacking its own cells) or may contribute to the formation of new one. If you feel joint pain or skin rash consult your physician immediately.

Histamine2 receptor antagonist: This interferes with the secretion of gastric acids by blocking the histamine actions which is a protein produced by body stimulates gastric acid secretion. There medicines are available in different forms like tablets, capsules, syrups and injections.

Antacids: Antacids give rapid pain relief by neutralizing the acids present in the stomach. Thus relieving or eliminating the wear and tear and pain to the stomach walls and ulcer sites. Meals and at bedtime only when acidity occurs. Medicines like aluminium hydroxide, magnesium trisilicate, calcium carbonate, sodium bicarbonate are taken orally in the form of pills and in the liquid forms.

Ranitidine: It is categorized under the drug name of histamine 2 blockers. Its main function is to reduce the amount of acid production in the stomach. It is used to prevent ulcers in both stomach and intestine. It is also used in Zollinger-Ellison syndrome (a condition in which hyperplasia of the islets cells of pancreas causes excessive production of gastric acid). It is also prescribed by in hurt burn and gastroesophageal diseases (condition in which acid reflux from stomach to oesophagus and causing burning sensation). People who consume ranitidine on daily basis over a long period of time are prone to pneumonia. Symptoms of pneumonia are fever, chest pain, shortness of breath and expectorating green or yellow coloured mucus. Avoid in case of allergy, liver or kidney diseases and porphyria.

Cyto protective agents: These agents protect the tissues that lines the stomach and small intestines. These are prescription-only medicines like prostaglandine analogues, which interfere with gastric acid secretion by direct action on parietal cell and promoting gastric and duodenal ulcers. Microprostol is one from them which is taken orally in the form of tablets. Along with chelates and complexes, also belong to this class. Chelates and complexes form a surface covering over the ulcer with the help of adherent complex protein, thus protecting it from further damage by acids and helping in healing. Sucralate is available in forms of tablets and suspensions.

5.1.1.7 Management of Peptic Ulcer

The bland diet is given in the peptic ulcer because it is mild diet and soft and does not cause any irritation in the stomach and it is easily digested, so the bland diet is recommended in the peptic ulcer.

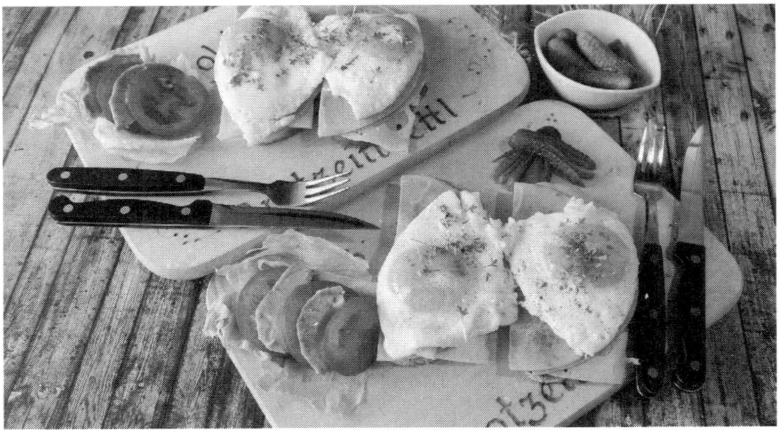

The nutrition is given to provide an adequate form and continuously neutralize the acid present in the stomach and also help to stop or minimize the secretion of gastric acid from the stomach. Nutrition reduces the irritation like chemical, mechanical in the stomach or small intestine.

Foods to be given: Foods in bland diet are juices, smoothies, milk and milk products, well cooked cereals and pulses, vegetables and fruits.

Foods to be avoided: Fried foods, strong spices, junk foods, fatty tough meats which are not easily digested, alcoholic and carbonated beverages, and strongly flavoured vegetables.

Bland diet and soft diet: Bland diet is a special diet which is recommended for the patient who is suffering from the peptic ulcer. The foods which are chemically, mechanically and thermally irritating to the gastrointestinal mucosa are restricted.

Chemically irritating foods increase the gastric juice flow and cause the stomach pain and irritability in the patient. Chemically irritating foods are meat extractives, fried foods, spices and condiments and some beverages like coffee, tea, alcohol, carbonated drinks and cocoa.

In mechanically irritating food the peristaltic action increases in the stomach because of the fibrous food, for example, skin and seed of vegetables and fruit as well as whole grain cereals and whole pulses.

Thermally irritating foods are either very hot or very cold and their consumption causes irritation in the stomach.

So, bland diets are recommended because they can decrease or neutralize the flow of gastric acid in the stomach. Frequent feedings are prescribed in the peptic ulcer. Fat is also allowed in moderate amount like the fats which are easily digested such as egg yolk, butter cream and fat of whole milk because it reduces the delayed emptying of the stomach and decreases movement. The food should be eaten in small amounts because to avoid overfeeling of the stomach as it causes pain. Fibre can be restricted in the meal but if given, only in one time meal.

Soft diet: It is the type of diet which consists of mildly season, tender and easy to digest food. It contains refined, low fibre food as well as processed carbohydrates. The consistency of this food is very soft, made up of very simple foods and easily digestible foods and it is easy to chew. Commonly, it is the diet used for old age people but it can be used in some gastrointestinal disorders. It is very easy to digest and absorb and it leaves very low residue. So this diet is prescribed in the some infections, post-surgery as well as some gastrointestinal disorders. Soft diet is nutritionally balanced and adequate and it supplies a proper amounts of protein, carbohydrate, fat and energy. The food in soft diet maybe chopped, pureed, mashed, ground as well as moist.

Foods allowed

- Pulses, vegetables and cereals.
- Refined cereals like semolina, biscuits, bread, pasta, rice and its products.
- Milk and milk products like cottage cheese curd and mildly flavoured and processed cheese.
- Fruits and vegetables can be in the form of purees, soups and juices.
- Soft fruits like mango, banana, papaya, grapes, etc. Hard food can be eaten after removing the skin and their seed.
- Eggs and white meat like fish and chicken.
- Fats like cream butter, vegetable oil, etc.

Foods avoided

- Whole pulses
- Fried foods, fatty and red meats, cake, pastries, etc.
- Spicy and highly flavoured food like pickles.
- Nuts and dried fruits
- Raw fruits and vegetables which have hard skin and seeds.
- High fibre vegetables like beans, peas, tomato, etc., can be avoided and it can be used in the form of fruits juices, etc.
- Whole grain cereals and their products are wheat and their products.
- Avoid alcohol and hard beverages.

5.1.1.8 Menu Planning for Peptic Ulcer

Early morning: Coconut water

Breakfast: Double toned milk + Besan Chilla + Coriander Chutney

Mid-morning: Mango juice

Lunch: Plain Dosa+ Vegetable Sambhar

Evening snack: Vegetable Soup

Dinner: Rice + Washed moong dal + Buttermilk

Post-dinner: Skimmed milk

Eating a healthy diversified diet rich in fruits, vegetables and fibres devoid of harmful aritificial preservatives is key to helping your body healing its wounds. Risk factors in peptic ulcers like cigarette smoking and drinking alcohol is also avoided. Polyphenols found in fruits and vegetable helps in digestion and brain health and gives other health benefits. Polyphenols has antioxidants which help in good stomach health. Commonly included foods are:

1. Apples
2. Grapes
3. Pomegranates
4. Green tea
5. Vegetables
6. Curcumin (present in turmeric)
7. Legumes, beans and lentils
8. Healthy fats (avocado and olive oil)
9. Drinking plenty of water(staying hydrated has lots of benefits and helps in health of digestive tract.
10. Whole foods fruits vegetables, whole grains has more fibre and absorptive power, which decreases the acid production in stomach.
11. Fermented foods like yogurt, curd, etc., inhibit the activity of *Heliconbacter pylori*.

A study was conducted on patients with active duodenal ulcers over a period of 5 weeks. Patients were divided into two groups; one was given regular hospital diet while other group was given bland diet. Both the diets were prepared keeping in mind the nutritional requirements of the patients. It was done so as to find the effect of different food products given in ulcers. From the study it was found that there was no significant difference in the response of the patients of both the diets. Patients on routine hospital diet ate and assimilated the food products not given to the patients on bland diet.

Foods to be included: Probiotic food (yogurt, kimchi, kombucha, miso, tempeh, sauerkraut and curt) is rich in bacteria that prevents any infection and inflammation of the gut. It is found to be helpful in ulcers as it fights against ulcer causing bacteria. Food rich in vitamin C, as it helps against fighting infection. Bell peppers are consumed for vitamin C. Food containing vitamin A, as it helps in reducing the size of wound. Sweet potato is a good source of vitamin A. Fibre rich food like apple, oats, peas are also helpful.

Foods to be avoided: Milk can help in relieving the symptoms, but it actually worsens the disease by increasing the acid production in the stomach. Alcohol is very harmful in ulcers as it further degenerates the protective lining of the stomach. Foods rich in fat are hard to digest, thus can cause bloating and pain in the stomach. Some spices irritate the wound to a further extent and delays the process of healing, so it is advised to avoid spices.

5.2 CONSTIPATION

Constipation woes are very common in everyone's life. Home cures and way of life changes can frequently help to settle it, yet once in a while, it might require clinical consideration. The obstruction can occur for some reasons, for example, when stool goes through the colon too gradually. The more slow the nourishment travels through the stomach related tract, the more water the colon will ingest and the harder the defecation will turn into. At different occasions, it might basically be because of an absence of fibre or water.

Pellet-like stool, may happen when hard stool breaks into smaller pieces. This breakage can occur during absorption, or it might happen in the butt preceding an individual has a solid discharge. It may be more hard to pass these little pellets than an ordinary stool, and an individual may strain to defecate. A great many people have a normal defecation design, passing stool from between three times each day to once at regular intervals. At the point when nourishment goes through the stomach related framework, the colon ingests a portion of water that the nourishment contains. Nourishment that passes more gradually than expected invests an excess of energy in the colon. Thus, the colon assimilates a lot of water, and the stool may turn out to be hard. Some different indications that an individual may involve with expansion to stone like stool include:

- Agonizing solid discharges.
- Stressing to crap.
- Stools that are too enormous to even think about passing the inclination that some stool stays deserted, considerably after a defecation.

5.2.1 Causes

5.2.1.1 Obstruction due to Food Intake

Obstruction is progressively predominant in geriatrics population because of the adjustments in muscle tone and sensory system work that ordinarily happen with expanding age. A more established grown-up who doesn't eat enough fibre or takes meds that may cause blockage has a significantly higher danger of hard stools.

Some other hazard factors for stoppage include:

Nervousness: Kids and babies may not defecate when there is a significant change in their home or washroom schedule. Kids who are under latrine training may decline to go to toilet if their folks or parental figures are corrective or excessively forceful with can preparing.

Medicines: Unnecessary utilization of obstruction drugs, for example, bowel purges and diuretics, may cause hard stool. Antidepressants and a few opiates may likewise slow assimilation, causing dry and pebbly stools.

Neurological conditions: A few conditions that influence the sensory system, for example, dementia, may make it hard for an individual to realize when and how to go to the washroom.

Gastrointestinal issues: Fractious gut disorder and different conditions that influence the stomach and digestion tracts may cause clogging. A few people with nourishment sensitivities likewise experience this side effect.

Physical wounds and disorders: Spinal line wounds, harm to the guts, and muscle wounds to the pelvic floor, for example, those subsequent from labor — may make it hard for an individual to have a solid discharge. This deferral can slow processing and cause stone crap. Numerous interminable sicknesses can cause blockage by influencing nerve or muscle work. Diabetes, hypothyroidism, and colon diseases may cause this side effect.

Sedentary lifestyle: An inactive way of life may expand the danger of blockage, particularly for individuals with other hazard factors.

Dietary factors: Low fibre diets may cause rock crap. A few people grow pebbly stools when they don't drink enough water.

Obstruction causes

- Trouble passing stool
- Stressing when passing stool
- Passing less stool than expected
- Dry, or hard stool

Different side effects include:

- Pain and squeezing in the stomach area
- Bloated
- Sickness
- Lost hunger

Stomach pain is a typical display of obstruction, so they regularly happen together. There are numerous reasons why individuals experience stomach torment and obstruction, running from certain way of life components to serious ailments.

The NIDDK characterizes obstruction as having less than three solid discharges for seven days.

Different indications of obstruction include:

- Stomach torment
- Trouble when passing stools

- Hard, dry, or uneven stools
- Indications of stomach torment
- squeezing torments
- loss of hunger

Pathophysiology: Blockage all alone can be awkward, however it commonly isn't hazardous. In any case, it can turn into an issue on the off chance that it is a side effect of an increasingly genuine fundamental condition, for example, colorectal malignancy, or in the event that it begins to create additional harm. Harm that can emerge because of extreme obstruction incorporates:

Rectal seeping subsequent to stressing

Symptomatic haemorrhoids (heaps), which are swollen, kindled veins in the rear end

Feral impaction happens when dried stool stagnates and gathers in the rectum and rear end, conceivably prompting a mechanical hindrance.

Other potential difficulties incorporate a diminished personal satisfaction and despondency.

Looking for clinical guidance for obstruction may help forestall difficulties.

Absence of fibre in the eating routine.

Role of fibre: Individuals with a high admission of dietary fibre are more averse to encounter blockage. This is on the grounds that fibre advances normal solid discharges, particularly when an individual consolidates it with appropriate hydration.

High fibre nourishments include:

- Natural products
- Vegetables
- Entire grains
- Nuts
- Lentils, chickpeas, and different vegetables

Low fibre nourishments include:

- High fat nourishments, for example, cheddar, meat, and eggs.
- Profoundly handled nourishments, for example, white bread, chips, and other pre-made nourishments.

5.2.2 Clinical Signs and Symptoms

Clogging frequently results from the eating routine and way of life. Eating certain nourishments can assist with improving the recurrence of defecations. The clinical network characterises clogging as a decrease in solid discharges or trouble passing stools.

Individuals who suffer from constipation may have:

1. Hard, dry, or knotty stools
2. Stools that resemble little stones or marbles
3. Inconvenience during solid discharges
4. A sentiment of being not able to exhaust the insides completely
5. Lost hunger because of a nonstop feeling of completion
6. A marginally swollen stomach

An individual may likewise see little dashes of splendid red blood in the stools or on the bathroom tissue in the wake of cleaning. Everybody's gut propensities are extraordinary, yet individuals who are clogged typically have less than three defecations for each week. Obstruction is extremely normal. In the United States, around 16 out of each 100 grown-ups have side effects of clogging. The danger of obstruction increments with age. Around 33 out of each 100 grown-ups beyond 60 years old in the U.S. have side effects of clogging.

5.2.2.1 Physical Inactivity

Low degree of physical action may likewise prompt obstruction. Some past investigations have discovered that genuinely fit individuals, including long distance runners, are less inclined to encounter clogging than others, despite the fact that the specific purposes behind this stay hazy. An examination from 2013 notes that expanding versatility may help improve obstruction among more seasoned grown-ups. Individuals who go through a few days or weeks in bed or sitting in a seat may have a higher danger of stoppage.

A few drugs can likewise expand the danger of clogging. These include:

- **Medicines help with discomfort medicates:** These incorporate codeine (present with acetaminophen in Tylenol #3), oxycodone (OxyContin), and hydromorphine).
- **Tricyclic antidepressants**: These incorporate amitriptyline (Elavil) and imipramine (Tofranil).
- **Certain anticonvulsants:** Examples incorporate phenytoin (Dilantin) and carbamazepine (Tegretol).
- **Calcium channel blockers:** These lower pulse, and specific sorts lower pulse. They incorporate diltiazem (Cardizem) and nifedipine (Procardia).
- **Stomach settling agents that contain aluminium:** These incorporate Amphoral and Basaljel.

- **Stomach settling agents that contain calcium:** One model is Tums.
- **Diuretics:** These expel overabundance liquid from the body. They incorporate hydrochlorothiazide (hydro distil) and furosemide (Lasix).

Iron enhancements: Doctors recommend these to treat iron insufficiency frailty.

5.2.2.2 Irritable Bowel Syndrome

Individuals with utilitarian intestinal trouble, for example, irritable bowel disorder (IBS), have a higher danger of blockage than individuals without the condition.

An individual with IBS may undergo–

- stomach torment
- swelling
- distension
- changes in the recurrence or consistency of stools

With IBS, obstruction can vary after some time. At the point when obstruction is absent, there may rather be free stools with looseness of the bowels.

5.2.2.3 Ageing

As individuals age, the commonness of obstruction, in general, increases. Up to 40% of more established individuals in the network and up to 60% of those in organisations may encounter obstruction. It might be that as individuals age, nourishment takes more time to go through the stomach related tract. Numerous individuals additionally become less portable, which may likewise add to stoppage. Ailments, prescriptions, and a low admission of fibre or water might be different variables that lead to clogging with age.

5.2.2.4 Change in Environment

At the point when an individual ventures, for instance, their typical routine changes. This can influence the stomach related framework. In an article from 2008, researchers got some information about the stomach related changes they encountered while going outside of the United States. The outcomes demonstrated that 9% of individuals experienced obstruction when they went to another nation.

5.2.2.5 Damages to Organs

A portion of these confusions can become dangerous. Consequently, individuals should converse with a medicinal services proficient before they begin utilizing purgatives. In the event that an individual overlooks the desire to have a defecation, the inclination may bit by bit leave until they never again want to go. Nonetheless, the more they delay, the drier and harder the stool will turn into. This will expand the danger of feral impaction.

5.2.2.6 Water – A forgotten Nutrient

Normally, drinking enough water can help lessen the danger of blockage. Other appropriate liquids incorporate normally improved natural product or vegetable squeezes and clear soups. Note that a few fluids can expand the danger of lack of hydration and aggravate clogging for certain individuals. For instance, the individuals who are inclined to obstruction should confine their admission of juiced soft drinks, espresso, and liquor.

5.2.2.7 Colorectal Problems

Some conditions that influence the colon can block and limit the section of stool, prompting stoppage. Instances of such conditions include:

- Carcinogenic tumours
- Hernia
- Scar tissue
- Diverticulitis
- Colorectal stricture, which is an unusual narrowing of the colon or rectum
- Different conditions

Some other ailments can likewise cause or add to stoppage. These include:

- **Neurological conditions:** Multiple sclerosis, Parkinson's illness, stroke, spinal line wounds, and interminable intestinal pseudo-block can prompt stoppage.
- Conditions that include hormonal capacity, electrolytes, or renal capacity: These incorporate uraemia, diabetes, hypercalcaemia , and hypothyroidism.
- **Intestinal blockage:** This can happen if a tumour squares or crushes some portion of the stomach related framework.
- **Conditions that influence the stomach related framework:** Constipation can happen with celiac malady, IBD, and other fiery conditions.
- **Malignant growth treatment:** Chemotherapy and narcotic help with discomfort prescriptions, can likewise trigger blockage.

5.2.3 Obstruction in Infants and Children

Stoppage can here and there influence youngsters and infants. On the off chance that an infant doesn't pass meconium, their first strong stool, inside 48 hours of birth, they may have Hirschsprung's ailment. This is a condition wherein certain nerve cells are absent from part of the digestive organ. Stool can't push ahead in the influenced territory of colon, which causes a reinforcement. A human services supplier will for the most part have the option to detect these side effects and suggest medical procedure as treatment. Much of the time, the standpoint is useful for babies brought into the world with this condition. In the event that a breastfed infant goes seven days without passing stool, this isn't generally an issue. Breastfed babies don't normally encounter clogging. All the more regularly, blockage can happen: At the point when a baby first beginnings taking recipe takes care of:

- During weaning
- During potty preparing
- Now and again of stress

During potty preparing, stoppage can happen if a kid feels focused, particularly if different changes are happening, for example, beginning at nursery. Giving the youngster a lot of time to exhaust their insides may help. Aside from not passing stool, a few manifestations that demonstrate stoppage in kids include a firm or expanded stomach area -

- Low vitality
- Diminished hunger
- Fractiousness

5.2.4 Pregnancy

As indicated by one source, around 40% of ladies experience clogging during pregnancy. This can result from:

- hormonal changes;
- physical changes, for example, when the uterus pushes on the digestion tracts;
- dietary or physical action changes; or
- Numerous ladies take iron enhancements during pregnancy. These can add to blockage.

5.2.5 Prevention and Management of Constipation

- Blockage normally settles itself without the requirement for remedy treatment. By and large, making way of life changes, for example, getting more exercise, eating more fibre, and drinking more water can help.

- Permitting time for defecation, without stress or interference, may likewise help. Individuals ought to likewise not overlook the inclination to have a defecation.
- Intestinal medicines can improve manifestations for the time being, yet individuals should utilize them with care and just when essential. This is on the grounds that a few diuretics can have serious unfriendly impacts.
- The Food and Drug Administration (FDA) encourages individuals to check with their primary care physician before utilising them, and to adhere to the directions on the mark with care.

On the off chance that stoppage continues, individuals should see a specialist. They may require more grounded prescription. The specialist may likewise test for any hidden conditions. Tracking solid discharges, stool attributes, and dietary and different components may help an appropriate treatment.

5.2.6 Role of Medicines

A few intestinal medicines are accessible over the counter, while others are accessible with a prescription. Individuals should possibly consider utilizing diuretics if making way of life changes has not made a difference. It is ideal to check with a specialist before use. Coming up next are a few purgatives and stool conditioners that may help ease blockage.

Fibre supplements: Also known as mass shaping intestinal medicines, these might be the most secure alternative. Individuals should take these with a lot of water. A physician can always refer these over the counter medications to treat or prevent constipation.

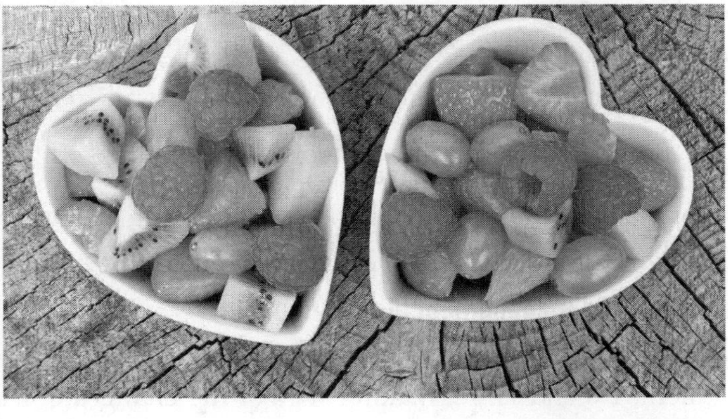

Energisers cause the muscles in the digestion tracts to contract musically.

Oils assist the stool move easily through the colon. One example is mineral oil (Fleet).

Stool conditioners dampen the stool.

Osmotic treatments bring water into the colon to hydrate the stool and ease the movement. Saline diuretics are a kind of osmotic.

Neuromuscular operators incorporate narcotic opponents and 5-HT4 agonists. They work at explicit receptors to control development through the gut.

5.2.7 Dietary Management

In the event that intestinal medicines don't work, a specialist may need to evacuate the affected stool physically.

In the event that stoppage doesn't react to treatment or if there are different side effects, a specialist may propose a stomach imaging study, for example, a CT filter, MRI output, or X-beam, to check whether there is a blockage because of a basic ailment process in the gut.

On the off chance that there is an individual may require explicit physician recommended drugs or medical procedure to determine it. Contingent upon the after effects of the tests and the individual's reaction to clinical or careful treatment, they may likewise require further treatment. Changing your eating regimen and expanding your physical movement level are the most straightforward and quickest approaches to treat and forestall stoppage. Attempt the accompanying procedures also.

Consistently, drink 1/2 to 2 quarts of unsweetened, decaffeinated liquids, similar to water, to hydrate the body. Breaking point utilisation of liquor and jazzed drinks, which cause drying out. Add fibre-rich nourishments to your eating routine, for example, crude products of the soil, entire grains, beans, prunes, or wheat oat. Your day by day admission of fibre ought to be somewhere in the range of 20 and 35 gm. Cut down on low-fibre nourishments, for example, meat, milk, cheddar, and prepared food sources. Focus on around 150 minutes of moderate exercise each week, with an objective of 30 minutes of the day at any rate five times each week. Have a go at strolling, swimming, or biking.

On the off chance that you want to have a defecation, don't delay. The more you pause, the harder your stool can turn into. Add fibre enhancements to your eating regimen if necessary. Simply make sure to drink a lot of liquids since liquids assist fibre with working all the more effectively.

Use intestinal medicines sparingly. Your primary care physician may endorse diuretics or purifications for a brief timeframe to help relax your stools. Never use diuretics for over about fourteen days without conversing with your primary care physician. Your body can get subject to them for appropriate colon work.

Consider adding probiotics to your eating routine, similar to those found in yogurt and kefir with live dynamic societies. Source have demonstrated that this dietary change can be useful for those with incessant clogging.

On the off chance that you despite everything experience difficulty with stoppage, your doctor may recommend prescriptions to help. These prescriptions work by expanding the discharges in your digestion tracts, making the stool simpler to pass.

Your doctor may likewise exhort that you quit taking certain drugs that may cause stoppage. Progressively extreme colon or rectal issues may require manual methodology to free the colon from affected stool, treatment to retrain moderate muscles, or medical procedure to evacuate the issue some portion of your colon.

5.3 DIARRHOEA

Diarrhoea is the passing of watery or loose stools with the increased frequency in a day more than the normal levels. Diarrhoea is a common ailment. But it can a symptom of a serious underlying condition also. The frequent episodes of diarrhoea can be symptom of disorders of the intestines. The ulcerative colitis, gastroenteritis, stomach infections, typhoid fever or attack of any pathogen on the gastrointestinal systems as happens in food poisoning.

5.3.1 Types of Diarrhoea

5.3.1.1 Acute Diarrhoea

Acute diarrhoea is defined as a short duration of loose or watery stools like for one day to one week but the patient defecates many times in a day. The most common cause is gastroenteritis or food poisoning caused by the attack of bacteria such as *Escherichia coli* salmonella or in enteric fever. Generally, it is harmless and does not require a lot of attention and can be treated easily with drugs and diets. But treatment should be started immediately so that dehydration can be prevented. Antimotility agents should be avoided in patients with bloody diarrhoea. Probiotics are mostly recommended for better recovery. The antibiotics are effective in the treatment of Shigellosis, Campylobacteriosis, *Clostridium difficile*, Traveller's diarrhoea, and protozoal infections. Prevention of acute diarrhoea is promoted through adequate hand washing, safe food preparation, access to clean water, and vaccinations.

5.3.1.2 Chronic Diarrhoea

Chronic diarrhoea is explained as the passing of watery or loose stools for more than 2-4 weeks and many times a day. It is often a prediction of serious underlying condition of gastrointestinal system. The weakened immune system is also a reason for this chronic illness and it can lead to increased mortality rates, specially in children. The reasons of chronic diarrhoea can be many: such as attack of parasites in the intestines such as parasites *Entamoeba histolytica, Giardia, microsporidia,* etc. The pathogens also have a major roles in causing chronic diarrhoea in people. The presence of bacteria such as *Aeromonas, Campylobacter, Clostridium difficile, Salmonella, Shigella,* etc., are major causes. The virus attacks are not to be forgotten like notavirus and rotavirus, etc. Although the reasons can be unknown also for onset of chronic diarrhoea. The other causes can be as under:

- Chronic pancreatitis, pancreatic enzyme deficiencies, cystic fibrosis
- Intestinal disorders such as ulcerative colitis, Crohn's diseases and irritable bowel syndrome
- Excess use of medications: hormonal or laxatives or antibiotics
- Food intolerance or allergies
- Disorder of the thyroid (e.g., hyperthyroidism)
- AIDS
- Tumours
- Reduced blood flow to the intestine

5.3.2 Dietary Management of Diarrhoea

Energy: An increased calorie recommendations can be made depending upon the digestive capacity of the patient. BRAT diet is given in chronic diarrhoea cases, i.e., banana, rice, applesauce, toast. These food products are very good for intestines and stomach.

Carbohydrates: The fibre is recommended at low levels and refined food products are being advised such as white breads, banana, buttermilk, custards, fruit juice mixed with glucose and salt.

Proteins: In chronic diarrhoea if the patient loses weight then it becomes a concern as proteins are very less digested in such patients. So protein foods such as dal and rice khichdi, curd, buttermilk, moong dal soup, creamy palak soup or chicken broth can be recommended. Milk is given if it is tolerated otherwise should be avoided.

Fats: Medium chain triglycerides are recommended such as coconut oil which are very easily digested by the gut.The fats are just given based on the tolerance by the GI system.

Foods to be completely avoided

1. Whole grains, pulses and cruciferous vegetables.
2. Pungent smelling foods such as onions, garlic, radish, etc.
3. Sweet food products such as bakery products, sweets, etc.
4. Caffeine-containing beverages such as coffee and tea can have a laxative effect.
5. Alcoholic beverages such as beer, wine and liquor can worsen diarrhoea.
6. Red meats and fried meat products such as bacon, mutton, etc.
7. Monosodium glutamate (MSG), a flavour enhancer, may exacerbate diarrhoea.
8. Dry fruits such as figs, dates, raisins, and prunes can have a laxative effect.

Eat low fibre foods

- Curd or greek yoghurt (unless you are lactose intolerant)
- Rice
- Noodles
- White bread
- Lean meats
- Cottage cheese
- 1–2 tbsp of vegetables at a time
- Refined grains

To prevent complications that can result from frequent bowel movements in chronic diarrhoea conditions. Follow instructions as follows:

- Watch and maintain a food diary and observe the foods which do not suit you
- Drink a lot of water during the day
- Enough amounts of water and electrolytes in the diet
- Eat small frequent feedings

5.3.3 How to Manage Dehydration

Dehydration is a condition that happens when an individual has lost such a lot of liquid that the body can never again work typically and creates signs and indications because of the loss of liquid. Adults should look for clinical consideration for associated drying out if encountering diminished creation with pee, fever more than 101°F, seizures, trouble breathing, or chest or stomach torment. Clinical treatment of lack of hydration in grown-ups may include drinking liquids that contain electrolytes and starches, notwithstanding water.

Lack of hydration is a condition that can happen when the loss of body liquids, for the most part water, surpasses the sum that is taken in. With lack of hydration, more water is moving out of individual cells and afterward out of the body than the measure of water that is taken in through drinking.

Restoratively, lack of hydration for the most part implies an individual has lost enough liquid with the goal that the body starts to lose its capacity to work ordinarily and afterward starts to create side effects identified with the liquid misfortune. Despite the fact that babies and kids are at most elevated hazard for drying out, numerous grown-ups and particularly the older have noteworthy hazard factors.

Individuals (and creatures) lose water each day in respiration while we breathe in and out, and as water in our perspiration, pee, and stool. Alongside the water, we likewise lose limited quantities of salts or electrolytes. Our bodies are continually rearranging the harmony among water (and salts or electrolytes) misfortunes with liquid admission.

The administration of lack of hydration commonly includes the utilisation of oral rehydration arrangement (ORS). We can likewise make it at home.

5.3.3.1 Management of Dehydration in Constipation

1. Drink a lot of water. Since obstruction is identified with drying out in the colon, you have to ensure you are drinking bunches of water. At the point when your body is appropriately hydrated, less water will be pulled back from the colon. This will keep the stool delicate and simple to pass. One of the best methods for curing dehydration in constipation is ORT.

   Reactions may incorporate regurgitating, high blood sodium, or high blood potassium. In the case of spewing happens, it is suggested that utilisation be stopped for 10 minutes and afterward continuously restarted.

   The prescribed plan incorporates sodium chloride, sodium citrate, potassium chloride, and glucose. Glucose might be supplanted by sucrose and sodium citrate might be supplanted by sodium bicarbonate, if not available.

2. Get your fibre through foods grown from the ground. There are two kinds of fibre, soluble and insoluble. Both are significant for keeping up ordinary solid discharges. Soluble fibre likewise keeps stool delicate in light of the fact that it assimilates water. Insoluble fibre adds mass to stool and furthermore acts like a sweeper, assisting with clearing things out of the digestion tracts.
3. Clogging has been related with a lack of dietary fibre in Western culture for a considerable length of time. A connection between expanding the day by day fibre admission and faecal load just as colonic travel time has been demonstrated. The suggested measure of dietary fibre is 20 to 35 gm for each day and this can be acquired from entire wheat bread, oats, citrus natural products, and vegetables. Insoluble fibre, for example, grain wheat, may cause stomach gas and swelling which results in uneasiness. In certain patients, these specialists additionally postpone gastric discharging and discourage hunger. To improve the resistance and adherence you may begin with low portions of fibre and increment their dietary fibre consumption continuously for long until ~20 to 25 g/d. On the off chance that the obstruction has not improved, at that point soluble fibre enhancements ought to be attempted.
4. Supplement your eating regimen with Omega-3s. Omega-3 oils help grease up your digestion tracts so things can travel through the colon effortlessly. Fish oil is by a long shot the best wellspring of omega-3, in any case, flax oil and hemp oil are quite acceptable also.

5.4 DUMPING SYNDROME

5.4.1 Introduction

Dumping syndrome is also referred to as rapid gastric emptying. Dumping syndrome generally occurs when the food (mainly sugars) move too quickly from the stomach into the small intestine. Dumping syndrome is a complex physiological response to the presence of larger (than normal) quantity of liquid and food in the proximal part of the small intestine. It generally occurs as a result of loss of gastrointestinal and systemic response to a meal and also due to loss of normal regulation of gastric emptying. Dumping syndrome may result as a result of total or subtotal gastrectomy. Therefore, dumping syndrome is very common after bariatric surgery or gastrectomy due to cancer of the stomach.

5.4.2 Causes of Dumping Syndrome

5.4.2.1 Surgeries

Bariatric surgery: Bariatric surgery is a procedure which is generally performed on the morbidly obese patients as a treatment option to help weight loss. International Guidelines for Surgical treatment for obesity among the Asian Indians suggest that – (i) surgery should be performed on the individual having BMI above 32.5 kg/metre sq. with co-morbidities such as obstructive sleep apnoea (OSA), Type II diabetes mellitus, hypertension, dyslipidemia, cardiovascular disease, stroke, gout, arthritis, etc., and (ii) surgery should be performed on individual having BMI above 37.5 kg/metre sq. without co-morbidity. Restrictiction and malabsorption are the two basic principles underlying bariatric surgery. Bariatric surgery involves modification of the digestive system either by decreasing the volume of the stomach (restriction) or by altering the path of the food particles causing an element of malabsorption. Types of bariatric surgery that usually cause dumping syndrome includes Laproscopic gastric bypass surgery.

Weight loss surgery patients often think dumping syndrome as a 'good thing' as it discourages the poor dietary choices and makes the patient feel full even after taking a small amount of food thus ,leading to rapid loss in weight.

Gatrointestinal surgeries: Dumping syndrome can also occur as a result of manipulation of the pyloric region of the stomach or due to Nissen fundoplication or Laproscopic Nissen fundoplication (a surgical procedure which is performed to treat gastroesophageal refles disease or hiatal hernia)

The incidence of dumping syndrome ranges from 5% (in case of minor surgery procedures) to as high as 40% (after total gastrectomy). After the surgery procedures where the portion of the stomach remains, there is a chance of the remaining stomach to somewhat increase in size over a period of several months.

Therefore, the newer surgical procedures which preserve the proximal and distal part of the stomach or create small stomach like reservoirs have helped to reduce dumping syndrome.

5.4.3 Classification of Dumping Syndrome

Based on time limit, dumping syndrome is divided into two forms.

5.4.3.1 Early Dumping Syndrome (30 min after eating)

Early dumping syndrome generally occurs within 30 min after the consumption of a meal. Along with the consumption of foods that are high in fats, sugars (table sugar or fruit sugar) and refined carbohydrates, it can also occur due to the consumption of foods that are too hot or too cold or by drinking water or other fluids with the meal. Symptoms of early dumping syndrome include bloating, vomiting, sweating, diarrhoea, dizziness, heart palpitations, rapid heart rate and nausea.

5.4.3.2 Late Dumping Syndrome (over time)

Late dumping syndrome is considered as a type of hypoglycaemia (low blood sugar). When an individual consumes too much of sugar, the newly formed small size stomach could not digest the food bolus properly so the small intestines absorb and deposits too much of it into the blood stream. Therefore the body compensates by releasing more amount of insulin which causes drop in the blood sugar. Symptoms of late dumping syndrome include anxiety, diarrhoea, dizziness, fainting, fatigue, heart palpitation, rapid heart rate, strong feelings of hunger, sweating, weakness, mental changes such as problems of concentrating or confusion.

Both the early and late dumping syndromes generally occur after the consumption of meal, that contains foods which are especially high in fats, refined carbohydrates or sugars (table sugars or fruit sugars that are found naturally in fruits).

5.4.4 Symptoms of Dumping Syndrome

Symptoms may occur in several stages, each one of these is related to the "dumping" of food and beverages into the small intestine but their mechanisms very. All the patients do not suffer the consequences to the same degree. Based on the stages of symptoms occurrence, dumping syndrome is divided into three further stages as describe below.

5.4.4.1 First Stage

Here in this first stage, patient may usually experience nausea and fullness of the abdomen within 10–20 min after consumption of a meal. The stage may generally be attributed to distention of the small bowel from foods and fluids. At the same time, patient may also suffer from flushing, rapid heart beat, faintness, sweating, etc. There is a need for the patient to sit or lie down in order to avoid the above-mentioned symptoms.

5.4.4.2 Intermediate Stage

In the intermediate stage, patients may experience increase in flatulence, bloating in the abdomen, diarrhoea, cramps and pain in the abdominal region, etc. These 'colonic' symptoms are most likely related to the increase in the malabsorption of carbohydrates and the other food stuffs. Also there occurs subsequent fermentation of the subtrates after entering the colon.

5.4.4.3 Late Stage

The late stage is related to reactive hypoglycaemia (low blood sugar), sometimes referred to as alimentary hypoglycaemia. It generally occurs from 1 to 3 hr after the consumption of meal. Patients may usually perspire, feel anxious, weak, trembling, hungry and face difficulty in concentrating. Rapid delivery, assimilation and absorption of the carbohydrates causes excessive rise in the insulin level which leads to subsequent decline in the blood glucose level.

5.4.5 Management of Dumping Syndrome

Severity of the symptoms vary from mild to relatively debilitating. The symptoms in dumping syndrome depend on the nature and severity of the surgery and the dietary practice of the individual. Long-term as well as short-term implications are numerous but dietary interventions can either eliminate or reduce the symptoms in most of the cases. On the other hand for those individuals in whom the symptoms of dumping syndrome persists even after the alterations of the dietary practice in such cases especially medications that slows down the motility should be advised.

5.4.6 Complications

5.4.6.1 Weight Loss

Patients who are symptomatic after the gastric surgery often lose weight. The loss of weight may occur due to lack of food intake. Intake of inadequate amount of food often results from the fear and anxiety which is often related to the confusing and often distressing symptoms. Most of the time, many patients often think that the symptoms of the dumping syndrome occur due to the act of eating rather than attributing them to specific patterns, volumes and types of food that is consumed. Sometimes the individuals can correctly relate the intake of food types with distress but they rarely can select appropriate foods based on their experience with foods or meals.

5.4.6.2 Problems in Digestion

In some form of the gastric surgery, in addition to dumping syndrome and hypoglycaemia, malabsorption and steatorrhea may also result. About 10% of these individuals have significant steatorrhea from clinical point of view, which is secondary to rapid transit, pancreatic and biliary insufficiency and loss of gastric lipase. Due to the disturbances at the time of entry of the food particles into the small intestine, efficiency of digestion may be reduced because of the disturbances in the release of intestinal hormones and enzymes. Lactose tolerant patients who were completely alright with lactose digestion before the gastric surgery, after surgery may relatively experience lactase deficiency either because the food enters the small intestine further downstream or because the transit time increases through the proximal small intestine.

5.4.6.3 Dietary Deficiencies

Due to the long term inadequate dietary intake and malabsorption, anaemia, osteoporosis and selective vitamin and mineral deficiencies may occur. Deficiency of iron is often associated with loss of acid secretion which mainly causes the reduction of the iron compounds, lowering their absorption, blood loss, rapid transit and diminished contact with the site of iron absorption. Deficiency of vitamin B_{12} causes megaloblastic anemia or pernicious anaemia. As the amount of gastric mucosa is reduced after the surgery therefore intrinsic factor may not be produced in sufficient quantities for the complete absorption of vitamin B_{12}. After gastrectomy patients generally receive prophylactic vitamin B_{12} injection or reservoirs because of the overgrowth of bacteria in the proximal small bowel or in the afferent loop which contributes to vitamin B_{12} depletion as the bacteria compete with the host for the utilization of the vitamins.

In patients with rapid emptying and dumping syndrome, somatostatin analogs are used in them for slowing gastric emptying. Acarbose is an alpha-glucoside hydrolase inhibitor which generally helps in the management of blood sugar level in type II diabetes mellitus, has been also used in some persons with dumping syndrome. Acarbose inhibits the digestion and absorption of starch, sucrose and maltose. Acarbose may oppose the alimentary hyper and hypoglycaemia related to dumpting syndrome but also has the potential to worsen the colonic gas and diarrhoea.

5.4.7 Nutritional Care for Patients with Dumping Syndrome

- High protein and moderate amount of fats with sufficient calories should be provided for weight maintenance or gain as required. Complex carbohydrates should be provided in tolerable amount.
- Small and frequent meals throughout the day result in increased absorption and less dramatic fluid shifts.
- Lying down and avoiding activity after an hour of eating helps in slowing the gastric activity.
- Adequate amount of fluids (with small amount at a time) should be taken throughout the day.
- Intake of fibrous food slows upper GI transit and increases viscosity. However to avoid obstructions, caution should be used with large particles and fibre supplements especially with oesophageal or gastric outlet narrowing or dysmotility.

- Lactose (milk sugar) may be poorly tolerated due to rapid transit and so may be avoided. Cheese, curd and yogurt can be better tolerated.

The primary objective of nutritional care in dumping syndrome patients is to restore nutritional status and restore quality of life. As the patients are not able to eat enough because of the accompanying problems such as diarrhoea, increased intestinal activities, etc. The patients become malnourished, underweight and frustrated.

Proteins and fats are hydrolysed slowly into osmotically active substances, therefore they are better tolerated than carbohydrates. Quantities of simple carbs such as lactose, sucrose and dextrose should be restricted as they are hydrolysed more rapidly. Complex carbs such as starches can be included in the diet.

Many patients have problem with tolerating liquids with meal as liquids enter the jejunum rapidly. Therefore patients with severe problems of dumping must limit the intake of liquids with meal or they can consume fluids between the meals without solid food. Lying down immediately after the meals may also decrease the severity of meals.

Several fibre supplements are beneficial in the management of the dumping syndrome as the upper GI transit time is reduced by them and the rate of glucose absorption is reduced therefore decreasing the insulin response. Pectin (present in many fruits and vegetables) and gums (present in guar, gum arabic, oatmeal, barley) are the soluble dietary fibres that are used for the treatment of the dumping syndrome. However, proper cautions must be exercised when amount have been taken in bulk, especially without sufficient amount of water.

Diets that especially aim to prevent the symptoms of dumping syndrome is basically higher in fat content, i.e., 35% to 45% of calories, low in simple carbs and high in protein (20% of calories) With the help of such diets patients can achieve and maintain optimal weight and correct the nutritional status.

After the gastric surgery as patients either can tolerate only small amounts (6 gm or less per meal) of lactose at a time or often cannot tolerate it. Therefore these individuals do better with cheese or unsweetened yogurt instead of the liquid milk. Hence Vitamin D and calcium must be supplemented as there is decreased intake of the dairy products. Lactose products are commercially available for people with significant lactose malabsorption.

In case of steatorrhea medium chain triglyceride (MCT) is a better option. When steatorrhea is a problem, formulas should be provided to the patients whose fat content is derived mainly from medium chain triglycerides as these may be tolerated better.

5.4.8 Conclusion

Diets of the patients suffering from dumping syndrome must be adjusted based on a careful dietary and social history from the patients.

Gastric surgery has long been considered the main cause of dumping syndrome. However, many recent studies have reported increasing number of cases of dumping syndrome not related to any previous gastric surgeries. This incidence has increased the importance of understanding the pathophysiology of dumping syndrome into more details in recent years. Dumping syndrome occurs because of the GI response to voluminous and hyperosmolar chyme, i.e., expelled rapidly from the stomach into the small intestine. It involves neural as well as hormonal mechanisms. Hence this review encompasses the symptoms, diagnosis as well as treatment approaches of dumping syndrome. Therefore there is a need to focus on the current research status of dumping syndrome.

5.5 GLUTEN INTOLERANCE (CELIAC DISEASE)

5.5.1 Introduction

Gluten intolerance is a lifetime condition in which intake of gluten results in damage to the intestines. Although gluten intolerance is commonly referred to as an allergy but it is actually an autoimmune disease which is triggered by the external factors such as diet (containing gluten). This disease results from an inappropriate T cell - mediated immune response caused by the ingestion of the gluten by the individuals who are genetically predisposed to celiac disease.

The prevalence of the celiac disease have been underestimated in the past and now it is considered to be about 1 in 133 individuals in the United States of America. Onset is usually from infancy to young adulthood, but about 20% of cases occur in adults above 60 years of age.

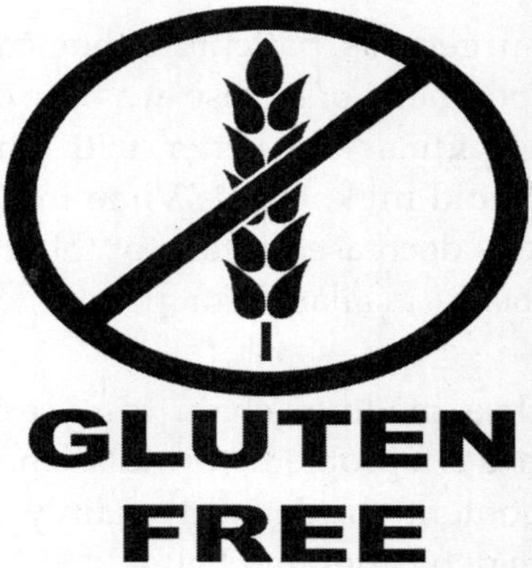

5.5.2 Gluten

Gluten is a group of proteins present in the cereal grains. Gluten proteins play an important role in determining the unique baking quality of wheat by conferring the capacity of water absorption, cohesivity, viscosity and elastic properties of the dough. Gluten proteins can be divided into two main fractions according to their solubility in aqueous alcohols, i.e., the soluble gliadins and the insoluble glutenin.

5.5.3 Pathophysiology

Celiac disease is often caused by reaction to the gliadin. The resulting damage for the intestinal mucosal villi causes the potential or actual malabsorption of many nutrients. Gluten refers to the specific peptide fraction of proteins which are found in wheat, rye, barley, etc. At the time of absorption these peptide molecules are modified to a form that triggers the local as well as the systemic immune response in many cases. Studies identified that the peptide fraction of gliadin is mainly responsible for the celiac disease. The overzealous inflammatory and immune response in the untreated cases response eventually resulting in the damage to the intestinal mucosa, altered neuro peptide secretion and the reduced digestive and absorptive functions. The villi cells becomes deficient in the enzymes such as disaccharidases and peptidases required for the digestion and also becomes carrier deficit which are required to transport nutrients into the bloodstream. Extent of the villous changes greatly varies and there is significant atrophy and flattening of the villi which leads to compromise in the absorption of the macro- and micronutrients.

Reduction in the release of peptide hormones from the small intestine results in decreased secretion from the gall bladder and pancreas leading be to indigestion. Celiac disease mainly affects the proximal and the middle portion of the small intestine (although distal portion may also involved). Again the symptoms of celiac disease vary greatly and non-specific therefore celiac disease may be misdiagnosed many times as irritable bowel disease or other GI disorders for years.

Gluten intolerance is generally considered chronic and it requires lifetime omission of gluten from the diet. Mortality and morbidity rates may rise in individuals who are either diagnosed very lately or in individuals who are not able to comply with the diet. Increased risk of lymphomas along with other malignancies influence the overall morbidity especially in those who continues eating gluten containing foods.

There are two other distinct conditions (which are not to be confused with celiac disease) in celiac gluten sensitivity. In these two conditions, reducing the amount of gluten in the diet will help whereas in celiac disease consumption of even little amount of gluten will lead to immune response activation, which will even lead to long-term and short-term complications.

5.5.4 Signs and Symptoms

There are many signs and symptoms related to gluten intolerance. But their presentation varies. Intestinal symptoms such as loss of weight, pain in the abdomen, fatigue, constipation, diarrhoea or vomiting are the most common. Other intestinal symptoms that are not usual includes infertility, miscarriages, delayed puberty, migraines, mouth ulcers, chronic liver disease, dermatitis herpetiformis. Presentation in the young children is most likely to include the more "classic" symptoms such as diarrhoea and steatorrhoea, abdominal bloating, abdominal pain, apathy and poor weight gain. In late onset, the first manifestation is more varied and it may include other inflammatory and autoimmune disorders, generalized fatigue, failure to gain or maintain weight, consequences of nutrient malabsorption including anemias, osteoporosis, or vitamin K related coagulopathy. Almost half of the coeliac patients however have few or no obvious symptoms and some may be overweight at presentation. The main point to be noted is that no matter what the manifestation of the disease is, the treatment remains the same.

5.5.5 Diagnosis and Clinical Features

Whenever there is suspicion of gluten intolerance, the most commonly recommended screening blood test done world wide is the 'tTG - IgA antibody'. However, the gold standard for diagnosis of celiac disease is the histopathology examination of the duodenal tissue taken endoscopically. The diagnosis of celiac disease is made by a combination of clinical, laboratory and histologic evaluations but small bowel biopsy is the final diagnostic end point. When the infant starts consuming gluten containing cereals the disease may become apparent or it may not appear until the middle age, when it will get triggered by the stress, GI surgery, pregnancy or viral infections.

Major clinical symptoms usually diminish in most of the individuals after the consumption of gluten free diets for 2 to 8 weeks. On the other hand it may take longer in some others. Levels of the specific antibodies usually become undetectable within 3 to 6 months with strict dietary control in most individuals whereas in others the recovery may be slower.

5.5.6 Medical Treatment

Following a gluten-free diet greatly reverses the process. However, some individuals require a long time or even years of diet therapy for the maximal recovery. The toxic peptide fraction of the cereals such as wheat, rye, barley should be avoided for the entire life. Refractory sprue may not entirely respond to the removal of gluten or it may only respond temporarily. However, many of these patients do show a response to steroids, azathioprine,. cyclosporine or other medications generally used in inflammatory or immunologic reactions. In some cases, treating the underlying causes of some other diseases may clear the symptoms.

5.5.7 Nutrition Therapy for Celiac Disease

Complete withdrawal of the offender from the diet results in the clinical improvement, i.e., the gluten proteins. No matter what the manifestation is, the treatment remains the same, i.e., removal of the gluten protein from the diet. The diet requires a major life changes on the part of the patient to adhere to it sufficiently for the quick recovery. Along with wheat (gliadin) the diet should also omit other sources of prolamines such as secalin in rye, hordein in barley as well as avenin in oats.

Finding out the hidden sources of gluten present in the diet is an important part of the management of the celiac disease. Some of the undoubted food items are soy sauce, malt vinegar, breakfast cereals such as cornflakes and rice crispies, spices such as hing, packaged soups and gravies.

For a gluten intolerant patient, the requirement of the macronutrient is similar to that of the RDA. The diet should be initially supplemented with vitamins, minerals and proteins in order to correct deficiencies and replenish the nutrient stores. Vitamin D administration as well as calcium supplementation is required to correct osteomalacia or osteoporosis. Due to steatorrhea vitamin A and Vitamin E stores gets depleted hence these two fat-soluble vitamins are required to replenish the depleted stores. Iron, folate or vitamin B_{12} helps to treat anemia depending upon its nature. In patients with purpura, bleeding or with prolonged bleeding time, vitamin K is prescribed for them. Fluid replacement and electrolyte balance is essential for those who have dehydration due to severe diarrhoea.

In case of malabsorption multiple vitamins and mineral supplements are required to meet the dietary reference intake (DRIs). In persons with steatorrhoea medium chain triglyceride (MCT) helps provide calories. Intolerance of lactose (milk sugar) and fructose (fruit sugar) occurs secondary to celiac disease. Initially a low lactose and low fructose diet helps in controlling the symptoms. Once the GI tract returns to more normal function , lactase activity may also return and a lactose ingestion trial can be tried. Products made from corn, potato, rice, soyabean, tapioca, arrowroot, amaranth, quinoa, millet and buckwheat can be substituted in the food products. While using the flours, it is also important that they are not to be contaminated with gluten containing flour during milling.

Freedom from symptoms after the consumption of gluten does not necessarily mean that cells of the GI tract are not damaged. The precipitating condition usually continues to exist and gluten causes the changes of the mucosa within hours. Adults who start and again stop a gluten-free diet for numerous times, eventually may reach a state in which they do not respond to the diet. There may also occur development of complications such as chronic ulcerative and extraintestinal manifestations may develop. Risks of malignant disease such as lymphoma increases and adherence to a gluten-free diet appears to reduce the risk.

5.5.8 Dietary Recommendations

Gluten-free diet should be started to follow only after the confirmation of the disease and not before that. Once confirmed a strict gluten-free diet is to be followed for the entire life even if the symptoms fade away completely and tTG level returns to normal. Treatment is simply avoiding the offending food such as gliadin in wheat along with other prolamines such as secalin in rye or hordein in barley. It is to be noted that all types and varieties of wheat such as bulgar, durum, spelt, kamut contain gluten and hence there is no safe variety of wheat available as yet.

Atleast 5 to 10 percent of gluten intolerant patients (no idea to determine who are those) have an adverse reaction to the protein avenin found in oats. Oats is therefore put on the unsafe list of the foods.

After the exclusion of the offending cereals, the gluten-free food items that should be included in the diet are – rice, bajra (pearl millet), jowar (sorghum), ragi (finger millet), cholai (amaranth), kuttu (buckwheat), corn, quinoa, arrowroot, sago (sabudana), singhara (water chestnut).

All the other food groups must be included in gluten-free diets as a part of the healthy diets besides permitted cereals. Hence, legumes and pulses, meat, fish, eggs, fruits and vegetables, seeds, nuts and oilseeds as well as fats are all on the lists of safe foods. During the early stages after diagnosis tolerant to milk may be compromised but yogurt, paneer and cheese are better tolerated in this stage. Sugar, honey or jaggery can be taken within the prescribed healthy limits.

5.5.9 Points for Remember

- First thing to highlight is that there are lots of naturally occurring gluten-free foods available. Therefore, it is perfectly possible to have a healthy gluten-free diet with variety. Example includes All pulses, fruits and vegetables, milk, curd, chicken, meat, eggs, fish and nuts.

- It is not just enough to use gluten-free flours or grains. Proper precautions while cooking, washing, storing and serving should be emphasized.
- There should be use of separate grinder for making flour, separate soap and sponges for dish washing, separate batches of oil for frying, as there is always high chances of cross contamination which can deny the benefits of a gluten free diet.
- When the packaged foods are part of the diet, reading the food labels is the another important thing hence looking out for the ingredients and additives is crucial. Use of the words in the food labels that definitely indicates the presence of gluten in the products such as hydrolysed wheat starch, wheat germ oil, durum, triticum or malt. Some other words which strongly indicate its presence such as crumbs, filler, thickener, wafer or breaded.
- Eating out can be a big challenge for the celiac patients. As gluten could be found in a number of food items that in general seems to be gluten free such as chicken butter masala or a drink. Therefore while eating out simple dishes most preferably rice based should be ordered. Fried food, gravies, etc., should be avoided.
- Celiac patients should reject the food immediately whenever they are in doubt.
- Presence of gluten in the medications and in the excipient or carriers should be taken care of. In such situation, the food or drug manufacturer must be contacted in order to confirm the source of the starch which could be either wheat/rice/potato/tapioca/corn. Starch source in medication containing sodium starch glycolate also require verification before use.

5.5.10 Guidelines for Gluten Content of Foods

The Codex Alimentarius Commission has laid the guidelines in order to ensure fair trade practices and to protect the consumers. 20 parts per million (ppm) or 20 mg of gluten per kg of food is generally considered gluten-free foods in India and many other parts of the world. The India's food regulatory body FSSAI, has formulated laws governing gluten-free foods through Food Safety and Standards (Food Standards and Food Additives) Second Amendment Regulation, 2016. There are two categories of products . They are (i) the gluten-free foods (either naturally gluten- free or the gluten content in the product is below 20 ppm or 20 mg per kg of food) and (ii) specifically processed foods in order to reduce the gluten content to a level ranging between 20–100 mg per kg of food.

5.5.11 Conclusion

A strict gluten-free diet for the whole life is the only treatment available for this condition. In the first 6 to 12 months after the diagnosis, supplements are required to treat the nutritional deficiencies that are present such as iron, calcium, folate and vitamin B_{12}. Medications for any associated conditions such as anaemia, osteoporosis, diabetes or any other conditions should be continued as usual.

5.6 GASTROESOPHAGEAL REFLUX DISEASE (GERD)

5.6.1 Introduction

Gastroesophageal reflux disease is a disease which brings up the food into the esophagus because of acidic stomach which causes heart burn. The pressure in the stomach is higher than the muscles which is found where the oesophagus and stomach join. GERD is chronic and it is non-progressive but in some cases it is progressive and causes complications.

5.6.2 Aetiology

GERD has the following reason to develop in the stomach because of muscle length decrease or there is no relaxation in the lower oesophageal sphincter, motility of stomach is reduced which allows the food to remain in stomach for a longer time. GERD can cause another stomach problem that is *hiatus hernia*. Factors which cause GERD are chocolate eating habit, alcohol, caffeine, spicy foods because of it the acids are secreted in the stomach and fatty foods remain in the stomach and it feels like the fullness of stomach. The reflux is caused because of gravity which works against digestion and which leads the reflux when patients lie horizontally or bend. GERD may worsen because of pregnancy or constipation because of increasing intra-abdominal pressure. Other causes are increased secretion states, disorders of connective tissue, blockage of stomach and it leads to ulceration and results in fullness of stomach and it takes longer time for emptying of stomach.

5.6.3 Symptoms

The symptoms of the GERD are the mouth taste become sour, feeling of burning in the heart, that is, heart burn, difficulty in swallowing which causes pain in the oesophagus, bring up wind frequently, it also causes sore throat, cough, feeling of fullness of stomach.

There are many short-term and long-term complications build up because of gastroesophageal reflux which increases severe problem of reflux. Some of them are bleeding in oesophagus which causes erosion in oesophagus and also causes ulcer in the stomach, oesophagitis, also leads to narrowing in the intestines. Sometimes it may cause one of the severe diseases in the oesophagus that is cancer in the oesophagus which is known as adenocarcinoma. Wrong kind of diet with high ingestion of soft drinks, cold drinks, sugar fat and processed foods results in GERD. Some people have habit of eating at inappropriate time or late eating is the reason behind gastroesophageal reflux. Sometime eating pattern is wrong, starvation lasts longer, stress, smoking and intake of alcohol cause GRED. Gastric acid can cause irritation in the in the oesophageal secretion. By this the high secretion of bile, pepsin, and pancreatic juice occur. There are low chance of clearance of acid from the oesophagus.

5.6.4 Oesophagitis

There are many oesophageal complication of gastroesophageal reflux disease which are oesophagitis, adenocarcinoma, Barrett metaplasia and stricture. Oesophagitis is a chronic disorder which is treated with the long-term process of anti-secretary therapy and it causes less effect of disease severity. There are another type of surgery to cure this type of disease that is laproscopic, anti-reflux surgery. There is main risk which causes from oesophagitis is adenocarcinoma. The adenocarcinoma originates from barrete metaplasia.

The cause of the oesophagitis are acid and pepsin. The acid and pepsin producing the burning sensation on the oesophagus that produce inflammation on the oesophagus. That's why acid and pepsin show the severity across the gastroesophageal reflux disease. Obesity is also associated with the gastroesophageal reflux disease, with the increase of weight there is increase severity for risk of gastroesophageal reflux disease.

5.6.5 Understanding the Anatomy of Oesophagus

The oesophagus is a hollow tube which is made up of muscles and arises from the pharynx to the stomach. The oesophagus is made up of both muscles that is smooth muscles and striated muscles. It is functionally divided in three portions:

- Posterior cricoids portion
- Oesophagus body
- LOS

Posterior cricoids portion: It is made up of striated muscles and it helps in the swallowing of the food material.

Oesophagus body: It is made up of the smooth muscles and it initiates the peristalsis movement of the body under the control or influence of extrinsic which is known as vagus and the intrinsic which is known as Auerbach's plexus.

The LOS (Lower Oesophageal Surface): It is the lower oesophageal surface and this is made by the phrenoesophageal ligament or membrane and this is formed by the fusion of endothoracic and endoabdominal fascia.

The muscles which is longitude in the oesophagus is shortens during the swallowing of the food and it also shortens the gastric cardia tents. The LOS is 4 cm long and 2 cm wide which lies in the oesophagus in intra-abdominally. The intrinsic part of the LOS is made up of the intrinsic muscles of the distal oesophagus and the proximal stomach in the cardia with sling fibers.

5.6.6 Transient Lower Oesophageal Sphincter Relax (TLESRs)

The transient lower oesophageal sphincter relaxations is the base of the lower oesophageal surface and are different from the swallow which is induced the LOS relaxation. It allows belching from the stomach. It means emit winds noisily from the stomach through the mouth. It shows the relationship between the majority of healthy persons and the patients suffering from the mild gastroesophageal reflux disease in the terms of reflux events.

Patients having the severe gastroesophageal reflux show some other factors like:

- Defective LOS function
- Low basal LOS pressure
- Hiatus hernia

With the severity of the disease, the proportion of the reflux with the transient lower oesophageal sphincter relaxation is inversely proportional to the disease occur that is gastroesophageal reflux disease.

5.6.7 Mechanics of GERD

The gastric acid which is present in the stomach, it is the combination of esophageal motility, gastric emptying (if the food is not taken at the appropriate time and the stomach feels fullness after long hours of eating is known as gastric emptying), LOS function. The coordination of the peristaltic moves delivers the food from the mouth to oesophagus. This movement of food from the mouth to the oesophagus is achieved by the pharyngeal which is also known as voluntary muscles and the oesophageal which is also known as involuntary muscles and it is coordinated by the Auerbach's plexus.

Peristaltic movement of the oesophagus can be achieved by:

- Primary: By swallow
- Secondary: It is initiated by the oesophagus because of the food which is reflux in oesophagus.
- Tertiary: Non-peristaltic oesophageal movements.

The LOS is relaxed when the completely swallowed ingested food passes. The LOS pressure is low and it is an important factor which determines the gastroesophageal reflux disease. The pressure of the LOS is decreased or reduced by the alcohol, smoking cigarette, and some of the foods like chewing gum which have the presence of peppermint in it.

The secretion of saliva in the adults is about 1000 to 1500 mL per day and it has the average pH is 7. The large volume of saliva secreted and it contributes in the buffering of the acid present in the stomach and it involves the primary peristalsis which is also called swallowing. The volume of saliva in the gastroesophageal reflux patients has the same value as compared to the healthy person. Sometimes it can be doubled or increased by the consumption of chewing gum and it is known as non-pharmacological treatment in the gastroesophageal reflux disease.

If the food is present in the stomach and it is not digested it shows the fullness of the stomach and from this it shows the effect of backflow pressure. Most of the patients having gastroesophageal reflux disease have long effect of the relaxation in the fundus because of the delay in emptying the stomach. Gastric emptying in the diabetes disease and the obstruction of the gastric outlet in the peptic ulcer disease, both diseases show the association with the gastroesophageal reflux disease.

5.6.8 Diagnosis of Gastroesophageal Reflux Disease

GERD is defined as the mucosal damage which is produced because of abnormal reflux of stomach or gastric contents in the oesophagus. The diagnoses are:

- Endoscopy
- Oesophageal manometry
- Ambulatory reflux monitoring
- Empiric therapy

5.6.9 Management and Treatment of GERD

The general instructions which are to be followed in the gastroesophageal reflux disease are to minimize the causes of gastroesophageal reflux, remove the acid concentration from the stomach, body weight should be normal.

Stay upright after eating because gravity is the important factor which keeps the food in the stomach for digestion and absorption. Burp of acid from the mouth is because of acid in the stomach. Eating more without feeling of hunger cause fullness of stomach and after lying down with the full stomach can cause the risk of the increase of the reflux or acidity in the stomach. The young and healthy person takes less hours to digest the food in the stomach after a complete and healthy meal but in the person who is old or suffering from gastroesophageal reflux disease can take more hours to digest. The stomach remains full because food is present in the stomach and it cannot be digested easily.

The treatment involved in the GERD is modification in the eating habits and living pattern or modification in the diets and the lifestyle, drug therapy, and sometimes surgery also. The diets should be made in the preference of individual food habits, that is, food tolerances, symptoms of the GERD may vary greatly from individual to individual. The diet may also be modified to remove the foods which can cause reflux in the stomach. The foods which can cause the reflux in the stomach or which reduce the lower oesophageal sphincter pressure are alcohol, caffeine, mint, processed or carbonated beverages, juices of citrus products and made from tomato, chocolate and the products which have chocolate, coffee (the presence of caffeine or without caffeine).

Avoid the food which has high content of fat because it reduces the reflux by decreasing the lower oesophageal sphincter pressure. Decrease of weight may be advised because with high weight the intra-gastric pressure in the stomach increases. Gap in the meals should be less because it decreases the gastric pressure while if large gap between meals can cause the reflux problem.

If the person has gastroesophageal reflux because of abdominal obesity then it is needed to prescribe a low energy content diet. If the patient has GERD but reason is not abdominal obesity then there is no need to prescribe low energy diet. The energy should remain same as it is prescribed for the normal and healthy person. The fat in the diet must be restricted because it triggers strong reflux in the duodenum and it causes fullness of stomach but in obese patients the lower intake of fat is advised. Vitamins and minerals are important in all diseases to reduce pain and decrease presence of disease in the body. If the patient is bleeding in the oesophagus and has other complications, intake of vitamins and minerals is prescribed like Vitamin C and B complex vitamins and iron.

Meals are the main source in the GERD because it causes the GERD symptom such as it stimulates the gastric acid production which causes reflux in the oesophagus. Meals should be eaten within 2 to 3 hours before going to bed because if meal eaten then at the same time going to bed increases acid in night time. Consumption of alcohol should be avoided because it can cause nocturnal reflux.

5.7 HIATUS HERNIA

The hiatus hernia disturbs both physiology and anatomy of a normal person's reflux mechanism. The effect of the hiatus hernia is that it reduces the length and pressure of oesophageal sphincter and it leads to the impair and increase of diaphragm expansion. The peristaltic movement of the oesophagus is decreased. By which cross sectional area of the oesophagogastric junction is increases and it act as reservoir reflux of hernia sac in the esophagus during swallowing. So the effect is theoverall increase of the acid exposure in the stomach and esophagus. The symptoms of the hiatus hernia are totally associated with gastroesophageal reflux disease which increase the risk or severity of the oesophagitis, adenocarcinoma or Barrett's esophagus. The treatment with proton pump inhibitor is not working in the case of both hiatus hernia and gastroesophageal reflux disease. Hiatus hernia favours gastroesophageal reflux disease in contributing the mucosal injury in the stomach.

The three types of the hiatus hernia are:

- Type 1
- Type 2
- Type 3

Type 1: This is the very common type.The widening of the diaphragm which have the muscular hiatal aperture with the phrenoesophageal membrane which allows the cardia of the gastic to move upward or herniated upwards.

Type 2: This defect is caused in the membrane which is known as phrenoesophageal membrane. The gastric oesophagus junction is fixed in the ligament of arcuate and the preaortic fascia and the gastric part of the fundus forms the some part of herniation.

Type 3: It is the mixture of type 1 and type 2 with the presence of more symptom and sliding effect of the type 2. It causes major damage to other organ that is cause herniated to the large defect to the pancreas and spleen.

5.7.1 Diagnosis of Hiatus Hernia

The large hiatal disease is diagnosed by:

- Endoscopy
- Radiology
- Manometric studies

Hiatal hernia involves upper abdomen and the protrusion occurs through the opening in the diaphragm between the stomach and the chest. The oesophagus passes through hiatus. Common symptoms include heartburn, reflux of acid and indigestion.

5.7.2 Dietary Management of Hiatal Hernia

The foods should be chosen carefully for the patients suffering from hiatal hernia. The foods should be bland and free of spices so that no irritation is caused to the lining of stomach. Further, the foods which have delayed gastric emptying should be avoided completely. Foods said to prolong gastric (stomach) emptying time include high fat foods, cream, ice cream, high fat cheese, red meats, cured meats, potato chips, and more. The foods should be taken to relieve the symptoms of GERD completely and high protein diet helps a lot. It is said that high protein diet helps to close the LES sphincter.

The sugary food products should be completely avoided such as ice creams, bakery products chocolate, coffee which relaxes the LES sphincters and it is also responsible to increase secretion of stomach acid content. Alcohol, mint, citrus fruit, tomatoes and carbonated beverages may cause irritation and further damage the lining of the oesophagus.

5.7.2.1 Other Lifestyle/Diet Changes

Being overweight has been associated with an increase in the incidence of GERD and hiatal hernia. Other diet tips known to lower the symptoms of hiatal hernia include:

Eat small frequent meals.

Drink plenty of water and sugarfree beverages.

Keep a diary/food log of triggers that lead to binge eating.

Chew your food thoroughly and eat slowly and drink lots of water during meals to promote proper digestion.

Do *not* eat right before exercising or bending over.

Eat foods high in probiotics (such as fermented foods kefir, sauerkraut, natto, etc.).

Avoid starvation or fasting to avoid release of gastric HCL.

5.8 DYSPEPSIA

Dyspepsia is the term given to a group of gastrointestinal symptoms associated with the ingestion of food, e.g., nausea, heartburn, epigastric pain, discomfort and distension. It is commonly known as indigestion. Dyspepsia may be functional or organic. In functional dyspepsia there is no change in any part of the GI tract. The symptoms may have a psychological basis or be due to intolerance to a particular food or due to faulty food habits such as intake of very spicy food, large meals, etc., organic dyspepsia may be due to chronic kidney disease or heart disease.

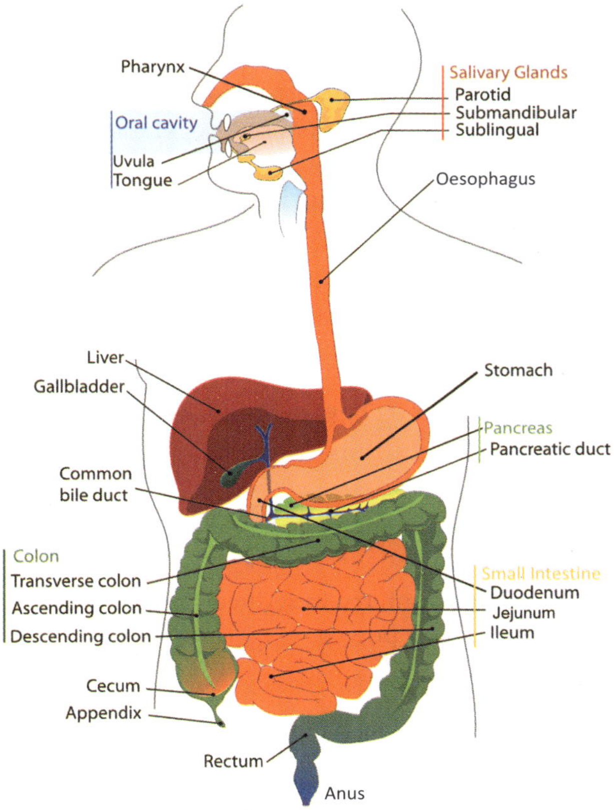

Dyspepsia is caused by certain medications. Lifestyle can contribute by consumption of greasy or spicy foods, improper food intake or high oily or junk food. The symptoms of nausea, heartburn, epigastric pain , discomfort and distension show after the indigestion problem in very bad condition when the person reaches, this is an emergency situation.

5.8.1 Medication

Some common medicines to prevent indigestion like antacids, H-2-receptor antagonists, antibiotics, antidepressants, these medicines reduce the stomach acid. But all these medicines have some other side effects which affect the body. Dyspepsia diet (indigestion diet) and high fibre food help in dyspepsia like banana is good source of fibre. It helps to prevent many GI infections.

5.8.2 Symptoms

The symptoms are very common like upper abdominal discomfort, indigestion, heart burn, bloating, fullness, nausea, and anorexia. These symptoms can also be seen in GI reflux, peptic ulcer disease and stomach cancer or pancreas and gallstone disease .

5.8.3 Diet and Feeding Pattern

The prescribed bland diets have reduced gaseous foods like whole pulses such as rajmah, chana. Strongly flavoured vegetables like radish, turnip, cauliflower, broccoli, beans and peas must be avoided. Lactose intolerance is a very common cause of dyspepsia. Lifestyle pattern also promotes irregular meals and lack of activity. Alcohol and smoking are major causes of dyspepsia as well.

5.8.4 Points to Remember

- Don't eat food which causes discomfort.
- Don't gulp the food and chew the food 32 times per slice.
- Don't eat right before bedtime. Keep a gap of 2-3 hours between food and sleep.
- Avoid taking antacids and anti-inflammatory drugs except under physician guidance.
- And last very important, try to reduce stress level. Take good sleep. It boosts your immune power.

5.8.5 Treatment

Obesity is a reversible cause of both reflux and non-reflux like dyspepsia. General lifestyle changes are of modest benefit. Other treatments in management of reflux are surgery based and work best in PPI responsive and volume reflux patients. The pattern of acid dyspeptic disorders changes functional dyspeptic syndromes less sensitive to acid suppression. Reflux like dyspepsia responds best to PPIs with a smaller response by pain predominant and little or none by dysmotility like dyspepsia.

The pattern of dyspepsia is changing. Recent guidance has emphasized the importance of early referral for new onset dyspepsia in the over 55s without a trial of treatment.

5.8.6 Flatulence

While eating or drinking normally, it's natural to swallow air. If you ventilate often, you can see that your stomach starts bloating. Maybe it could also cause burping. Often this is due to the release of more air than usual. This is also seen due to the GI system malfunction and age factor is one of the reasons.

The major reasons are:

- Smoking
- Carbonated drinks
- Eating very fast
- Elevated junk foods intake
- Increased intake of uncooked food products
- Unhealthy food eating
- Consumption of alcoholic products
- High intake of protein products

Some type of dietary foods (rich in high protein), like rajma rich in high protein, lentils also good source of protein, some vegetables like cabbage, apple, raisins. Some types of high fructose fruit also cause this situation. It takes too much time to digest food, due to which various types of gases are produced in the stomach. Some foods are also not completely absorbed by the body, it means that they pass from the intestine to the colon without being completely digested. In the colon it contains large amounts of bacteria. These bacteria help in the food digestion. Bacteria break down the food and release gas. The build-up of this gas causes flatulence/gas.

5.9 FOODS TO IMPROVE DIGESTIVE SYSTEM

5.9.1 Digestion

The digestive system comprises of the alimentary canal and some glands for the process of gastrointestinal tracts. It is a process of ingestion, digestion, absorption and ejection or elimination. The alimentary canal starts with the mouth, transits across the thorax, stomach, intestine and ends in the anus. The food is digested with the help of various enzymes present in the gastrointestinal tract to absorb the essential substances from the foods like amino acids, protein, vitamins and minerals. The body absorbs these nutrients to provide raw materials for the synthesis of new cells or generation of new cells, enzymes and hormones and it also provides the energy required in the body for the important processes in the body.

The digestive system is divided into five processes:

- Ingestion
- Propulsion
- Digestion
- Absorption
- Elimination

Ingestion is the process by which food has been eaten from the mouth and taking the food in the alimentary canal. This is the process by which food is moving with the other contents in the alimentary canal.

Digestion consists of two processes of digestion: **(a) mechanical breakdown** is the process by which the food is mechanically broken down. For example, chewing (mastication). **(b) chemical breakdown** is the process by which food is broken down with the help of various enzymes secreted from the accessory organs and the glands in the digestive system.

Absorption is the process by which food is absorbed in the body by the cells with the help of capillaries of the lymph and the blood which is circulating in the body.

Elimination is the process by which the eaten food is not absorbed in the body and considered the waste. So the unabsorbed food is excreted from the body as a waste material like stool or feaces.

5.9.1.1 How the Food is Digested

The food is ingested in the mouth and by the action of saliva and teeth it is swallowed. Saliva breaks carbs into simpler sugar. With the help of oesophagus the food enter the stomach. In the sphincter, the food passes and is mixed with the gastric juices. The stomach churns the food and breaks down it with chemically as well as mechanically. The food enters into small intestine through the duodenum. There are enzymes secreted from the pancreas and the bile juice from the liver. Food is digested in the parts of small intestine, that is, jejunum and ileum. The absorption of the nutrient occurs in the small intestine. Liver breaks down the fat with the help of bile juice and filters the impurities from the body. The nutrients are absorbed in the small intestine and the undigested food or waste is passed to the large intestine. The waste is stored in the rectum and ejected out with the help of anus from the body. Some people suffer from many digestive issues as they do not take proper diet or we can say, balanced diet. The proper diet contains vitamins, minerals, carbohydrates, protein and many organic as well as inorganic molecules.

If the food is not digested properly it can cause many issues:

- Diarrhoea
- Constipation
- Bloating
- Vomiting
- Abdominal pain
- Heartburn
- Acidic reflex action, that is, presence of gas in the stomach

- Gastro-oesophageal reflux disease
- Irritable bowel syndrome
- Crohn's disease

Avoid foods which is rich in refined carbs, food additives like many chemicals, saturated and trans fats which are found in many processed foods and they are not good for digestive health. Artificial sweetener also not good for digestion.Include food which contain high fibre like papaya, apple, beetroot, etc.

The foods which improve digestion

1. **Ginger (*Zingiber officinale*)** is well known and ancient example for improving digestion. It is famous in the form of ginger ale or ginger stick. Sometimes it is consumed during travelling because it helps to improve the motion sickness.

   It also helps in the prevention of vomiting which occurs during pregnancy and post-operative vomiting. It was used as a medicine in the ancient times for improving the digestion health.

   Ginger is consumed both in fresh and dried form.

   Fresh ginger are combined with brown sugar and it produces normal stool within 4 days and cures patient up to 70%. It also helps to remove toxins and control vomiting. Dried ginger is also used to improve digestion and absorption in the gastrointestinal tract. Ginger tea is common home remedy.

2. **Cumin (*Cuminum cyminum*)** is used as a nutritional supplement as well as food ingredient. It was used in ancient times as a food additive. Cumin enhances the flavour of the food.

   It helps to increase the activity of various digestive enzymes for enhancing the digestive process. It also helps to release the bile juice from the liver which helps to digest the fat and various nutrients and minerals in the stomach. Cumin is an important herb that removes digestive problem like vomiting, diarrhoea, formation of gas, irregular bowel movement, etc. Cumin is also known as a natural laxative.

3. **Yogurt or curd:** Yogurt is an useful ingredient to maintain digestion. It is a fermented or cultured milk product which is thickened by adding probiotic or acid cultures in the milk. The probiotic which is used to make yogurt are *Lactobacillus acidophilus, Lactobacillus bulgaricus, Lactobacillus casei*, etc.

   Yogurt is also useful for the people who have lactose intolerance. Lactose are also present in yogurt but is digested properly because of presence of certain bacteria.

It may also improve gastrointestinal diseases:

- Diarrhoea
- Constipation
- Inflammatory bowel disease
- *H. pylori* infection in the small intestine

4. **Carom seeds (*Trachyspermum ammi*)** are also improve the digestion. One substance present in carom seeds is thymol which has anti-bacterial property and it can fight against bacteria present in the digestive system. It can also help to cure acid reflux or gas present in the stomach and cure many small intestinal disorders.

   Carom seed is a natural herb which cures diarrhoea. Boil one spoon of carom seed in a glass of water and allow it to cool and strain water. Consume twice a day. This is the best method to cure the digestive problems. It will also help in the acid reflux. Carom water shows the result in a few minutes.

   It also helps in relieving the peptic ulcer which is the inflammation of the small intestine. It also improves the activity of various digestive enzymes which improve the digestion and it helps in high secretion of bile juice. It is the best ayurvedic medicine as well as household remedy for improving digestion.

5. **Mint (Mentha)** is the best herb or ingredient for digestion. It contains antioxidants and some phytonutritions that work for the stomach. The mint contains menthol which helps the enzyme to improve the digestion. It also contains various volatile oil like menthone, methyl acetate and menthol. It also contains anti-inflammatory as well as antibacterial property. Rosmarinic is the antioxidant present in mint. It is also known as stomach soother as well as breath freshener and cooling of stomach or provide cooling sensation.

   It improves the following digestive disorders:

   - Bloating
   - Stomach pain
   - Vomiting
   - Acidic reflux
   - Changes in bowel habits
   - Upset stomach

6. **Kefir** is a traditional as well as popular beverage. Kefir is the Turkish word which means good feeling. Kefir is the grain which looks like a small clump of cauliflower or coral. It contain various types of

bacteria like lactobacillus, lacto cocci and aceto. It contains yeast also both non-lactose fermenting as well as lactose fermenting yeast. Yeast present in the kefir is the friendly yeast which is also present in the yogurt.

Fermentation of milk with the kefir grain which is known as kefir. Kefir can be made with the various types of milk such as goat or sheep milk, cow milk, buffalo milk, coconut milk, soya milk, rice milk but cow milk is most commonly used.

Kefir contains many compounds such as minerals, vitamins and essential amino acids which help to maintain the function of the body as well as the digest complete protein. Kefir is also known as natural probiotic and it contains live bacteria. The microorganisms in the kefir help to digest the proteins and absorb the lactose and the person with lactose intolerance can also consume kefir.

7. **Kiwi** has its medicinal properties and has been used since ancient times. It contains many fibre protein vitamins as well as healthy minerals. It also contains fructose, glucose and small amount of sucrose and it is a good source of vitamin A, vitamin K and vitamin E. It also contains flavonoid antioxidant like beta carotene, xanthin as well as lutein. It also helps to improve immune system.

   Kiwi also helps to improve digestion as it contains many proteolytic enzymes like actinidin, the protein dissolving enzyme which helps digestion of protein and it may help to digest a meal just like the papain in the papaya and bromelain in the pineapple. The property of the insoluble fibre is that it adds bulkiness to the stool which improves the digestion in the digestive tract or gastrointestinal tract.

8. **Whole grains** contain all part of the grain that is the endosperm, germ and bran. Whole grain are known for their high content of dietary fibre, fermentable carbohydrates as well as grain fibre like wheat, barley, oats, rye that help to increase the stool weight and its speed of the intestinal transit, etc. Wheat bran is known for its effective reaction, that is, increasing the stool weight by the ratio of 5:1.

   Whole grains provide many necessary dietary fibers, oligosaccharide and resistance starch to the diet. Wheat is the most common whole grain which is consumed and it is a rich source of oligosaccharides and it is accepted as a prebiotic.

   Dietary fibres mainly come from the plant that is not easily digested by the small intestine. It can be metabolized by the bacteria present in the stomach. Fibre is mainly pectin cellulose hemicellulose, gum mucilage, and lignin. It helps to slow the passage of food in the intestine and it increases the fecal bulk. Wheat bran and whole grain are rich in the insoluble fibre and some vegetables are also good sources.

Insoluble fibre make the stool soft and bulky binding with water. So it is found mainly in the whole grain products. Whole grain is helpful in the treatment and prevention of constipation, diverticulosis, haemorrhoids. Diverticula is the pouch in the small intestine which can become painful and inflamed.

Sources: The dietary fibre is only found in the plant source like vegetables, fruit, grain as well as nuts but not in a source of meat. The removal of peel seeds reduces the fibre content. For example whole tomato has high fibre content than peeled tomatoes.

5.10 INFLAMMATORY BOWEL DISEASE (IBD)

The stomach related tract includes the mouth, throat, stomach, small digestive tract, and internal organ. This is only responsible because of inadequate nourishment, deficiency of essential supplements, and difficulty in excreting any unwanted material and waste items from the body. Irritation can be caused at others parts also along the stomach related tract which may upset the ordinary functioning of the body. IBD can be agonizing and problematic, and moreover it might even cause death. Ulcerative colitis (UC) and Crohn's disease (CD) together are known as the inflammatory bowel diseases (IBD).

The normal functioning includes our stomach digestive system runs from your mouth to our anus. In this functioning and our stomach digestive system is working efficiently, nourishment moves easily through our stomach digestive systems and then out of our body. Our body ingests various supplements that are needed from nourishment of our digestive system, and the waste material is excreted out from the body in form of stools.

If a person has IBD, some part of your stomach digestive tract is damaged. After some time, the irritation can cause serious sufferings, looseness of the bowels, and once in a while bleeding stool. IBD symptoms can occur and can disappear for some time. And this results in the irritation in your stomach from IBD. Your body can't assimilate the essential supplements it needs. This can only occur due to lack of healthy diet, and it may also result in several medical issues, for example anaemia.

Some of the ecological variants those attach them with the body's surface and disturb the functioning of the system. A point reaches when the intestinal functioning does not occur appropriately, then many white blood cells amass in the inner covering (mucosa) of the gut then these cells at that point discharge some allergic compounds that lead to tissue injury (irritation). This aggravation of the mucosa can cause looseness of the bowels, which is the most important recognized side effect of ulcerative colitis and Crohn's infection, with or without the intestinal complication.

The two types of IBD are ulcerative colitis and Crohn's disease.

5.10.1 Ulcerative Colitis

It is a disease of idiopathic origin; it develops in the form of acute and chronic ulcerinfiltrating colitis. It mainly affects the mucosa and sub-mucosa lining of the rectum and the descending colon. In rare cases, it may affect the entire length of the large intestine. Ulcerative colitis affects only colon and the disease in all the cases extends from the rectal part. In this disease major part of the large intestine is either inflamed or is ulcerated. Bloody diarrhoea or rectal bleeding is common in this disease. The motility of the bowel in the large intestine increases with increase in inflammation, this is due to the enhanced secretions. Because of enhanced secretions, bowel movement takes place almost all day long and thus patient gets diarrhoea.

Some terms related to colitis, which we need to study:

- Ulcerative procitis: It is the mildest type of ulcerative colitis. Only rectal part gets inflamed.
- Universal colitis: It is also known by the name pancolitis. It is a severe type of colitis as it affects the whole colon.
- Proctosigmoiditis: In this type of colitis, inflammation affects only the lower end of colon along with the rectal part.
- Distal colitis: In this type, inflammation reaches up to the left colon starting from rectum.
- Acute serious ulcerative colitis: It is the most severe type of the colitis. In this type whole colon gets affected with severe manifestations and complications. It is caused by a not so common variable.

5.10.2 Crohn's Disease

Inflammation in any part of the gastrointestinal tract, starting from buccal cavity up to anus is considered Crohn's disease. Inflammation can either be in patches or can be continuous. In this disease all mucosal layers are affected and are inflamed.

- **Diet:** Dietary habits and ulcerative colitis are directly related. Diet plays a key role in the course of bowel inflammation; it can either increase or decrease the severity and time period of inflammation.

From a study it was found that people whose dietary intake composed more of solid food had reduced the risk of ulcerative colitis by 79 per cent. Gluten intolerance or sensitivity is common in irritable bowel disease. Gluten intolerance is also associated with chronic pain. Gluten intolerance accounted for 23.6 and 27.3 per cent cases of Crohn's disease and ulcerative colitis respectively. People who consume high protein diet, particularly rich in protein from animal origin are at a greater risk of getting inflammatory bowel disease or any other gastrointestinal disorder. Vitamin D doesn't affect human health by maintaining calcium homeostasis and bone metabolism but also acts as an immune modulator and is very potential as an anti-inflammatory vitamin. Consuming diet rich in fats and refined products also contribute to the development of IBD.

- **Hereditary factors:** Family history and genetics play a key role in the development of a disease. In case of IBD, it has been found that heredity and the disease are directly linked. IBD is more commonly seen in patients whose parents or siblings are affected; this originates because of the inborn error which diminishes epithelial cells barrier function. Chances of getting IBD increases by 3 to 20 folds in case of prior infection in close family. Monozygotic twins are at a 50 per cent risk factor of getting IBD.
- **Smoking cigarette:** Smoking tobacco or cigarette is one of the leading causes of Crohn's disease. From certain studies it has been found that smoking may help in relieving pain because of ulcerative colitis, but will eventually worsen the condition in the long run.
- **Non-steroidal anti-inflammatory medicines:** These medicines increase the risk of getting IBD or can intensify the infection in patients already suffering from IBD. This group of medicines includes medications which are commonly used and are available over the counter. These medications include diclofenac sodium (present in most pain killers, Voltaren), naproxen sodium (Aleve) and ibuprofen (Advil, Motrin IB and many more).
- **Environmental factors:** The locality or area where you live also plays an important role in the early development or delaying of the IBD. People living in industrialized area are more prone to the development of IBD. From various studies conducted all over the world it has been found that people who reside in the northern atmosphere are at more risk of getting IBD than those residing in southern atmosphere. Other environmental factors which affect the development of IBD include mode of birth (normal delivery or C-section), pre-mature delivery or

normal healthy baby delivery, breast-feeding and consumption of medicines.

- **Other factors:** Mental and psychological state of the individual, lifestyle (sedentary or active), exercise, alcohol, eating pattern, exposure to microbes and antibiotics also contribute directly or indirectly to the development of IBD .
- **Stress:** Stress is the cause behind the development of many diseases in the modern world. Stress plays a major role in the development of IBD. Stress causes immense amount of pressure, which, in turn, leads to hormonal as well as neurological changes in the individual. Stress can either aggravate the disease or at least elevates the manifestations of the disease.
- **Effect of medications:** With increase in the number of IBD patients, scientists had keen interest to look for the causes which may be linked with the consumption of certain medicines or drugs. It has been found that exposure to different types of medicines increases the risk of getting IBD. Some antibiotics are found to be the culprit behind the development of IBD and particularly Crohn's disease. Some other medications like oral contraceptives are linked positively with the development of IBD and Crohn's disease.

5.10.3 Path-Physiology of Inflammatory Bowel Disease

Crohn's disease, inflammatory bowel disease and ulcerative colitis are considered to be of idiopathic origin. These diseases affect the gastro-intestinal tract. These diseases are often viewed together because of various reasons including aggravation of gastrointestinal tract, obscure aetiology and recurrence of manifestations over and again. Though these diseases have different side-effects as well as intestinal attributes. Despite much advancement in the medical field, Crohn's disease requires surgery either in early or late stages of the disease. Surgery is used for treating intractable disease or its complications like haemorrhage, fistulas, strictures and abscesses. Though there is an increasing demand for the non-surgical method of treatment. Despite the emergence of new drugs and non-invasive method of surgeries the patients are treated using traditional methods. Proper treatment of ulcerative colitis is safe and viable. It also provides personal satisfaction to those patients whose illness can't be therapeutically overseen.

- Proctocolectomy along with ileostomy is used as an alternative in patients who are unsatisfied with the therapeutic methods. Patients undergoing colostomy are the key to revolution in therapeutic methodology.

- **Liver disease** Like fatty liver, cirrhosis, auto-immune hepatitis occur in about 3-5 per cent people. Though slight abnormalities are common in liver function test (LFT). Some of these conditions like primary sclerosing cholangitis can act as predecessor of IBD. In this case IBD can be at its full swing by the time of diagnosis.
- Disorder that occurs as a consequence of disrupted physiology of the bowel: These disorders are commonly seen in Crohn's disease, particularly in the small intestine. Malabsorption is the most common consequence of the disease. Malabsorption of fat soluble vitamins (A, D, E and K), vitamin B12 and many minerals leads to various deficiencies like hypomagnesaemia, hypocalcaemia, bone demineralization and thickening issue.
- **Osteopenia:** Decrease in bone mass is considered osteopenia. It can occur either at the initiation of IBD or may be because of corticosteroid consumption. As 90 per cent of the pinnacle bone mass is gained during early years of life, it is very common to get pediatric IBD because of osteopaenia. Failure in attaining desired bone mass increases the risk of getting fractures. Corticosteroids and low bone mineral density are directly linked. Corticosteroids reduce the amount of calcium and phosphorous absorption. Other contributing factors of low bone mineral density are aseptic or vascular necrosis, it is rarely seen. Aseptic or vascular necrosis is also associated with the use of corticosteroids. Persistent joint pain particularly in hips and knees are the prompt consideration of the related complication. In growing children, adolescents and young adults malabsorption hinders development and repair.
- **Renal disease:** Nephrolithiasis occurs as oxalate calculi in Crohn's disease and as uric corrosive calculi in ulcerative colitis. Hypercalciuria is a side effect of consuming corticosteroids, and may be fatal. Optional amyloidosis is very rare but has been accounted for Crohn's disease. Because of urethral compression by inflammatory masses or entrance of inflammatory masses in vesicular fistulae leads to obstructive complications.
- **Delayed puberty and physical development in children:** Growth retardation (characterized by decrease in the speed of development, decrease by every year for age, decrease in height and age ratio) and diminished sexual development can also be a complication of Crohn's disease in children.
- **Risk associated with people suffering from cancer:** People having Crohn's disease or ulcerative colitis along with cancer are at an

increased risk of getting colorectal malignant growth when compared to others. Colorectal disease frequently occurs within 8-10 years of diagnosis of IBD. The complication progresses with the age.

- **Risk for getting blood clot diseases:** Individual suffering from IBD has a greater risk of getting deep vein thrombosis (formation of blood clot in the blood vessels of the body) or pneumonic embolism (unexpected breakage in lung artery because of blood clot) by three folds. Blood thinners are prescribed to the patients with any sign of blood clot in blood vessels.
- **Risk of getting primary sclerosing cholangitis (PSC):** It is a type of serious and aggravated scarring in the bile duct or bile channel. Around 75 per cent of the PSC patients are suffering from IBD also. PSC is more dominant in patients with ulcerative colitis when compared to patients suffering from Crohn's disease. PSC is more common among men than females. Signs of the PSC include weight loss, tingling, sickness and jaundice. About 5 per cent patients suffering from ulcerative colitis and 1 per cent with Crohn's diseases are at the risk of developing PSC. No medication has been discovered yet for PSC. Liver transplant is done for treating the condition.

5.10.4 Dietary Management of Irritable Bowel Disease

5.10.4.1 Role of Diet

There are many disputes on the effect of different food products in the treatment of IBD. Many nutritionists considered ignoring entire food group or a few specific foods. But with new researches it has been found that food which either increases the inflammation or worsens the symptoms of the disease are to be avoided. It is advised to restrict as few foods as possible so as to maintain normal diet and proper supply of all the nutrients. Proper nutrient intake helps in maintaining normal body functions particularly of digestive tract, thus maintaining overall well-being.

In recent times, healing mucosal membrane has become the major therapeutic goal for the doctors around the globe. Treating mucosal membrane helps in preventing the complications of IBD. Mucosal healing relies on naturally occurring cellular events which help in repairing the epithelial layer. Repaired epithelial layer ensures restoration of cellular integrity as well as physiological functions of the colon which include water absorption and barrier function. Also, the nutritional status is generally hampered during or after an inflammatory episode of the intestinal wall. These episodes occur as a result of catabolic action of pro-inflammatory cytokines.

Consuming a diet rich in protein helps in repairing of epithelial tissues after an inflammatory episode. It depends on the type of protein consumed as well as the type of protein synthesized by the body. Balance between essential (not synthesized by the body, consumed through diet) and non-essential (synthesized in the body) amino acids help in the early recovery. Endogenous protein helps in healing the mucosal lining as they are available in the blood supply, while dietary proteins are acted upon in the colon by the gut microflora and are used in healing.

With studies it has come to notice of the scientists that buffalo milk contains many bioactive peptides which have been used to prevent various diseases. During the gastrointestinal digestion of the milk and products, these bioactive peptides are released into the gut. Recently new peptides have been identified in buffalo milk and its products (MBCP), these novel peptides have the potential of reducing hydrogen peroxide induced oxidative stress in the epithelial lining of the intestine as well as in erythrocytes.

5.10.4.2 Dietary Recommendations for Ulcerative Colitis

To minimize loose stools and stomach ache, low calorie diet is prescribed. Avoid foods which can cause stool excretion, particularly new products of soil, juices and prunes. Some desserts like candies, ice creams and sodas when eaten during inflammation cause watery stools which reduce the water movement in to the gastrointestinal tract. Alcohol and alcohol based beverages are completely avoided. Add more of omega-3 unsaturated fatty acids in the diet. Omega 3 fatty acids help in relieving symptoms and in easy bowel movement. It is found in fishes like salmon, herring, mackerel and sardines. Small and frequent feeding pattern is helpful with the patients. Eating small meals helps body fight against inflammation and further damage by proving all variety of nutrients. Supplementation is prescribed in case of anorexia and if food sources are not endured well in the body.

5.10.4.3 Dietary Recommendations for Crohn's Disease

Low calorie diet is recommended as it helps in relieving pain and improves bowel movement. If on stricture, say no to nuts, beans, seeds and small meals. Food low in temperature helps in reducing loose stools. Stay away from food which can increase bowel movement like leafy vegetables, cold drinks, soda and prunes. Follow lactose-free diet if suffering from lactose bigotry. Lactose intolerance can cause bloating, cramps, gas and even diarrhoea within 30 to 90 minutes of consuming food containing milk in various forms. Breath hydrogen test is used to validate premonitions of lactose intolerance. Fat malabsorption can cause sleek and putrid stools. During fat malabsorption, low fat diet is prescribed. Littler and progressive meals are better tolerated, with the betterment in health quantity of dietary intake can be increased.

Foods recommended to a patient on IBD are turkey, fishes (salmon, herring, sardines and mackerel), chicken, egg, mashed potatoes, noodles, rice, bread (white or sourdough), apple sauce, oatmeal, diluted juices, canned fruits, red meat, liver, spreads, breakfast cereals and fortified foods.

Vitamin D has a significant role in maintaining gastrointestinal barrier integrity, keeps a check on the microflora and fauna of the gut and finally checking inflammatory immune response.

Fibrous food is restricted but some fibrous foods can be well tolerated by the body. Foods like tender cooked vegetables, cooked fruits, canned fruits and starchy food like cereals, tortillas and whole wheat noodles. Vegetables, fruits, lean protein, low or zero fat dairy products and whole grains are well tolerated and given to the patients.

5.10.4.4 Role of Medication

IBD is chronic in nature and is recurring disease. It affects ileum, colon or both and is commonly associated with systemic manifestations. It is idiopathic in nature but many factors trigger immune components leading to manifestation of the disease. Two major types of IBD include Crohn's disease and ulcerative colitis.

Other manifestations which are extra intestinal in both Crohn's disease and ulcerative colitis include fever, arthritis, hepatitis, oral ulceration, uveitis and dermatitis. These manifestations can either shoot up or can even depress to almost neutral.

Drugs used in treating IBD are corticosteroids, 5-amino salicylic acid, immunosuppressants and TNF gamma inhibitors.

Moderate to serious cases of IBD are commonly treated with cholestyramine, corticosteroids (prednisone) and 5-ASA mixes (sulfasalazine). Though these medicines have wholesome reactions, before consuming these medicines do contact your physician.

- **Cholestyramine:** It reduces the absorption amount of fat soluble vitamins namely A, D, E and K. It also hampers the absorption of calcium, iron, folate and vitamin B12.
- **Corticosteroids:** These include prednisolone, prednisone and budesonide. These medicines affect the body's ability to maintain and correct the inflammatory process. They keep the immune activity in check. They are very effective in short-term flares. They are not at

all recommended for long term use as they have very severe side effects. Side effects include weight gain, bone loss, infection, skin fragility, mood swings, sleep disturbances and cataracts.

- **Prednisone:** It reduces the amount of calcium and phosphorous absorbed from small intestine. It also causes degradation of zinc, potassium, calcium and vitamin C in the body. With prolonged use of this medicine bone health can be disrupted. People on prednisone require 1200 mg calcium per day. It also increases the rate of protein catabolism, so increased protein intake is provided.
- **Sulfasalazine:** It interferes with folate absorption in the body. People who are prescribed this medicine are additionally prescribed with 1 mg folate supplementation per day.

All the above medications should be taken under medical supervision.

5.10.5 Complications of Inflammatory Bowel Disease

Complications of Crohn's disease and ulcerative colitis are:

- Malabsorption due to impaired absorption of fat, vitamin B_{12}, proteins and electrolytes from the diseased small bowel.
- Fistula formation may occur in long standing cases. These may be internal fistulae between the loops of the intestine, or external fistulae such as enterocutaneous, rectal and anal fistulae.
- Stricture formation may occur in chronic cases due to extensive fibrosis in the affected bowel wall.

5.11 DIVERTICULITIS

Diverticulitis is a predominant gastrointestinal issue that is related with noteworthy morbidity and health care costs. Entanglements of diverticulitis, for example, stomach sepsis, are more averse to happen with ensuing occasions. A few hazard factors, a large number of which are modifiable, have been recognized including corpulence, diet, and physical inertia. Diet and lifestyle could influence danger of diverticulitis through their belongings on the intestinal microbiome and aggravation. Investigations have discovered that the capacity of the gut microbiome varies between people with diverticulitis versus without diverticulitis. Hereditary variables, just as modifications in colonic neuromusculature, can likewise add to the improvement of diverticulitis. Randomized preliminaries of haemodynamically stable patients who require pressing medical procedure for intense, convoluted diverticulitis that has not improved with anti-infection agents give proof to help essential anastomosis versus sigmoid colectomy with end colostomy. In spite of these progresses, more research is expected to expand our comprehension of the pathogenesis of diverticulitis and to explain treatment calculations.

Pathophysiology of diverticulitis may be understood as a negative effect on intestines leading to the diverticulum sac; therefore, causing second rate irritation, blockage and further obstruction by bothering the mucosa. Additional naming of diverticulitis includes convoluted and uncomplicated. The portrayal of confounded diverticulitis is by abscess development, check, fistulas and perforation. A noteworthy though during diverticulitis administration includes the choice between hospitalizing the patient and not doing so. American Society for Colon and Rectal Surgery (ASCRS) suggests that this choice is affected by a number of factors including the inability to tolerate administration by oral means, the level of torment, mainly comorbidities, along with social help at home. A development has been seen in the recent years in the ordered characterization of diverticular ailment of the symptomatic kind. These are inclusive of segmental colitis related with diverticulosis (SCAD), interminable intermittent diverticulitis and symptomatic uncomplicated diverticular infection, or SUDD.

Segmental colitis associated with diverticulosis (SCAD): The present perception of SCAD is as that of a particular substance. It may be termed the indistinct segmental irritation in the sigmoid colon skirted by numerous diverticula. The diverticular orifice doesn't necessarily have to be included in this. Incorporating the risk factors are males of more than fifty years. Introduction during initial stages is marked by frequent seeping of the rectum, accompanied by stomach pain and loose bowels in some.

5.11.1 Epidemiology

The lifetime danger of diverticulitis in an individual with diverticulosis was accounted for to go from 10% to 25%.10 Be that as it may, these appraisals originate before the normal utilization of adaptable endoscopy and, subsequently, a precise evaluation of predominance. Moreover, the analysis of diverticulitis was made on clinical grounds. Diverticulitis is more typical in men than women until the sixth decade, when it turns out to be progressively basic in women. The predominance of hospitalization for diverticulitis in the United States is most prominent in whites comparative in African Americans and Hispanics, and most reduced in Asians. Individuals living in urban zones are more prone to be hospitalized for diverticulitis than those in rustic areas. Diverticulitis is increasingly basic in developed nations, yet could be expanding in different parts of the world. After migration, non-Western people have a less danger of hospitalization for diverticular sickness than Western locals, despite the fact that hazard increments with time since movement.

5.11.2 Classification

1. **Asymptomatic diverticulosis:** Asymptomatic diverticulosis is frequently a coincidental finding in patients experiencing imaging for other indications. Be that as it may, the clinical noteworthiness of such discoveries is hazy as there is no sign for treatment or further line up for patients with asymptomatic diverticulosis.
2. **Diverticulitis:** Aggravation of a diverticulum prompts diverticulitis. It can present as either an intense or constant procedure. Diverticulitis is the most well known inconvenience of diverticulosis, which happens in about 10% to 25% of patients.
   - Obesity, and focal stoutness specifically, expands the danger of diverticulitis.
   - Smoking is likewise connected with an expanded danger of diverticulitis – especially confused diverticulitis.
   - On the other hand, dietary fibre admission and judicious weight control plans (high in natural products, vegetables, and entire grains) lessen the danger of diverticulitis.
   - Nuts and seeds don't seem to build a hazard, and in a huge availability, nuts and popcorn were related with decreased danger of diverticulitis.
   - Physical movement (especially enthusiastic movement, for example, running) is related with diminished risk.
   - Liquor: It isn't certain whether liquor influences danger of diverticulitis.

Immunosuppression is thought to build danger of diverticulitis. The hazard related with corticosteroids is all around characterized. Be that as it may, investigations of different types of immunosuppression, for example, chemotherapy, organ transplantation, renal failure are examples of immunosuppression and related hazards for diverticulitis.

5.11.3 Pathogenesis

The pathophysiology of diverticulitis is not entirely comprehended. Long standing yet problematic speculations propose that diverticulitis results from obstacle and injury to a diverticulum with ensuing ischemia, microperforation, also, infection. This hypothesis prompted across the board conviction that patients with diverticulosis ought to abstain from eating nuts and seeds, and the broad utilization of anti-infection agents for diverticulitis treatment. In any case, later examinations demonstrated that nut and seed utilization don't expand danger of diverticulitis, and that anti-toxins may not hurry recuperation or improve outcomes.These discoveries have prompted models of diverticulitis pathogenesis that include incessant irritation and changes in the gut microbiome.

The pathogenesis of the diverticular disease is multifaceted and has been comprehended bleakly. A few factors with the likes of structure of the colonic divider, colonic motility, qualities that are inherited, admission of fibre, levels of Vitamin D, physical movement and obesity have been studied and known to affect the pathogenesis of the disorder.

Structure and motility of the colonic divider: Diverticula of the colon are defined as mucosal herniations in the divider muscle layer of the colon through more vulnerable purposes of vein sections through the wall of the colon. Furthermore, in the western world, they are usually found in the sigmoid colon.

Inheritance: Association of ecological hazard factors like diet has been made with the pathogenesis of the diverticular disease to a great instant, it has been pointed by the later epidemiologic information that hereditary factors, if committedly working, improve the diverticular disease. Investigations on relocation of population have further recommended that changes may not ensue in the rate of diverticular disease upon the reception of new natural elements by the population.

Two enormous, Scandinavian twin or family contemplates gave proof that hereditary components influence hazard for diverticular disease. In these examinations, the chances of creating diverticular illness if a co-twin had the malady was essentially higher among monozygotic twins than dizygotic twins and higher in non-twin kin than everybody. Factual displaying assessed that hereditary variables represented 40%- half of hazard for diverticular disease. These investigations could not plainly recognize diverticulitis from diverticulosis.

5.11.4 Adjustments in Colonic Neuromusculature

Restricted high-pressure zones in the colon were initially accepted to prompt development of diverticula at feeble spots in the colonic musculature. This may represent the perception that diverticulosis happens most of the time in the sigmoid, where the colon is less distensible, than the proximal colon and rectum. Moreover, diverticula are most certainly not found in the rectum, which works as a store, is exceptionally distensible, and is the place the tenia coli flare to make an extra, circumferential muscle layer. Modifications in the enteric sensory system, connective tissue, smooth muscle, what's more, colonic motility are accepted to add to the improvement of diverticulosis just as useful side effects in the setting of diverticulosis. It is less clear if these neuromotor variations from the norm are associated with the advancement of diverticulitis. Beginning stage diverticulosis happens in patients with connective tissue issue, supporting a job for connective tissue absconds in the arrangement of diverticulosis. Alterations in collagen structure and substance just as connective tissue digestion have been distinguished.

Administration of dietary fibre: A large point of view worldwide about improvement in diverticulosis is aimed at higher intra-colonic pressures being characterized by a low dietary fibre intake. However, this perception has an increased aura of questionability to it. Analysis of the connection between intestinal behaviour and admission of dietary fibre resulting in the improvement of diverticulosis of the asymptomatic kind was done by Peery et al., to find that fewer solid discharges and harder stools decreased the risk of diverticulosis. No relationship between the administration of dietary fibre and development of asymptomatic diverticulosis could be worked out. A lower intake of dietary fibre showed higher occurrence of diverticular disease with symptoms. When combined, there is limited and unsatisfactory proof for dietary fibre insufficiency leading to an improvement in diverticulosis, which is controversial. Still, there exists an advantage to increased fibre consumption for the decrease of symptoms of diverticulosis.

Role of Vitamin D: A lower serum vitamin D level can pose a higher danger of entangled diverticulitis; further indicating the chance of vitamin D deficiency linked to the pathogenesis of diverticulitis, although this remains just a guess.

Obesity and an active lifestyle: The diverticular disease has picked up pace in the recent years wherein obesity has also been on a high. Various gastrointestinal diseases have been linked to increased body weight, including diverticulitis. A positive relationship between the risk of diverticulitis and factors like body mass index (BMI), waist to hip ratio and waist length has been worked out. However, similar to vitamin D, this risk factor hasn't yet been characterised plainly and remains in the greys.

Chronic inflammation: A few investigations have related diverticulitis with a incessant fiery state. The most persuading proof, although circuitous, is that many hazard factors for diverticulitis are related with interminable, foundational irritation. For model, obesity, physical latency, and a Western eating regimen are hazard factors for different illnesses accepted to be brought about by constant irritation, including cardiovascular illness and diabetes—these hazard factors increment levels of biomarkers of inflammation. Increased articulation of grid metalloproteases and histamine, which are related with intestinal irritation, have likewise been connected to diverticulitis. Intestinal mucosal aggravation seen in patients with segmental colitis related with diverticular infection has morphological and clinical cover with IBD.

Modified microbiomes: Modifications in the gut microbiota are involved in the pathogenesis of numerous intestinal issue. Diet and lifestyle variables may incite adjustments in the gut microbiome that lead to mucosal aggravation and diverticulitis. Several lines of proof help a job for gut microbiota in diverticulitis. Intense diverticulitis includes smaller scale or macroperforation with translocation of commensal microscopic organisms over the colon mucosal hindrance, at times bringing about straight to the point contaminations, including sore arrangement and peritonitis. The standard treatment for diverticulitis is antibiotics. Diet and way of life hazard factors for diverticulitis influence the gut microbiome. For instance, stoutness and a Western dietary example are connected to diminished microbial variety in the digestive tract and changes in the microbiome arrangement and its functions. Dietary fibre is a significant well spring of vitality for intestinal organisms, which use complex sugars into short-chain unsaturated fats (SCFAs). SCFAs increment the creation of bodily fluid and antimicrobial peptides what's more, intervene insusceptible homeostasis, intestinal obstruction work, and legitimate degrees of cell proliferation.

5.11.5 Risk Factors

It has been confirmed that the role of diet and other lifestyle factors are linked to diverticulitis. Western dietary examples may be used to relate to higher risk factors, such as consumption of red meat, fat and refined grains. Patients with IBD are progressively inclined to the improvement of harm. People with Crohn's disease are at a higher risk of danger and death. There are numerous reports about sub-parts of IBD, one of them depends on protein level assessment. In the body, proteins are in a complex association that any little changes in every individual may prompt dysfunction of the entire system. Protein-protein interaction analysis can provide useful information for many diseases such as those related to digestive system

Genetic factors: Family history is implicated in the aetiology of IBD due to following reasons as there are about 3-20 times higher incidence of occurrence of IBD in first degree relatives. This is due to genetic defect causing diminished epithelial barrier function, also there is approximately 50% chance of development of IBD in monozygotic twins.

Microbial factors: At different times, role of a variety of microbes in initiation of inflammatory response by the body has been suspected. Accordingly, several microorganisms have been suspected but without definite evidence: mycobacterium tuberculosis, salmonella, shigella, helicobacter, clostridia, bacteroidesetc

Immunological factors: The examination of IBD pathogenesis has revealed that in a normal individual there is lack of immune responsiveness to dietary antigens, particularly the T cell reaction. Some researchers have shown proof that the dysfunctions of intrinsic and versatile pathways add to the abnormal intestinal reaction in patients with IBD. Immunological examinations have as of late centred around the mucosal natural insusceptible reactions, for example, epithelial lining respectability, intrinsic microbial detecting, autophagy and unfolded protein reaction.

5.11.6 Nutrition and Diverticulase

Research has found that an eating routine that limits nourishments that are high in FODMAPs — fermentable oligosaccharides, disaccharides, monosaccharides, and polyols — can profit individuals with bad tempered bowel disorder. Specialists have recommended individuals with diverticulitis may likewise profit by this eating regimen.

Some instances of nourishments high in FODMAPs include:

- Certain fruits, for example, apple, pear, and plum
- Dairy nourishments, for example, milk, yogurt, and frozen yogurt
- Fermented nourishments, for example, sauerkraut or kimchi
- Beans
- Cabbage
- Brussels grows
- Onions and garlic

Nourishments high in sugar and fat: A standard eating routine high in fat and sugar and low in fibre might be connected with an expanded frequency of diverticulitis. Research recommends that keeping away from the accompanying nourishments may help forestall diverticulitis or diminish its indications:

- red meat
- refined grains
- full-fat dairy
- singed nourishments

5.11.7 Diet plan: Diverticulitis

Calories: 1478 kcal

Protein: 62.1 g

Carbs: 223.8 g

Fats: 54.3 g

Food exchanges	No. of exchanges	Energy	Protein	Carbs	Fats
Milk	2.8	232	15.9	23.9	8.4
Meat	3	150	19.9	3	19.9
Pulses		-	-	-	-
Cereal	11.3	373	10.6	90.2	2.3
Veg A	1	73	3.3	13.1	0.7
Veg B	4.2	87	5.1	15.5	0.3
Fruit	1	331	5.1	74.5	1.4
Fat	5	232	5.2	3.2	23.4
Sugar	-	-	-	--	
Total		1478	67.1	223.7	54.3 g

Exchange	Total no.	Breakfast	Mid morning	Lunch	Snacks	Dinner
Milk	2.8	0.6	-	-	1.4	0.8
Meat	3	-	3	-	-	-
Pulses		-	--	-	-	-
Cereal	11.3	2.5	-	5	-	3.8
Veg A		-	-	-	-	1
Veg B	4.2	1	-	1.2	1	1
Fruit	1	1	-	-	-	-
Fat	5	5	1	1	-	--
Sugar						

Breakfast	Food exchanges	Food items	Amount	Menu plan
	Cereals Veg B Milk Fruit Fats	Suji Peas and carrot Tea or coffee Peach Peanuts Mustard oil	50 g 50 g 150 mL 1 pcs 20 g 5 g	Suji upma And fruit Tea or coffee Peach
Mid-morning	Meat Fruit	Egg Orange	3 2	Scrambled egg and orange juice

Lunch	Cereals Veg B Fat	White rice Potato Green beans Mustard oil	40 g 60 g 60 g 5 gm	Steamed rice and aloo beans
Snacks	Milk Fruit	Curd Banana	200 gm 1	Banana and curd
Dinner	Milk Cereal Veg B Veg A Fat	Skim milk Daliya Peas and carrots Tomato Mustard oil	200 mL 60 g 50 g 4 pcs 1 tsp	Veg daliya, tomato soup and skim milk

CASE STUDIES

1. TO PLAN A DIET DAY FOR FEMALE AGED 55 YEARS SUFFERING FROM GERD AND SEVERE NAUSEA

Nutritive Values

Nutrients	Recommendation	Modified
Energy	1900 kcal (from RDA)	1950 kcal
Protein	20% of energy	95 gm
Fats	15% of energy	31 gm
Carbohydrates	60 % 0f energy	285 gm

Meal time	Menu	Ingredient	Amount	Energy	Protein	Cho	Fat
Breakfast	Egg white Porridge	Egg white Rice flakes Skim milk Honey	50 gm 70 gm 200 mL 15 gm	85 172 58 47.8	7 3.2 5 0.04	- 38.6 9.2 11.9	7 0.5 0.2 -
Mid-morning	Fruit salad	Papaya Sapota Melon Dates	100 gm 100 gm 50 gm 20 gm	32 98 8 63.4	0.6 0.7 0.1 0.5	7.2 21.4 1.65 15.16	0.1 1.1 0.1 0.08
Lunch	Khichdi + Grilled chicken	Rice Chicken Mung dal Carrot Lemon Peas oil	150 g 70 gm 50 gm 20 gm 20 gm 10 gm 10 gm	523 76.3 174 9.6 5.4 9.3 90	12.75 18.13 12.2 0.18 0.14 0.72 -	116.1 - 18.9 2.12 1.14 1.59 -	0.9 0.21 0.6 0.04 0.02 0.01 10
Evening snack	Boiled channa Coconut water	Bengal gram Coconut water	100 gm 100 mL	180 24	8.55 1.4	30 4.4	2.65 0.1

Dinner	Rice + Dal	Masoor dal Singhi Potato Ridge gourd Oil	30 gm 50 gm 50 gm 100 gm 5 gm	102 62 48.5 17 45	7.53 11.4 0.8 0.5 -	17.7 3.45 11.3 3.4 -	0.18 0.3 0.05 0.1 5
			Total	1981 kcal	91 gm	315 gm	34 gm

2. TO PLAN A DIET DAY FOR FEMALE AGED 35 YEARS SUFFERING FROM DYSPEPSIA AND CHRONIC GASTRITIC

Nutritive Values

Nutrients	Recommendation	Modified
Energy	RDA	1950 kcal
Protein	20%	95 gm
Fats	20%	42 gm
Carbohydrates	60% of energy	285 gm

Meal Time	Menu	Ingredient	Amount	Energy	Protein	Cho	Fat
Breakfast	Oats upma	Rolled oats Black gram Cashew Carrot Peas oil	40 gm 30 gm 10 gm 60 gm 20 gm 5 gm	151 104 59.6 28.8 18.6 45	5.26 7.2 2.12 0.54 1.44 -	27.08 17.88 2.23 6.36 - -	2.60 0.42 4.69 0.12 0.02 5
Mid-morning	Coconut water	Coconut water	200 mL	48	2.8	8.8	0.2
Lunch	Roti Sabji Dal soup Grilled Chicken	Refined flour Potato Raw banana Arhaar dal Chicken Oil	50 gm 100 gm 100 gm 20 gm 100 gm 5 gm	174 97 89 69 109 45	5.5 1.6 1.1 5.64 25.9 -	36.95 22.6 23 11.32 - -	0.45 0.1 0.3 0.12 0.6 5
Evening snack	Yogurt Sweet potato	Sweet potato yogurt	100 gm 40 gm	120 23.6	1.2 4	28.2 1.44	0.3 0.16
Dinner	Khichdi	Rice Moong dal Oil	60 gm 50 gm 5 gm	209 234 45	5.1 17.15 -	46.44 41.9 -	0.36 0.84 5
			Total	1903	86.5	277.1	51.06

B. DIETARY MANAGEMENT IN GASTROINTESTINAL SURGERIES

5.12 HERNIA

5.12.1 Possible Complications and Risks

Possible risks in the intestinal surgery are most commonly seen in many patients. It's not like the kind of symptoms. It is usually seen risks and symptoms which make a person feel uncomfortable and also the risk factors level are high. Patients who have undergone an abdominal surgery are closely monitored for potential complications and risks, which may include but are not limited to

- Scar tissue
- Pain
- Bleeding
- Infection
- Shock
- Paralytic ileus or temporary paralysis of the bowel
- Uncomfortableness

These are the major complications and the risk factors which we can see easily in any of the intestinal surgery patient. By this a doctor gets to know that the person has this kind of the problem by then they find the solution and the treatment for this. There are many more types of these solutions like inguinal hernia surgery, exploratory laparotomy, cholecystectomy, appendectomy.

Most of the patients experience certain symptoms that prompt them to seek medical attention. These typically include pain, diarrhoea, constipation, and any sudden change in bowel movement. In this problem a patient can survive easily and can face the death easily both are available in this. If the problem is severe than the chances of death are high but when the problem is in the nascent stage then the patient can easily survive.

That is why they prefer normal and balanced diet in this period so that they will not face any other problem regarding the abdominal surgery. They should also be careful that their diet is good for digestion. Keep your follow-up appointments to make sure your recovery goes well.

Post-operative complications

- Vascular complications
- Respiratory complications
- Haemorrhage

- Muscle atrophy and imbalance
- Poor healing
- Gaping of incision
- Incisional hernia

We can have vegetarian and non-vegetarian foods. The main thing is the intake of good protein.

If you have difficulties while eating consider supplementing your diet with protein powder, which can be added to drink such as smoothies.

Morning meal is really a important part of our life. Nowadays many people skip the morning diet because of the busy schedule but it affects body. It is really a bad habit. We should not skip the breakfast, lunch, and the dinner too. We should take proper meal everyday for the better and the healthy life so that in future we will not get ill and any kind of disease.

5.13 HAEMORRHOIDS

It is defined as swelling and inflammation of the veins in the rectum and anus area, which causes displeasure and bleeding. These are also defined as symbolic growth and distal displacement of the normal anal cushion. It is an abnormal mass of exposed and clogged blood vessels in swollen tissue that forms internally in the anal canal or around the anus, causing bleeding, pain, or itching. When it occurs internally, it often bulges out of the external sphincter of the anus, and when it appears externally, it can lead to thrombosis, also known as piles.

5.13.1 Management of Haemmorhoids

Haemorrhoids can be managed or treated by following various steps such as diagnosis, treatment, dietary management and taking precautions necessary. Consulting a doctor should be the first step of it all so that he/she can tell which method of treatment is best for a person according to the physical condition of patient and stage or type of haemorrhoids. The doctor can also guide the patient about the risks involved so that patient can make a fair choice.

5.13.2 Diagnosis

The doctor looks at the bottom. He might put a lubricated gloved finger or an instrument inside the anus. An *anoscope* is a hollow, lighted tube for viewing the several inches of the rectum. A *proctoscope* works like an *anoscope*, but it lets the doctor see more of the rectum.

Sigmoidoscopy refers to looking at the lower colon, or sigmoid, and colonoscopy looks at the entire colon. Both use a light, flexible viewing tube that enters the rectum.

A barium X-ray can also be used to show the outline of the entire interior of the colon. First, the patient receives a barium enema, and then a technician will take X-rays of the lower gastrointestinal tract.

Colonoscopy is a procedure in which the doctor looks at the whole colon with a long, flexible tube called colonoscope. They can also take tissue samples or treat other problems they find.

5.13.3 Treatment at Home

- Ease pain and itching
- Soaking

Fill a bath with a few inches of warm water and soak in it for almost 15 minutes in one go. Do this twice or thrice a day and mostly after every bowel movement. Use unscented soap and avoid scrubbing while washing the area. Pat the area gently to dry.

5.13.4 Dietary Management

Soluble fibre diffuses in water to form gel-like substance. Stools formed are soft, and are preceded without constipation, and maybe a little irritation.

Insoluble fibre is also called "roughage." It doesn't dissolve. It helps to keep things moving through and out of the system and to balance the chemistry in the guts.

Many "high-fibre" foods have both kinds.

Diet should have an objective for 25-30 gm or more of fibre daily. About one-third of that should be soluble.

Too much fibre can cause gas and bloating, so add a little bit of it to the diet at a single time. Drink more fluids to help the body use up that fibre completely: 8-10 large glasses (at least a half-gallon) of water each day.

5.13.4.1 Beans, Lentils, and Nuts

Half cup of beans such as kidney, or black beans cover about one-third of the daily needs. It has between 7 and 10 gm of fibre (containing both soluble and insoluble fibre), depending on what variety of it is chosen.

Almost 20 almonds or pecans have around 3 gm of fibre each and 1/2 cup of edamame also have the same amount of fibre with about half the calories only.

Instead of using meat in soups, one can add or alternate beans. Beans and nuts can also be used in salads. Try incorporating Indian and Middle Eastern recipes, which often call for beans, lentils, and peas.

5.13.4.2 Grains

Switch white breads, pastas, and crackers for similar things made with whole-grain flours, buckwheat, stone-ground cornmeal, or rye to increase the amount of insoluble fibre. Cooked oats and barley can provide a good amount of soluble fibre as well.

Prefer no-butter popcorn while craving for some munchies. One can put oat bran or wheat germ on salads and soups.

5.13.4.3 Fruits and Vegetables

There is no plant foods that are harmful in this disease. Eat with the skins on and when they're thin, like on apples, pears, plums, and potatoes. That's where the insoluble fibre is present in plant foods, along with compounds called flavonoids that help in controlling haemorrhoid bleeding.

Fruits with bright colours such as berries, grapes, tomatoes, and kale and some other dark, leafy greens are rich in flavonoids. And the fresher these foods are, the better are for the body. Try to ingest them as a whole unit without causing any damage to the skins or leaves until they are ready to eat. Do not cook to the point at which their colour fades or is lost.

A serving of fruit can provide a good amount, i.e., at least 10% of daily fibre which is usually 3 to 4 gm. A cup of leafy greens, broccoli, brussels sprouts, winter squash, or green peas give about 4 to 5 gm of fibre.

Few vegetables and fruits have fibre along with a lot of water. Cucumbers, celery, mild bell peppers, and watermelon mostly contain a lot of water which is about or more than 90%).

Add some fruit or vegetable to any daily meal, like any of the berries or banana in cereal, apple chunks on salad, spinach in omelet, etc.

Munch on dry fruits like figs, apricots, and dates. Switch sugary baked desserts with fresh fruit such as having raw strawberries rather than strawberry pie.

5.13.4.4 Others

In the absence of necessary intake of fibre then he/she maybe advised to have some fibre supplements along with their meals.

5.13.5 Precautions

By following these steps one can prevent haemorrhoids from occurring and also reduce symptoms or irritation of existing haemorrhoids.

Foods with very little or no fibre can be the reason for constipation (and therefore worse haemorrhoids), so it's best to limit or avoid how much you eat of them.

Below is the list of some foods that should be avoided:

- White bread and bagels
- Milk, cheese, and other dairy
- Meat
- Processed foods such as frozen meals and fast food

Restrict the amount of salt as it can cause the body hanging on to water, which ultimately puts more pressure on the blood vessels which leads to higher pressure on the veins in bottom that can be the reason of causing hemorrhoids.

Iron supplements can cause or worsen constipation and some other digestive problems as well. Consultation from a doctor is necessary before taking them.

Do not sit for very long periods and losing weight should be priority if the patient is overweight.

The patient should avoid taking medications that can cause or worsen constipation.

5.14 BARIATRIC SURGERY

Bariatric surgery is a surgical treatment of obesity with high risk problems which can be fatal. As we all know that obesity is itself a disease and a major cause of many diseases as well. Now let us know what exactly the obesity is.

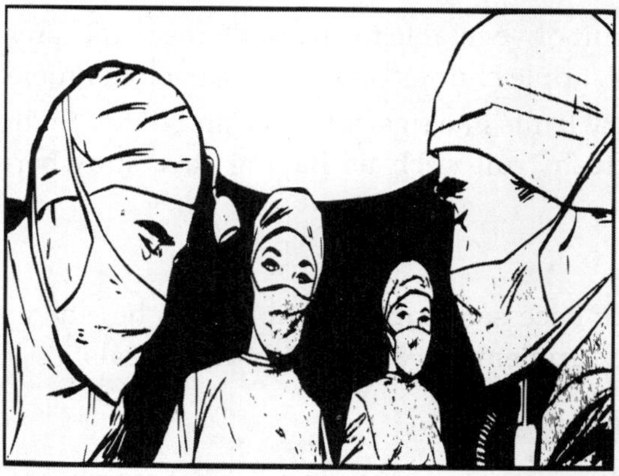

5.14.1 Obesity

When we come to define obesity we understand that it is a disorder of the nutrients in the body. The macronutrients fat is the one which leads to this defined set of problems causing impairment in the functioning of the biological system of body. In the western world obesity is the leading cause of all diseases. Due to the readily available, packed and highly caloric market food is one the major reasons of obesity. It is most seen in the people of high strata where availability of nutrients is much more. Although the human body composition has enough fat distribution all over the body which is either in the form of 'storage fat' or in the form of 'essential fat'. When we see at the ratios we conclude that the ratios are higher for the females that is 18-30% whereas lower for the males comparatively that is 10-25% as the females require more amount of fat during pregnancy and lactation time.

Now when the total fat deposit in the body is increased to 20% or more than that of the ideal body weight of the individual then the condition of obesity prevails in the body. The excess amount of fat starts accumulating in the body in various regions and the fat distribution in the various regions of the body refers to the adiposity of the body. Males and females differ in the total fat ratios and also the adiposity which is inherited from the genes of the parents and their ancestors. The males are often seen with a big fat tummy which is often called the pregnancy tummy and the body's shape changes to the shape of an apple This type of fat accumulation around the trunk region is referred to as the android fat distribution and is an indicative of disease like high blood pressure often called hypertension which even leads to strokes in the heart due to deposition of fat in the inner regions of the arteries and also causes high lipids in the blood called hyperlipidemia.

Now that we have covered what is obesity let's talk about the hazards of the obesity.

The excess body fat not only increases the weight but is also responsible for the mental pressure. The unhappiness gained from the rejection from the society due to body shape and figure leaves a harsh impression in minds leading to depression.

The obese people are lazier and lethargic due to the increased amount of oxygen in the body as the body is unable to filter the air properly and that the exchange of the gases in the air bags does not take place efficiently due to the extra fat layer around it blocking the porosity of the air bags. Therefore, breathing problems arise and the person is unable to breathe properly and the problematic breathing starts over.

The diseases occurring due to obesity are not for a short term but are chronic in nature like diabetes mellitus, osteoporosis, a wide range of cardiovascular diseases, the high levels of bad cholesterol that is LDL (low density lipids) and VLDL (very low density lipids) with low levels of good cholesterol HDL (high density lipids).

5.14.2 Obesity and Bariatric Surgery

According to WHO (World Health Organization), the method by which we measure the obesity is the use of BMI (body mass index) which is calculated through a person's body weight in kilograms to the height of the person in square of metres.

In Asians, the BMI equals to 25 or more than that is referred to as obese class and in the western countries the BMI ranges are 30 or above that due to the changes in the body structure of the individuals. Not every obese is eligible for bariatric surgery. Bariatric surgery is recommended only for those with severe obesity conditions, that is, difficulty in breathing and walking which are major concerns of the body and cardiovascular diseases which do not allow adequate blood flow in the body. Bariatric therapy is an excellent boon for the morbidity of the obese patients. This surgery is majorly for class 2 and class 3 obesity. Class 1 obesity involves BMI ranging from 30 to 35, class 2 obesity involves BMI ranges from 35 to 40 and the class 3, the highest risk involves the BMI ranges from 40 and above. The severe classes of obesity cannot be treated at home by both exercise and diet as the patient is unable to digest and assimilate properly.

Bariatric Surgery

The initial research was laid down by a team of medical surgeons with Drs. Arnold Kremen and Richard Varco at the University of Minnesota that defined the disease obesity as a dangerous disease for surgery on it. The main motive behind this treatment was based on the "short gut" syndrome which is actually a disease caused by the site of absorption and assimilation of nutrients in the digestive system. Inadequacy in the absorption also called malabsorption occurs in the small intestine in this syndrome. The surgeons were inspired to develop the bypass of the small intestine in which the food material does not come in direct contact with the major part of the small intestine. The three distinct parts of the small intestine are the duodenum, the jejunum and the ileum.

The jejunocholic anastomosis was the procedure followed initially where the end-to-end connection by surgery was made between the side to side blood cells, the parts of the intestine and the other parts of the body, that is, the large intestine. This was done in the year 1956 for morbid obesity. This was then modified to the jejunoileal procedure which was more convenient and acceptable due to the metabolic complications following the jejunocolic anastomosis. This was called the intestinal bypass. Here the length of the jejunum was shortened to 14 inches that is 36 cm in length with the length of the ileum shortened to 4 inches that is 10 cm in length. This procedure though provided weight loss which could be better predicted beforehand and was even tested and performed over 30,000 operations but the complications aggravated due to this procedure could not be defied. The significant weight loss which was visible after the surgery returned back and produced several complications which were difficult to cope the problems included the kidney system, that is, the renal failure - both acute and chronic, deficiencies of minerals - the micronutrients were observed which lead to decreased immunity in the patients and also the patients were prone to cirrhosis, that is, the fibrosis processing of the tissues of the liver. Patients observed fatigue, diarrhoea and anorexic feelings postoperatively and that the weight loss was extreme till the two years of the surgery performed between the years 1965 to 1975 and in some of the patients the surgery was even revised but not acceptable much.

The second advancement seen in the treatment of the dangerous disease to achieve weight loss was by a member of Minnesota group, Dr. Edward Mason, who by careful examinations and investigating the disease concluded and also documents two new procedures for the weight loss which were far more safer and efficient than the previously used intestinal bypass which were overtaken by the two gastric procedures - the gastric band and the other one was the gastric bypass. In the gastric band the usage of small gastric pouch was made which allowed only limited intake as well as the limited exclusion from it. The other was the gastric bypass which is a surgical treatment in the stomach is divided into to two pouches, namely - the upper small pouch and other one is the larger one and the lower leftover part and the small intestine is thus attached to the stomach pouches. These two procedures or the basic operations introduced by Dr. Edward Mason are still prevalent forms of bariatric procedures. The gastric bypass involves interference with digestive system excluding food from the actual size of the stomach. Furthermore new interventions were allowed to come in the procedures in which the gastric banding came with an improved version with adjustability led by Scopinaro et al., with extended biliopancreatic bypass in which the normal procedure digestion is made into variation by making the stomach smaller that is reducing the area of digestion and the gastric juices working on the food. In the biliopancreatic bypass the part of the stomach is completely removed reducing the surface area of the stomach and that part is connected to the lower portion of the small intestine, that is, the ileum which has villi on it. Another Hess et al., added a new edition of it by introduction of biliopancreatic diversion with duodenal switch in which different part of the stomach is cut and removed and the lower region of the stomach, that is, the pylorus is left intact as the food passes from the pylorus through the pyloric sphincter to the duodenal region of the small intestine. In the more recent days, the sleeving or cutting down a sleeve portion and 2/3rd portion of the stomach is cut which becomes the first step of the biliopancreatic bypass surgery. It is a more efficient and acceptable form of achieving the goals of reduced weight in the severely obese patients. The removal of the 2/3rd part and the left 1/3rd part maintains the gastric curve although which is less in curvature but is in the continued form due to this procedure. The pyloric sphincter or the valve remains attached to the duodenal region of the small intestine whereas the second part of the duodenal is entirely separated from the small intestine leaving behind the attachment of the duodenal to the lowest part of the small intestine. The left out second and third segments are altogether bypassed the majority part of them. This is done to achieve no dysfunction of the small intestine but reducing the surface area of the section of the small intestine arrangement where the mixing of food with digestive enzymes takes place. Meanwhile the resolution of diabetes type 2 was taken out by Moo and Rubino's investigation extending further the benefits of gastric bypass for treatment of diabetic patients who do not fall under the category of obesity. In this procedure they used the duodeno-jejunal bypass. Other trials involve the joining of the lowest part of the small intestine, that is, the ileum to the ligament of Treitz by dislocating the ileal ideal position, which also helps in resolving diabetes type 2.

The third venture in the world of treating obesity was the follow-up section for more than 16 years of the treatment as documented by Pories et al., and MacDonald et al., with tremendous work in following up the operated patients up to 95% which concluded that the gastric bypass reduced the weight of the patients to the extent of 110 pounds. and also the associated risk of the chronic diseases like diabetes reduced leading to higher life expectancy.

Earlier the gastric bypass surgery was performed by opening of the belly, that is, open surgery but the fourth and new further advancement was the introduction of laparoscopic approach in performing the gastric bypass as the earlier was risky and was difficult surgical operations of the abdomen involving a large cut. The new approach of laparoscopy is on the safer side and involves less traumatic exposure.

5.14.3 Groups of Bariatric Operations

Traditionally, the bariatric operations have been classified into three major categories that are:

(a) restrictive,

(b) malabsorptive, and

(c) mixed.

- These three types differ in the procedures followed in the operations. The first one is the restrictive type which means restriction of something and in this case the food intake is restricted as in the case of gastric banding. This involves constriction of the stomach so that the feeling of fullness occurs even if the person eats a meal in quantity less than usually taken when in normal condition that means early satiety occurs as the stomach is constricted. An inflatable band at the top of the stomach that only limited quantity of food can enter in the stomach and that the feeling of fullness comes early.
- The second one being the malabsorptive meaning that the part of the digestive system, which involves the absorption, is interfered with that is the small intestine, the intestinal bypass where the parts of the small intestine are bypassed or cut short to lower the absorption surface area.
- The third is the mixed one in which both interference with the digestive system along with the limiting intake of the food in the stomach is taken into consideration. One such method or procedure is the gastric bypass with duodenal switch which involves cutting small pouch of the stomach and attaching the pyloric valve to the last segment of the small intestine and some part of the duodenal area.
- This classification is although very clear in biological cutting and joining of various parts but they too have effect on the hormones such as the hunger hormone – "ghrelin" which sends signals to the brain of the hunger and the person then seeks out for food. It is produced in the gut and carried out by bloodstream to the brain telling that the person is hungry. The control of this hormone plays a key role in the control of pangs of hunger. Being produced in the stomach when the stomach remains empty, it directly affects the hypothalamus region of the brain which is the control centre for the hormones and appetite. Their higher level leads to more and more hunger and the person tends to have more calories in the diet whereas the lower the levels, the more full the person feels and the low calorie intake takes place.

  Therefore the mechanism of the bariatric surgeries is still unknown as the gastric sleeve process also restricts the food intake due to the small size of the tube but the longitudinal gastrectomy inhibits the production of the hunger hormone from the stomach that is the source is discarded.

5.14.4 The Open and the Laproscopic Bariatric Surgery

In open surgery the abdomen of the patient is cut open by the surgeon. Mostly a large cut is enough to perform the operation. The open surgery causes severe pain, a big scar is therefore marked on the abdominal region of the patient and also the rate of recovering from the open surgery is way longer. But it is helpful in high level of obesity or having had a surgery involving before the bariatric surgery.

The laparoscopic surgery is safer and is now in more use. This involves small cuts with usage of thin surgical rods for the surgery. Every action performed is recorded in the camera which inserted with small scope attached to it. The pictures taken up by the camera attached to the small scope are projected onto a video monitor through which the surgeons see the procedure going on and nowadays these videos are even made available as a proof for safe surgery by the surgeons and produced to the patients and his or her family members. It involves less scarring of the abdominal region of the patient and involves lesser risk of life as compared to the open surgery. The amount of pain involved is also less in comparison with the open surgery.

After both types of bariatric surgeries the patients require rest for a period of time to recover properly. The follow-up procedures are different for the type of surgery performed on the patient.

5.14.5 Bariatric Operations Widely in Use

5.14.5.1 Roux-en-Y Gastric Bypass (RYGB)

The most common form of bariatric surgery performed worldwide is the RYGB. It is often referred to as the golden standard for weight loss surgery. This procedure involves two parts. Initially, a small pouch is made in the stomach of 30 cc in size or 30 milliliters or one ounce in volume to be clear. In the upper portion is divided leaving behind the leftover stomach area. The upper portion divided is the small pouch which is about the size of the ball used in the golf game. This division is done by using the staples or divisions in the stomach. To make clear divisions, the pouch which is proximally made now drains all of its contents into the Roux-en-Y. Roux-en-Y is created with the help of the small intestine in which its first portion is divided and the left over proximal part of the small bowel 100 cm below the point where the division takes place. The second part of the small intestine, that is, jejunum is divided 30 cm below the ligament pf Treitz and the distal end is made in contact of the small pouch of the stomach by gastroenterostomy of about 1 cm in diameter. The completion of the procedure is when the top end portion of the small intestine along with the distal end of the small intestine are connected together with the newly formed small pouch of the stomach and the bypassed stomach's role in this is served by mixing together of the digestive juices from various organs and the acids in the stomach mixing with the first portion of the small intestine well automatically.

This procedure is quite in use these days due to the considerably small size of the stomach created in the procedure which allows only limited amount of food which means the small the size the lesser the calories consumed. Now that the segments of the small intestine are connected to the stomach's small pouch and that the mixing of the food and further absorption of nutrients takes places in the joint form single tube so the food no longer passes through the original small intestine, therefore, less calories and nutrients are absorbed in the body through reduced digestive system. Furthermore, the re-system created by this surgery also brings about changes in the hormones of the gut and the person feels more full and the early satiety prevails which also further inhibits the major cause of onset of diabetes type 2 due to suppressed hunger pangs.

The procedure is also performed by varying the sizes and the capacity of the small intestine by increasing the conditions where more energy expenditure is required and thus maintenance of more than 50% of the excess body weight is maintained favourably. The use of plastic rings is also one of the factors to limit the outflow and the limbs of the Roux-en-, displacement of the small intestine further either in front behind. Colon of the large intestine is new advancement even with creation/performing of the gastrojejunostomies.

5.14.5.2 Adjustable Gastric Band (AGB)

In this procedure, a band is used with an inflatable cuff has attached to it. This band which allows the air to be filled in is wrapped around the upper portion of the stomach to again produce a small pouch of the stomach. The band is actually the shape of bracelet creating small pouch same size as that of the one created in the Roux-en-Y surgery. The leftover stomach is placed below the band. The size is further adjustable which is why the name adjustable band comes. The portion of the cuff is filled with sterile saline, which is injected accordingly with the help of a port. The port is placed under the skin through which it is filled with sterile saline. The degree of fullness depends on the opening between the two divided portions of the stomach made by the gastric band. The size of the opening is adjustable by the amount of sterile saline filled in the cuff of the band which is gradually being filled time to time with further sittings. This surgery allows the digestion and absorption is proper and involves no malabsorption of nutrients and the regulation process takes place. Although it reduces the carrying capacity of the stomach. No cuts are made in the procedure.

5.14.5.3 Biliopancreatic Bypass with Duodenal Switch (BPDS)

In this procedure a small pouch is made of the big stomach and the second thing done is the bypass of the large segment of the small intestine. The surgery uses the investigational bariatric procedure.

5.14.5.4 Sleeve Gastrectomy

The last segment of the stomach where the stomach ends is the pylorus and the duodenum which forms the first portion of the small intestine is divided 2 cm below the stomach ending and further as similar to the Roux-en-Y surgery, a Roux-en-Y anastomosis which means the end to end connection of the cut parts and in this the small pouch is anastomed with to the distal jejunum which is the second part of the small intestine and also this procedure involves the size of the small bowel significantly smaller than the gastric bypass in Roux-en-Y surgery. In this the distal part of the small intestine which is, then with surgery, brought upwards and anastomed to the new outlet of the small pouch of the newly created stomach. This allows the food to directly reach the last segment of the small intestine through a direct tubular structure. Only 1/3rd of the portion of the small intestine is left after the bypass. The bypassed portion of the small intestine carrying essential enzymes as bile and from pancreas are then reconnected to the last portion of the small intestine which is connected to the new stomach which reduces the calorie and nutrient intake efficiently.

5.14.6 Nutritional Contraindications

Although bariatric surgery is an effective way to lose excess fat from the body gradually reducing weight but the nutritional condition of the patient is adversely affected after this treatment and the follow-ups thus become utmost important for the patients to succumb the adverse effects of the surgical operation. The nutritional as well as the hormonal complications aggravate after the surgery which can produce severe deficiency of macronutrients such as protein and fat malabsorption in the body. The counselling sessions should be conducted for such patients who have undergone bariatric surgery and also their mineral and micronutrient supplementation such as of the vitamin B12, thiamine, calcium, iron, vitamin D and folate continues lifelong. The multivitamins and mineral supplements received by the patients lack iron, vitamin B12 and fat soluble vitamins, therefore, prophylactic supplementation till death are provided to the patient.

5.15 LACTOSE INTOLERANCE

Lactose intolerance is a disorder of inability of metabolization of lactose in the body due to absence or meagre amount of lactase enzyme. Lactose is not digested and the patient suffers from diarrhoea, flatulence and other allergy symptoms.

Lactose is a sugar found only in milk and also in its products. The person suffering from lactase deficiency is said to have milk allergy in which all milk and its products are prohibited.

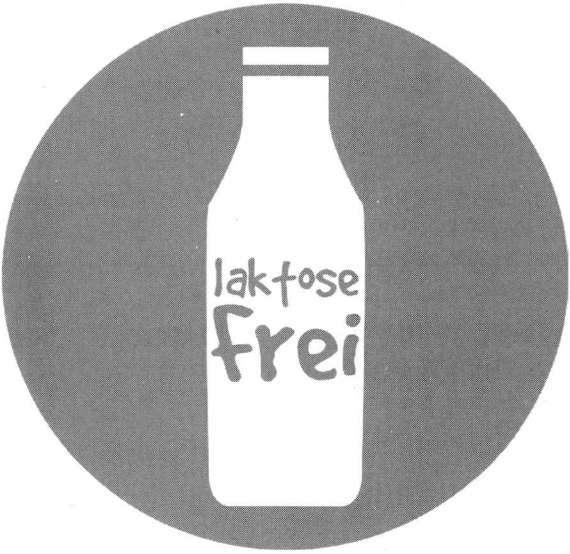

The symptoms after consumption of milk are bloating, abdominal pain, flatulence, nausea, diarrhoea, etc. in the people having lactose intolerance.

5.15.1 Diagnosis

Some tests which detect lactose intolerance are:

Hydrogen breath test: The patient is told not to eat 12 hours and then is given a lactose solution in the next early morning. Hydrogen concentrations in exhaled air are measured. High levels of hydrogen indicate lactose intolerance.

Lactose tolerance test: The patient takes a lactose solution in prescribed amounts and glucose levels in the blood are measured. If blood glucose levels remain the same, this indicates that glucose has not entered the blood. This is because the lactose has not been successfully broken down into glucose and galactose. In a milk tolerance test, the person drinks milk instead of a lactose solution.

5.15.2 Management of Lactose Intolerance

The best way to avoid lactose intolerance is not to drink milk and eat milk products. Other food products such as soyabean milk or almond milk are recommended to such patients. The dairy products are excluded from diet. Curd may be given but after testing its digestibility, and small amounts can be given.

CASE STUDY

1. TO PLAN A DAY'S DIET FOR FEMALE, 35 YEARS OLD SUFFERING FROM LACTOSE INTOLERANCE AND CVD.

Personal Information

Age: 35 years old
Sex: Female
Physiological condition: Lactose intolerance and CVD
RDA: 1600-1700 kcal/day
CHO: 55% of total energy requirement = 220 g/day
Protein: 14% of the total energy requirement = 56-63 g/day
Fat: 11-12% of the total energy requirement = 19-21 g/day

Principal Diet

Low calorie, high protein, low carbohydrate, low fat and high fibre

Comprehensive Exchange List

Food group	Exchange number	Protein	Carbohydrate	Fat	Energy
Milk	1	8	12	10	170
Meat	2	14		2	140
Pulses	3	19	51		300

Cereals	6	12	90		504
Veg A	5	5	17.5		100
Veg B	3		21		120
Fruits	2		20		80
Fats	2			10	90
Sugar	3		15		60

Distribution from the Table

Food group	No. of exchange list	Bed-tea	Breakfast	AM snack	Lunch	PM snack	Dinner	Post-dinner snack
Milk	1		1					
Meat	2			1		1		
Pulses	3		1		2			
Cereals	6		3		2		1	
Veg A	5		2		2		1	
Veg B	3			1	2			
Fruits	2		1					1
Fat	2		1		1			
Sugar	3			1	1		1	

Meal	Quantity	Food item	Energy (kcal)	CHO (g)	Proteins (g)	Fats (g)
Bed-tea	1 glass	Sugar-free garlic tea	-	-	-	-
Breakfast	1 glass	Yoghurt	150	12	8	3.2
	1 bowl	Wholewheat pasta	320	60	8	--
	1 small bowl	Berries	60	15	-	-
	1	Fish sandwich	230	160	22	2
Mid-morning	7-10	Almonds	12	-	-	4
	1 glass	Lemon water	-	-	-	-
Lunch	3 serving	Brown rice	240	45	6	-
	2 small bowl	Mixed vegetables curry	7.6	5	3.5	5
	1 large bowl	Carrot and broccoli salad	-	-	-	-
	1 glass	Garlic water	-	-	-	
	1 glass	dal	200	30	12	-

Evening tea	1 small bowl	Baked tuna	110	-	14	6
	Green tea	-	-	-	-	-
Dinner	2 medium	Chapattis	160	30	4	-
	1 large bowl	Unripe mango and cucumber salad	-	-	-	-
	1 small bowl	Mixed vegetables	7.2	2	-	5
Post-dinner	1 cup	Apple	60	15	-	-

QUESTIONS

1. Define peptic ulcer. Give causes, symptoms and dietary management of peptic ulcer.
2. Write about different types of peptic ulcers and discuss about their dietary management.
3. What are the differences between diarrhoea and constipation?
4. How does the rehydration therapy works for patients suffering from diarrhoea and constipation?
5. Describe celiac disease. Plan a day's diet of patient with gluten intolerance.
6. Describe flatulence and dyspepsia. Discuss about foods that can help in improving the digestion.
7. What is inflammatory bowel disease. Mention aetiology, symptoms and management.
8. Write short notes on dietary management of the following:
   (i) Gastrointestinal reflux disease
   (ii) Diverticular disease
   (iii) Lactose intolerance
   (iv) Hernia
9. Describe haemorrhoids. Give causes and dietary management.
10. Describe bariatric surgery along with precautions to be taken after the surgery. Also discuss about the dietary management that should be done after the surgery.
11. Plan a day's diet for a female patient of age 20 years suffering from lactose intolerance.
12. Plan a day's diet for a child of 5 years suffering from diarrhoea.

6

Renal Disorders

6.1 HUMAN KIDNEY

There are 2 kidneys in the human body. Each of them weighs 150 gm in an adult person. They are situated in the lumbar region of the abdominal cavity on either side of the vertebral column. The kidneys is bean shaped. The dimensions of the kidneys are as follows: 10 cm in length, 5 cm in width, and 2.5 cm thick. Due to the presence of liver on the right hand side, the right kidney is slightly lower than the left kidney. The kidney can be distinguished into the outer cortex and the inner medulla. Minor calyces join together to form the major calyces which ultimately terminate into the ureters.

Nephron is the smallest unit of the kidney. It is also the functional unit of the kidney. The kidney is made out of 1-1.3 million nephrons. The length of each nephron is 45 to 65 mm.

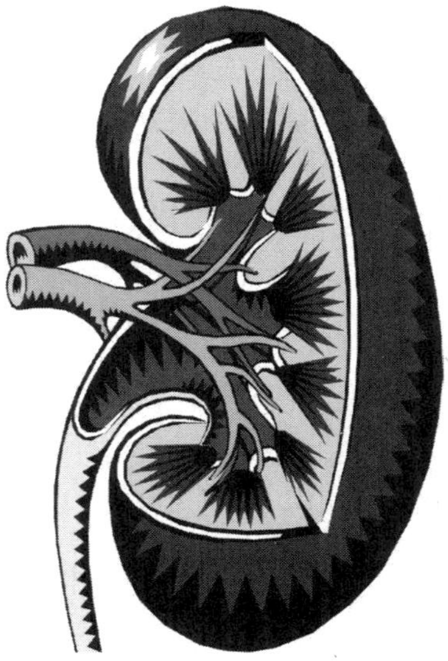

Kidney

Nephron can be differentiated into the following parts:

1. Bowman's capsule
2. Glomerulus
3. Proximal convoluted tubule (PCT)
4. Distal convoluted tubule (DCT)
5. Loop of henle
6. Collecting duct

Bowman's capsule and glomerulus together are known as the malpighian corpuscle.

The nephrons of the kidneys filter blood which is brought in the kidney by the afferent arteriole. Water in high amount is filtered which is then reabsorbed later and urea is removed through blood which is the major waste product of kidney.

6.1.1 Main Functions of Kidney

1. To form urine by the filtration process of blood and secretion of urine from the kidneys.
2. Production and secretion of hormone erythropoietin that helps in formation and secretion of red blood cells.
3. It also helps in formation and secretion of rennin hormone that helps in maintenance of blood pressure.

6.1.2 Microscopic Structure of Kidney

On viewing the microscopic structure of kidney the gross structure visible are the renal pelvis that gives striped appearance to kidney, the renal pyramids, and the collecting tubules that join together to major ducts known as collecting ducts that pass urine from kidney to ureter. The renal pelvis is a funnel-shaped structure that contains number of distal branches which are known as calyces. These act as pathway in conduction of urine from the kidney.

6.1.3 Disorders of the Kidney

Kidneys are a vital organ of the human body as we can see in the above paragraph that they perform a wide variety of functions that are necessary for the body to keep healthy and keep going. Due to poor lifestyle habits, the kidneys start deteriorating. There can be other causes for the same too which shall be discussed in the aetiology of kidney disorders.

Disorders of the kidneys can be categorised into the four following types:

1. Glomerular disorders can be chronic and acute as well.
2. Tubular disorders are mostly acute.
3. Interstitial disorders
4. Vascular disorders

Initially, the disorders of the kidneys focus on one part of the kidney, example glomerulus or tubules or the vascular parts, etc., but eventually in the end, all lead to end stage renal failure.

Two major pathological syndromes of the kidneys are:

1. Acute kidney failure
2. Chronic kidney failure

Azotaemia refers to the increase in the levels of BUN (blood, urea, nitrogen) and creatinine, while uraemia refers to the presence of signs and symptoms due to azotaemia.

6.1.4 Acute Renal Failure

6.1.4.1 Introduction

It refers to the syndrome in which there is rapid renal dysfunction leading to oliguria or anuria and sudden increase in metabolic wastes in the blood causing uraemia. The tubules are engaged in active secretion as well as resorption. These processes demand a lot of energy and therefore are vulnerable to ischaemic injuries, such injuries lead to damage of these tubules which ultimately causes metabolic trauma to the body and makes the situation life threatening. It is characterised by sudden decrease in the glomerular filtration rate (GFR).

6.1.4.2 Aetiology

Causes of acute renal failure can be classified as:

1. Pre-renal
2. Intra-renal
3. Post-renal

Pre-renal causes: They include the causes that lead to lesser amount of blood going to the nephrons leading to renal ischaemia. Such a situation is caused due to low cardiac output or hypovolemia.

Intra-renal causes: Intra means inside, therefore the causes that cause damage to the kidney tissue itself are termed intra-renal causes. Such causes include the damage to arteries and arterioles of the kidneys, and acute tubular necrosis due to less blood or ischaemia, damage of glomeruli or effect of a nephrotoxin.

Post-renal causes: These are due to the obstruction of the passage of urine through the distal renal tract to the collecting ducts. This is due to formation of a mass in the lumen of the wall of the tube.

6.1.4.3 Clinical Features

These depend on the stage of the disease the patient is in, but basically there are 3 patterns that can be seen in the patients.

They are as follows:

1. **Syndrome of acute nephritis:** Results in excessive proliferation of epithelial cells of the glomeruli that lead to decrease in the glomerular filtration rate and increase in the permeability of glomeruli.
2. **Syndrome in which tubular pathology occurs:** This happens when acute renal failure is caused due to proliferation of the tubules. It can be further categorised as:
   (a) **Oliguric phase:** This occurs from 7 to 10 days. In this phase, the urine output is as less as 400 mL per day. This further leads to accumulation of metabolic wastes and water in the human body causing hyperkalemia, hypernatremia, hypervolemia, and azotemia and metabolic acidosis as well.
   (b) **Diuretic phase:** This phase marks the beginning of the healing of tubules. The urine output begins to slightly increase and therefore is better.
   (c) **Phase of recovery:** In half of the patients full recovery of the tubular cells happens while in the rest death of epithelial cells occurs.
3. **Pre-renal syndrome**: This occurs in the patients of acute renal failure who have not undergone any damage to the glomerulus or tubular cells.

   This occurs due to ischaemia, hypovolemia, hypotension and cardiac insufficiency.The blood flow to the kidneys is very less, therefore it results in low glomerular filtration rate or GFR.

6.1.4.4 Dietary Management of Acute Renal Failure

Principles of dietary management

1. Maintaining the fluid-electrolyte balance
2. Reduction of endogenous protein catabolism
3. Help in wound healing
4. Help in fighting from infections and build immunity.

In the initial stages of acute renal failure, catabolism is the major process that occurs in the body of the patient. There is a lot of tissue destruction. Also the person does not feel like eating and therefore there is loss of appetite. Gastric troubles like vomiting, diarrhoea or gastric stasis may be present as well. Keeping in mind the loss of appetite and gastric troubles and inability of the body to accept the food, enteral or parenteral feeding is well suited and employed in most conditions. Early dialysis may also help the patient to cope up well and survive. It is really a very critical situation as stress accompanies various physiological conditions, hence it is necessary to carefully balance energy and protein.

Energy: 30-40 kcal/kg ideal body weight is the recommended energy requirement for the patient if acute renal failure.Carbohydrates have a protein sparing action, thus are required and helpful in such conditions.

Proteins: Patients cannot tolerate oral feedings due to the gastric troubles such as diarrhoea, nausea and vomiting therefore intravenous feedings and enteral feedings are given to such patients. 0.5-0.8 gm protein/kg/day are to be given to the patient of ARF.

Fluid and sodium: Depends upon the condition such as diarrhoea or vomiting. 500 mL/day is the basic allowance for a patient. Sodium 20-40 mg/day.

Potassium: The recommended intake is 30-50 mg/day in the oliguric phase.

6.1.4.5 Enteral Nutrition in Acute Renal Failure

According to recent researches it has been found out that enteral nutrition is considered safe for acute renal failure patients and in some cases parenteral amino acid supplementation helps a lot.

6.1.5 Chronic Kidney Failure

6.1.5.1 Definition and Introduction

It is a syndrome in which the renal parenchyma is destroyed. It is an irreversible disorder, also it is a progressive disorder. It takes place gradually and over a longer period of time than acute renal failure. It occurs when the number of nephrons in the kidneys is insufficient and therefore unable to perform the vital functions. Uremia develops and azotemia is also significant. Also, acidosis is a common trouble that is experienced in the chronic renal failure syndrome. The most commonly found form of kidney disorder is chronic kidney disease. It is a disease that persists for a longer period of time and takes a longer time to get cured as well. The major cause of this form of disease is due to the increased blood pressure. This condition is dangerous for the kidneys as it increases the pressure that is exerted on the glomerulus of the kidneys. Glomeruli consists of many tiny vessels and when the pressure in the glomeruli increases due to the increase in the blood pressure the vessels get damaged. This leads to a decrease in the function of the kidneys. When this condition progresses and leads to a condition where the kidneys totally become unable to perform their function the patient may have to go for dialysis, which acts as artificial kidney and filters the waste materials from the blood and purifies the blood. Another treatment that the patient has to go for in this condition of chronic kidney disease in extreme conditions is kidney transplant. Diabetes is a major cause of this disease as it increases the blood sugar level. This increased level of sugar levels in the blood causes major damages to the blood vessels of the kidneys if the high blood sugar levels persists for a long time. This leads to the condition where the kidneys become unable to filter the blood properly, and this leads, to a higher accumulation of toxins in the blood.

6.1.5.2 Aetiology

All the disorders of the kidneys in the long run without proper treatment lead to chronic renal failure.

The causes can be basically categorised into two groups:

1. Those causing glomerular damage.
2. Those causing tubular and interstitial or tubulointerstitial damage.

But as the disease progresses, it does not remain confined just in the glomerulus or in the tubules or interstitial spaces. All the parts are affected and damaged.

1. **Those causing glomerular pathology:** The glomeruli get destroyed due to immune mechanisms. Therefore the destruction of glomeruli leads to less filtration processes in the body and therefore leads to nephrotic syndrome. Nephrotic syndrome further leads to proteinuria, that is, presence of protein in the urine, hypoalbuminemia and oedema.

   There are basically 2 types of glomerular diseases that cause the chronic renal failure syndrome, they are as follows:

   (a) **Primary glomerular pathologies:** These include various kinds of glomerulonephritis. Chronic glomerulonephritis is the primary cause of chronic renal failure. The various types of glomerulonephritis are: Membranoproliferative glomerulonephritis, membranous glomerulonephritis, lipoid nephrosis, anti-glomerular basement nephritis.

(b) **Systemic Glomerular Pathology:** There are some changes that occur outside the nephrons but have a direct impact on them. Such conditions come under systemic glomerular pathology. These include systemic lupus erythematosus and diabetic nephropathy. Such conditions are also responsible for chronic renal failure syndrome.

2. **Diseases causing tubulointerstitial pathology:** Such pathology is related to the tubules of the nephrons including proximal convoluted tubule, distal convoluted tubule, and loop of henle. These diseases lead to proliferation or damage to these tubules that leads to disturbances in the secretion and resorption of various substances from the urine which leads to an extremely diluted urine. Therefore all the waste products cannot get out from the human body and accumulate there itself and cause heavy damage to the organs. Such tubulointerstitial diseases occur due to four main reasons.

   (a) **Vascular reasons:** Chronic hypertension and cardiac diseases lead to disturbances in the renal arteries and arterioles that further lead to nephrosclerosis or whitening of the nephrons. This further leads to ischaemia due to hypovolemia which leads necrosis of the nephrons.

   (b) **Infectious agents:** Chronic pyelonephritis is an example of an infectious disease that causes chronic renal failure.

   (c) **Toxic causes:** High doses of analgesics like aspirin and phenacetin lead to tubular damages that lead to defects in the kidneys which causes chronic renal failure over a long time.

   (d) **Obstructive causes:** Blood clots, tumours, and lumps lead to obstruction in the urinary tract that leads to fluid back pressure. This causes heavy damage to the kidneys and over a long run cause chronic kidney failure.

6.1.5.3 Stages of Chronic Renal Failure

The chronic renal failure syndrome passes gradually through four stages over a long period of time. The four stages are as follows:

(a) **Decreased renal reserve:** This is the first or primary stage of chronic renal failure. The kidneys can be seen in normal shape. They also function normally. The renal parenchyma is not much damaged and appears fine. However, symptoms can be seen in stressful conditions. The glomerular filtration rate is however half of the normal one. The creatinine levels are normal and the levels of blood-urea-nitrogen (BUN) are also on the normal side. The patient remains asymptomatic most of the time except during periods of stress.

(b) **Renal insufficiency:** This is the second stage. In this stage, the renal parenchyma is destroyed as much as seventy- five per cent and is in a very poor condition. The glomerular filtration rate also declines at a very high rate and is about twenty-five per cent of the normal one. The creatinine levels in the serum rise along with the blood urea nitrogen levels or BUN levels. Symptoms begin to appear in the patient and interfere with the everyday normal life. The symptoms include polyuria or excess urination and nocturia or urination in the night.

(c) **Renal failure:** Most of the parenchyma of kidneys is damaged by now and the glomerular filtration rate has dropped to ten per cent of the normal value. The kidneys have become non-functional. The tubules are also excessively damaged. There is no sodium-water balance present in the body now which leads to accumulation of water in the body of the human which is known as oedema. Metabolic acidosis occurs as a result of this and uremic symptoms begin to appear. Also there is deficiency of calcium in the blood serum levels. This condition is known as hypocalcemia.

(d) **End stage kidney disorder:** The glomerular filtration rate is five per cent of the normal value and symptoms of uremia are very clear. End stage kidney disorder is termed uremia.

6.1.5.4 Pathophysiology of Chronic Renal Failure

The clinical features of chronic renal syndrome can be easily studied by classifying them into two main types:

1. Primary uraemic manifestations or renal uraemic manifestations or intra-renalmanifestations.
2. Secondary uraemic manifestations or systemic or extra renal manifestations.

Primary uraemic manifestations or renal uraemic manifestations or intra-renal manifestations: These occur in the kidney itself and occur as a result of slowly degenerative kidney. These occur as symptoms in the diseased person. They include hyperkalemia, metabolic acidosis, sodium-water imbalance, hyperuricemia, and azotaemia.

(a) **Hyperkalemia:** Hyperkalemia refers to the excess amount of sodium in the blood serum. This occurs due to the disturbed sodium water balance in the body due to chronic renal failure. Metabolic acidosis worsens this situation.

(b) **Metabolic acidosis:** This is the condition in which acid-base balance is disturbed in the body and there is excess of hydrogen ions in the body and less of bicarbonate ions. This leads to acidosis. It further leads to hyperkalemia and hypercalcemia.

(c) **Sodium and water imbalance:** Sodium and water get retained in the human body due to their inability to pass through the bowman's capsule. This leads to imbalance between sodium and water. As the glomerular filtration rate declines, the juxtaglomerular apparatus secretes renin that further causes retention of sodium and water in the body.

Hyperuricemia: Hyperuricemia is the condition in which uric acid gets deposited in the human body. This is due to the inability of the human body to get rid of it due to low glomerular filtration rate. This uric acid can get deposited in the joints and cause gout and arthritis.

Azotaemia: Due to reduced glomerular filtration rate, the various proteins, nitrogenous wastes like urea, uric acid, and creatinine cannot be excreted out of the body leading to azotemia. The secondary uremic manifestations are related to the toxic effects of such accumulated metabolites in the body. They are as follows:

Secondary uremic manifestations or systemic or extra renal manifestations: These occur due to the above-mentioned primary manifestations like fluid-ion imbalance and azotaemia, etc.

6.1.5.5 Complications Associated with Chronic Renal Failure

Anemia: As the kidney has an important role in the secretion of erythropoietin, a hormone required for the synthesis of red blood cells, the body faces anemic situations as the functions of the kidney are hampered due to the end stage renal failure. Hence the person is anemic.

Integumentary system: Urochrome a colored pigment in the urine that gives urine its characteristic yellow colour gets deposited in the skin to give it a yellow colour also. Also, sweat and plasma now have more urea content than before.

Cardiovascular system: As the glomerular filtration rate declines the RAAS mechanism gets activated that causes the heart to overwork and therefore may lead to congestive heart failure as well.

Respiratory system: As the volume of blood increases and chances of heart failure increase, this leads to a back pressure on the respiratory system causing pulmonary edema and pulmonary congestion.

Digestive system: The presence of excess waste products in the blood serum level may cause ulcerations in the mucosal lining of the alimentary canal which may lead to nausea, vomiting and diarrhoea and bleeding. Bleeding may aggravate the already existing anemic condition.

Skeletal system: Joints develop gouty arthritis due to accumulation of uric acid crystals which do not filter out in the urine. There are two main types of disturbances that occur in the skeletal system due to end stage kidney disease. They are as follows:

Osteomalacia: As the kidneys are responsible for the synthesis of vitamin D3 in the body, this function also gets hampered and therefore the bones become weak and fracture easily.

Osteitis fibrosa : This occurs due to increased parathormone in the body. So as we see, how the chronic kidney failure syndrome affects the whole of the body and ultimately leads to the death of the patient due to multiple organ failure. It is a very serious condition and should be dealt with carefully and seriously to avoid mishaps

6.1.5.6 Dietary Management of Chronic Renal Failure

Objectives of diétary management:

1. To correct the fluid and ion balance
2. To get rid of acidosis
3. To prevent protein catabolism

Energy: Adequate carbohydrates need to be provided as they help in protein sparing action and also help in providing adequate energy to the body. 35 kcal/kg ideal body weight is the recommended daily allowance for energy in individuals with glomerular filtration rate less than 25 mL/min.

Protein: Around 0.6-0.75 gm of protein/kg body weight is the maximum amount of protein that can be given to the person. High biological value protein foods such as egg should be given.

Sodium: Recommended level of sodium is 2 g/dL in such a disease.

Vitamins: Fat-soluble vitamins like vitamin A and vitamin E are to be avoided as they can have toxic effects on the body. Also, vitamin D and K are not to be given as vitamin D cannot be converted into its active form and thus become a load on the kidneys.

Water: Should be balanced with the urine output of 24 hours.

6.1.5.7 Other Nutritional Administrations

Erythropoietin is also given to the patients of chronic renal failure as this hormone is used for the production of red blood cells and this is not present in the patients which makes them anaemic.

Iron supplements are also administered to the patients of chronic renal failure so that their iron deficiency can be monitored and make them return back to their normal status.

Along with all these medicines, statins that help decrease the cholesterol levels in the human body are given to the patients so that their risk of congestive heart failure is reduced.

Protein restricted diets along with keto/amino acids

From time immemorial, kidney patients are put on low protein diets as protein may put a load on kidneys as they are unable to filter excess nitrogenous wastes, hence to prevent their accumulation protein is restricted. Only that much amount of protein is given in the diet that can present the wear and tear of body tissues and maintain the structure of the body. A recent research shows that malnutrition, atherosclerosis and inflammation have a link to chronic kidney failure and are strongly associative.

6.2 NEPHROTIC SYNDROME

Nephrotic syndrome is a disorder of kidneys and the function of the kidneys is disrupted. It is shown by the symptoms of presence of proteins in urine and high cholesterol levels in the blood. The other signs are oedema in the proximities of the body such as legs, feet, ankles and also face. The patient may experience weight gain, fatigue and foam in urine.

6.2.1 Aetiology

The most common reasons for nephrotic syndrome are focal segmental glomerulosclerosis (FSGS), diabetes mellitus and hypertension.

6.2.2 Complications

The main symptoms of nephrotic syndrome are high albumin levels in the urine. Albumin functions to remove extra fluid from the blood and the excretion of albumin in the urine makes body deficient of proteins. The result is swelling of feet, ankles, face due to water retention.

The nephrotic syndrome results in high levels of cholesterol, and heart diseases develop. Nephrotic syndrome can also cause other serious health problems such as anaemia, heart disease, high blood pressure, fluid buildup, acute kidney injury, end-stage renal disease (ESRD) or kidney failure.

6.3 GLOMERULONEPHRITIS

Glomerulonephritis is a group of sicknesses that harm the part of the kidney that channels blood (called glomeruli). Different terms used are nephritis and nephrotic disorder. At the point when the kidney is harmed, it can't dispose of squanders and additional liquid in the body. On the off chance that the sickness proceeds, the kidneys may quit working totally, bringing about kidney disappointment.

Glomerulonephritis can come from nowhere (intense) or step by step (interminable). Glomerulonephritis happens all alone or as a major aspect of another ailment, for example, lupus or diabetes. Serious or drawn out irritation related with glomerulonephritis can harm your kidneys. Treatment relies upon the kind of glomerulonephritis you have. Glomerulonephritis (GN) is irritation of the glomeruli, which are structures in your kidneys that are comprised of minor veins. These bunches of vessels help channel your blood and expel overabundant liquids. In the event that your glomeruli are harmed, your kidneys will quit working appropriately, and you can go into kidney disappointment.

There are two sorts of glomerulonephritis—intense and ceaseless. The intense structure grows out of nowhere. Different occasions, your kidneys may stop working except if the correct treatment is begun rapidly. The early indications of the intense sickness are:

- Puffiness of your face in the first part of the day
- Blood in your pee (or dark coloured pee)
- Urinating not exactly common.

Early signs and side effects of the incessant structure may include:

- Blood or protein in the pee (hematuria, proteinuria)
- High circulatory strain
- Swelling of your lower legs or face (oedema)
- Frequent evening time pee
- Very bubbly or frothy pee

Side effects of kidney disappointment include:

- Lack of hunger
- Nausea and regurgitating
- Tiredness
- Difficult dozing
- Dry and bothersome skin
- Nighttime muscle cramps

6.3.1 Aetiology

Numerous conditions can cause glomerulonephritis. Once in a while the infection runs in families and here and there the reason is obscure. A few types of nephritis have not many inconveniences. However, most individuals have nephritis have atleast one of the accompanying issues:

- Blood in the urine (haematuria) can make urin pink or cola shading
- Protein in the urine (albuminuria or proteinuria) can cause forthyurine
- High blood pressure (hypertension) can harm the channels whenever left untreated
- High cholesterol
- Reduced kidney capacity
- Swelling of feet, legs and hands (oedema)

Tiredness is the most well known manifestation of ceaseless nephritis and doesn't generally have a basic clarification. Growing may likewise happen as the diminished capacity of the kidney meddles with the limit of the kidney to get rid of the ordinary heap of the salt and water. This growing might be increasingly observable in your legs after you have been standing, and in the tissue under your eyes when you first get up toward the beginning of the day.

Paleness becomes basic when the kidney work is decreased to about 33% of a typical level. Iron deficiency implies that there are insufficient red platelets in the blood and can cause tiredness and brevity of breath. As a rule, the specific reason for glomerulonephritis is obscure. It is imagined that the condition is regularly brought about by the insusceptible framework, the body's common resistance framework against diseases and contamination.

A significant number of the body's own synthetics, for example, proteins, can be like those found on living beings that cause contamination, for example, microbes and infections. Your resistant framework can confuse these proteins with a disease and assault the cells that convey them. This causes sickness.

Glomerulonephritis can be brought about by either irregular antibodies or lymphocytes, or both. The specific reason for some sorts of glomerulonephritis isn't known. In any case, in such cases, the reason is known to be identified with the insusceptible framework working strangely.

The kinds of glomerulonephritis that are brought about by the insusceptible framework responding against the body's own proteins and different synthetics are:

- Systemic lupus erythematosus: Where the resistant framework assaults huge numbers of the body's tissues and organs.

- Anti-glomerular cellar film malady, otherwise called Goodpasture's sickness, Where antibodies assault the layers of the glomeruli.
- Immunoglobulin A nephropathy, otherwise called IgA nephropathy and Berger Illness: Where a development of a counter-acting agent considered immunoglobulin A harms the kidneys.
- Membranous nephropathy (when not brought about by prescription, malignant growth or certain contaminations): Where the layers of the glomeruli thicken, harming the kidneys.
- Vasculitis, for example, Wegener's granulomatosis: Where the invulnerable framework assaults the veins in and around the glomeruli.

In spite of the fact that it isn't sure, the invulnerable framework may likewise assume a job in causing:

- **Minimal change infection:** Where the glomeruli are harmed yet the harm must be seen with an extraordinary high-power magnifying lens (this sort is increasingly basic in youngsters).
- **Focal and segmental glomerulosclerosis:** Where there is aggravation and scarring of the glomeruli.

6.3.2 Vasculitis

- **Polyarthritis:** This type of vasculitis influences little and medium veins in numerous pieces of your body, for example, your heart, kidneys and digestive organs.
- **Granulomatosis with polyangiitis:** This type of vasculitis, once in the past known as Wegener's granulomatosis, influences somwhat veins in the lungs, upper aviation routes and kidneys. The glomerulus is a minor, ball-formed structure, and it is a piece of the nephron. A nephron comprises of one glomerulus.

6.3.3 Acute Glomerulonephritis (GN)

When an immune system problem causes GN, doctors prescribe steroids and other drugs that help suppress the immune system. Antibiotics can treat a bacterial infection. Some people may need a treatment to clean the blood using an artificial filter, called dialysis, if their kidneys are greatly and irreversibly damaged.

To deal with uncomfortable symptoms, doctors may give medicines to lower blood pressure or help the kidneys make pee and get rid of waste. A person might need to drink less fluids than usual and eat a diet that's low in protein, salt, and potassium.

6.3.4 Chronic Glomerulonephritis

There's no specific way to treat chronic glomerulonephritis. To help healing and prevent more damage to the kidneys, a doctor might recommend that someone:

- eat a healthy diet with less protein, potassium, phosphorus, and salt,
- get plenty of exercise (at least 1 hour a day),
- drink less fluids,
- take calcium supplements, and
- take medicines to lower high blood pressure.

6.4 RENAL CALCULI (KIDNEY STONES)

Human body is a complex, technical machine that work all over the lifetime. This machine needs food as a fuel. As a machinery part, our body consists of organs that collaborate with one another to maintain the balance and work efficiently. Each organ has its specific functions and procedures to maintain homeostasis of the body. The nutrients are absorbed from the food we intake and the leftover is removed in the form of waste as faeces from the anus. The waste products of nutrients mainly the metabolism of protein that is urea with excess amount of water, and mineral compounds such as sodium, potassium, etc., are removed as a mixture in the form of urine.

The urine is formed in the kidneys, which consist of 1 million nephrons that are structural and functional units of kidney. These nephrons filter waste from the blood that compose to form urine. Urine comprises 96% of water, 2% urea (waste product of metabolism of protein), and other 2% uric acid, creatinine, ammonia, sodium, potassium, chlorides, phosphate, sulphate, and oxalate. These are the solute components that form urine. When any of these concentrations of these solutes disturb, it show its effect and cause disturbance in metabolism.

6.4.1 Pathophysiology

When there is disturbance in any of this structure or component, it causes damage to kidney and its function. When there is disturbance in the solute component of the urine mainly in oxalates, phosphates, urates and uric acid, it forms stones. These stones are known as renal stones or renal calculi. Calculi mean 'stones'. It is also known as 'nephrolithiasis'. And if these stones are found in ureter or urinary bladder, it is known as 'urolithiasis'. It is the hard insoluble crystallized mineral salts that are formed out of the filtrate produced by nephrons.

6.4.2 Classification of Kidney Stones

6.4.2.1 Calcium Oxalate

It is the most common type of a kidney stone found in 80% of the population. It forms due to increase in high level of calcium and oxalate ions in the urine because of decrease in water content in urine. Calcium and oxalate ions are present in urine and if they combine they form stones, so to inhibit the formation of stones there are inhibiting factors such as citrate, magnesium, etc., it is common as 1 in every 10 person gets kidney stones. The reason is they do not drink plenty of water. Water acts as a solvent for the urine. And the mineral components are the solutes. These minerals are taken from the food as much as is essential for the body. And the excess amount is filtered from the blood by the nephrons and then form urinary solutes and excreted in the form of urine. When there is less intake of water, the concentration of solute increases as the minerals binds with each other. So the oxalate ion gets struck to the calcium forming calcium oxalate stones during urine formation.

It is the second most common type of kidney stone. 8 to 15% population is affected by this type of stone. It is a mixture of about 30% of calcium oxalate stones. It is the result of calcium forming with phosphoric acid. This crystal formation results in alkaline medium of the urine. These are radio opaque stones. Calcium phosphate is wedge shaped prism crystals. These may be dirty white and spiked porcupine shaped. Similar to calcium oxalate stones, these calcium phosphate stones are also caused by hyperparathyroidism and hypercalcemia condition which disturb the amount of calcium absorption and amount in blood. As these are even calcium stones. Another cause for these stone formation is the renal tubular acidosis. So in renal tubular acidosis, there is problem in acidifying of urine which causes the alkaline medium of the urine and it predisposes calcium phosphate stones.

6.4.2.1.1 Aetiology of Calcium Oxalate Stone Formation

Formation of these stones can be due to several reasons that are in combination with the outcome of several diseases.

(a) **Dehydration or decrease in water level in body:** The most important reason for the formation of stones is the decreased level of water in our body, that is, decrease in solvent level of urine. It increases the chance for the particles to bind and form crystals. A normal 2-3 litres of water is required by the body on the daily basis. If this level decreases then the urine gets alkaline and leads to formation of crystals of calcium oxalate. So it is important to drink enough water so that concentration of urine can be maintained. Drinking of water makes the urine thin that helps in maintaining the electrolyte balance in the kidney.

(b) **Maintaining the protein intake:** Increasing the intake of protein at a higher level can be a risk factor for the proper metabolism of kidney. As increased protein leads to more urea formation which may increase the rate of solute in urine and leads to formation of crystals by binding of mineral particles.

(c) **Taking high intake of salt:** Salt contains sodium. So taking high intake of may lead to demineralization of bones. Sodium leads to removal of calcium from bones and mixes it into blood. This filters through the blood and mixes in urine. And high amount of calcium as solutes leads to formation of stones.

(d) **Taking vitamin C supplements:** Taking supplements or tablets of vitamin C without the recommendation of your health care expert. Excess of vitamin C can cause oxalate in urine.

(e) **Obesity:** Obesity comes with the various diseases. It can impair the secretion of insulin and resist and cause hyperinsulinemia, that causes metabolic disturbance in which cause imbalance and lead to calcium formation.

(f) **Inflammatory bowel disease:** During this disease, metabolic imbalance such as diarrhoea, and dysfunctioning of glands that interrupt the regulation of absorption of salts. These salts get mixed in the blood and pass to kidney where they affect the calcium re-absorption and form stones.

During this disease the absorption process of the fats get affected, due to which fat binds with the calcium and the remaining oxalate is moved to the kidney where it forms stones.

(g) **Hyperparathyroidism:** Hyperparathyroidism is caused due to increase in hormone parathyroid that is present in a good amount in our body. As in the normal conditions, this hormone is responsible for maintaining calcium level in blood and in our bones. So there is disturbance in this gland, it disturbs the level of hormone secretion which leads to loss of calcium.

(h) **Renal tubular acidosis:** It is the acidification of body due to inability of the kidney to acidify urine. Type 1 RTA that is distal tubule renal tubular acidosis is responsible for causing calcium phosphate stones. It is due to decreased citrate excretion and hypercalciuria. It is even affected due to high consumption of salts that more likely precipitate at higher pH.

6.4.2.2 Struvite Stones

These are magnesium ammonium phosphate stones. These are also radio-opaque stones which are large horny staghorn calculus. These stones account to almost 15% of the total cases. These stones are hard stones composed of minerals like calcium, magnesium, phosphates, ammonium. These stones are more common in women as compared to men. These stones are mainly bacteria infected stones that are caused during urinary tract infections. Bacteria responsible for the formation of struvite stones are proteus, pseudomonas, klebsiella, staphylococcus. Struvite stones are responsible in blocking the urinary tract pathways. These stones are removed by the surgical method. These stones grow rapidly and are responsible in damaging the kidneys.

Urinary urea is converted into ammonia and carbon dioxide by the help of urease enzyme

$$\text{Urea} \longrightarrow 2NH_3 + CO_2$$

Ammonium produced in the upper reaction then combines with water and forms alkaline ammonium.

$$NH_3 + H_2O \longrightarrow NH_4^+ + OH^-$$

6.4.2.2.1 Causes for Struvite Stones

Urinary tract infections: The main cause for the struvite stone is the bacteria that affect the urinary tract by causing the urinary tract infections. These bacteria convert protein metabolized waste product urea into ammonia. This struvite stones are produced in the alkaline medium which is due to urinary tract infections. These bacteria change the concentration of the urine by changing the concentration of solutes.

6.4.2.2.2 Treatment of Struvite Stones

Struvite stones are life threatening and should be removed from the kidney as soon as possible. If these stones are left in the kidney for a longer duration they can damage the kidney. Doctors treat these stones with the advanced method known as the shock wave lithotripsy (SWL) and percutaneous nephrolithotomy (PNL).

PNL method is used when the stones are larger in size and cannot be removed through the shock wave lithotripsy method. During this surgical process, the surgeon puts a cut on the back and put an incision inside and take the stone out. This process is painful so the patient is provided with anaesthesia.

Shock wave lithotripsy method is used to break down large crystal particles of stones inside the body itself. These shock waves convert big crystal particles into tiny small stones that come out of the body with urine through urinary pathway. If these crystals are present in large numbers, then this procedure is applied more than one time.

If these cases become complicated, if PNL and SWL aren't the options, then an open surgery has to be done. In this process, the surgeon puts a large incision on the abdomen and removes the stones from the kidney. If this process gets delayed, then it increases the chance of kidney getting damaged.

6.4.2.3 Uric Acid Stone

It is one of the major kidney stones. There is one in every ten person with this type of stone. Its rate in India is almost 10% in population suffering from uric acid crystals stone. These uric acid stones are formed when urine is highly acidic in pH. This leads to increase in uric acid concentration in urine. There are more chances of male to be suffering from uric acid stone disorder as compared to women. When pH level (below 5.5) is retained on the regular basis, it becomes a reason for the occurrence of uric acid stones.

Rise in acidic level in urine may be due to the following reasons that result in uric acid formation.

It depends on the intake of protein that is inherited and how the body possesses the uric acid concentration. This result in acidity of urine. As such condition on gout, where there is increased concentration of uric acid in bloodstream, this results in deposition of uric acid that causes severe pain in joints.

Digestion of purines leads to uric acid formation. So diet rich in purines such as animal protein like beef, fish, egg, poultry and pork. Richest source of purines are organ meats such as liver and fish. Intake of these foods and their nutrient breakdown may lead to formation of uric acid. This uric acid gets mixed into the blood, the filter through kidney and forms uric acid kidney stones. Sometimes these uric acid stones get mixed with calcium and form bigger stones.

- Person with chemotherapies is in higher risk of developing these uric acid stones.
- People suffering from diabeties and obese people are in higher risk for uric acid stones.

6.4.2.4 Cystic Stones

These stones are reoccurring stones. 'Cystinuria' a rare disorder causes this stone formation. Cystinuria is the phenomena in which the natural substance known as cystine gets mixed into the urine. Excess amount of cystine in urine leads to formation of crystals known as cystic stones. These stones can be controlled but not cured. It becomes a lifelong disease. Cystinuria is a inherited disorder. These can be inherited to future generation through genes. Every 1 in 7000 have cystinuria. Studies describes that the stones occurring in children that may be cystic stones is about 8-10%. And even 30-40% of the cystic stones are developed in the teen age. These stones show their symptom of occurrence by paining in abdominal region, blood in urine (haematuria), vomiting, nausea, etc.

6.4.3 Sizes of Kidney Stones

Renal calculi can be of different sizes. It may vary from a minute small sized crystal to a large size stone as a size of a golf ball. Its size may be from less than 2 mm to 2 cm. Stones of size more than 5 mm are considered to be larger stones. It is possible that the stones formed in the kidney migrate from to the ureter or urinary bladder and get stuck there. Being large in diameter these stones cannot pass through the kidney on its own and cause pain and irritation. These stones take larger time to get eradicated from the body, may be up to 1 year or may be more than that. These stones have higher risk of complications as they cannot be easily removed naturally from the tract.

6.4.3.1 Small Calculi

These are smaller in size and can pass easily through the urinary tract. But if these stones get intact in the tract they may cause damage by causing blood in urine. These smaller calculi cause damage to epithelium of urinary pathway causing fibrosis. It even leads to stricture. During contraction, this is an extreme pain condition by which the stones are passed to urinary bladder through ureter which is then passed thorugh urine. The sizes ranges from 2 mm to 7 mm.

6.4.3.2 Larger Calculi

These stones are formed in kidney by the combination of many smaller calculi. These are such big in size that they can cover calyces of renal pelvis. The size ranges from 7 mm to 2 cm. These stones if not treated may lead to further complications such as renal failure, tumours, hydronephrosis, etc.

6.4.4 Symptoms of Kidney Stones Formation

- Most people complain of pain in the mid back that radiates to one side or spreads to your groin.
- Nausea
- Vomiting
- Urge to often urination

- Pain during urination
- Pink/red urine

It is important to know that pain caused by kidney stones can come in waves with periods of time in between with no pain. If you feel or experience these symptoms, immediately call your doctor or run for emergency if you have kidney stone symptoms associated with:

- Fever
- Trouble passing in urine
- Inability to urinate
- Blood in urine (haematuria)
- Severe pain not relieved by over the counter medications

Passing of kidney stones can be extremely painful. The good news is that most of the kidney stones are passed by the intake of pain medication and drinking lots of water. In the cases with larger size crystals depending upon the situation and location of the stone in the patient surgery may be required. The most important factor in influencing the treatment of stones are the symptoms.

6.4.5 Management /Treatment of Renal Calculi

6.4.5.1 Surgical Methods for Removing Kidney Stones

Some stones are larger in size and may simply roll around the kidney and cause a nagging intermittent back pain. Still others may only be detected when the urine test is done showing blood in the urine. These stones are removed by surgical methods according to the size of the stones. The methods for removing the stones depend on the situations as follows.

Shock wave lithotripsy: One of the most effective means of treating stones in a stable patient is a procedure known as lithotripsy. It involves the use of high energy shock wave to break kidney stones. Shock waves are generated in a number of different ways by a typical machine. A large spark plug is used to create shocks that travel through different fluid medium. These individual shock waves spread out and then are focused or targeted on the selected kidney stones. Individual shock waves travel through the body to the stone does not cause damage to the body. Targeting of kidney stones with lithotripsy is done with the assistance of x-ray or ultrasound. Eventually, the shock waves meet together at their target to meet kidney stones. The stone absorbs the accumulated energy of the shock waves and this energy breaks the stone apart. In most cases the stone is broken into tiny pieces and each of these passes harmlessly through the body in the urine flow. Lithotripsy can be used to treat most stones in the kidney and the ureter. As a general rule, lithotripsy is an elective or non-urgent procedure used to treat stones in patients who are not in severe pain and you have no infection. In certain situations, lithotripsy may be ineffective or unsafe. For very large stones lithotripsy may be unable to effectively completely break the stones and multiple treatments may be required which may still be unsuccessful. Some medical conditions may require cautions with lithotripsy. Patients with large aneurysms and dilated arteries in the abdomen may not be candidate for lithotripsy. Pregnant women must not undergo lithotripsy. Successful rates of this procedure are generally about 80%.

6.4.6 Dietary Management in Kidney Stones

Stones are formed due to inappropriate mineral deposits in the kidney during filtration of urine. Nutritional management or diet therapy always plays a major role in prevention of any type of disease up to a major extent. By providing a balanced diet required by our body that can easily be adapted, we can prevent many diseases. Taking renal calculi in concern, the stone formation takes place due to mineral deposits and forming crystals. To maintain the balance of nutrient in body diet has to be taken that is specified from person to person.

1. **Hydration status of the body:** One of the best ways to prevent the formation of stones in our body is to drink plenty of water. Water helps in filtering the urine formed in the kidney and in maintaining the normal pH balance of urine. Water acts as the solvent in the urine and the minerals and waste products contribute to solute particle of the urine. If the solvent level increases, then the passage or flow of urine will be good. Daily recommendation of water for the body is 2-3 litres. It counts to almost 8-12 glasses of water per day.

   To prevent various types of stones the dietary measures to be taken in concern are:

2. **Low oxalate foods:** It is due to increase in oxalate and calcium level in urine. So to prevent the formation of calcium oxalate stone in we need to limit the amount of oxalate intake. But as we know oxalates are naturally occurring nutrient. It is present in foods including vegetables and fruits, nuts and oil seeds, legumes, grains, tea and even in chocolates. Foods rich in oxalate are peanuts, rhubarb, spinach, beetroots, swizz chard, sweet potatoes and chocolates. Those who have increased rate of formation of these calcium oxalate stones should limit the amount of intake of these foods.

3. **Avoid taking calcium and oxalate rich foods together:** If we consume calcium rich foods such as milk, cheese and various other dairy products with the combination of oxalates can reduce the formation of forming stones in the kidney. As their combined intake will bind these minerals in the stomach itself so that they would not reach to kidney and form stones.
4. **Maintaining the calcium intake normally:** It is a myth that the main reason for the formation of calcium oxalate kidney stones is calcium. But the fact is if we reduce the daily requirement of calcium intake in our diet, this can become the reason for formation of kidney stones. So the daily requirement of about 1000-1200 mg per day should be maintained. This amount of calcium can be served daily as 3 servings in the form of dairy products such as milk, cheese, paneer, curd, yoghurt, etc.
5. **Reduce the sodium intake:** Sodium leads to demineralization of bones causing removal of calcium from bones and mixing it into blood. Calcium travel to kidney and gets filtered into urine which binds further with oxalates and forms stones. The transportation for sodium and calcium is the same so if the intake of sodium is more then the amount of calcium in the urine will be increased. So it is better to reduce the sodium content in diet. It is better to prescribe low sodium foods. Restricted amount of sodium also helps in maintaining blood pressure that helps in reducing the rate of heart diseases.
6. **Restricting the intake of purines in diet:** Purines are the naturally occurring compounds present in foods. These purines on further digestion convert into uric acids. The uric acid then mixes with other minerals and forms uric acid stones. Foods rich in purines are mainly animal proteins like red meats, organ meats such as liver and fish, beef, shell fish, pork, etc. Intake of these foods increases the load to kidneys for excretion. Due to increase in high level of uric acid in urine the acidic level rises. So to prevent the formation of uric acid crystal stones, avoid or restrict the intake of purines. Beers and alcoholic bevereges too contain high amount of purines in them. Flavored sweetened products or drinks that have high fructose level should be avoided.
7. **Taking moderate amount of protein:** Protein on digestion forms urea. So increasing the amount of protein may lead to pressure in kidneys that can be harmful not only in case of stone formation but also for other diseases as well. It can also lead to formation of

ammonium that can be a factor in causing struvite stones. High protein intake leads to more calcium excretion.

8. **Avoiding vitamin C supplements:** Daily recommendation of vitamin C is 60 mg per day. If we increase the intake of vitamin C up to 500 mg per day then the production of oxalates in the body increases and causes pressure in kidneys that may result in calcium oxalate crystal formation.

Food recommended for the kidney related patients are:

1. Bell peppers
2. Blue berries
3. Garlic
4. Fish
5. Egg whites
6. Red grapes
7. Strawberries
8. Olive oil

6.5 DIALYSIS

Dialysis is recommended to the patients where kidney's function is lost to 85-90 percent. Dialysis is meant to substitute the natural function of renal system. The role of urinary system is to remove waste products from the system but in cases of renal failure dialysis is required.

6.5.1 Types of Dialysis

The three types of dialysis are as follows:

- Intermittent haemodialysis (IHD)
- Peritoneal dialysis (PD)
- Continuous renal replacement therapies (CRRT)

6.5.1.1 Intermittent Hemodialysis

A special machine is required to carry out intermittent dialysis with special filters which function as to move blood outside the body. The tube is inserted in the vein and blood is taken out through catheter. The special filters in the dialysis machine remove the waste products. The waste products are removed through the filters and then filtered blood is returned to the system of the patient via a separate catheter.

The patients undergo surgery before haemodialysis so that their veins can be dilated to insert catheters. The duration of haemodialysis is 3-4 hours per sitting and every 2- 3 times in a week.

6.5.1.2 Peritoneal Dialysis

The peritoneal dialysis works through diffusion technique. In this type the a sterile dialysate solution, rich in minerals and glucose, is run through a tube into the peritoneal cavity, the abdominal body cavity that surrounds the intestine. It has a semi-permeable membrane, the peritoneal membrane. Peritoneal dialysis uses natural filtering ability of our peritoneum and using the internal lining of abdomen the filtration process is carried out. The solution called dialysate is left in the peritoneal cavity for absorption of waste products of the body and then they are removed through tube and discarded.

This type of dialysis can be carried out many times a day and can be done overnight. The waste water is removed by a process of ultrafiltration in which osmosis occurs. The solution of dialysis has high glucose concentration and it moves to lower one. The pressure causes the fluid to move from the blood into the dialysate. As a result, more fluid is drained than is introduced.

Before starting peritoneal dialysis, the patient needs a small surgical procedure to insert a catheter into the abdomen. This is kept closed off, except when being used for dialysis.

6.5.1.3 Continuous Renal Replacement Therapy (CRRT)

The two types of dialysis are intermittent or continuous. Intermittent dialysis ends in 6 hours while continuous is a process of 24 hours and is done in ICU. The types of CRRT involves filtration or diffusion. The intermittent or slow dialysis results in hypotension and some other complications.

Kidney disease is a serious condition. In people with chronic kidney failure, the kidneys are unlikely to recover, but dialysis can enhance well-being and prolong life for up to 20 years or more.

6.5.2 Dietary Recommendations for Dialysis Patients

Energy: A normal energy requirement is as per the RDA. The patients feels weakness and lethargy so a light, bland and adequate calories are recommended.

Proteins: The proteins are increased to 1-1.2 gm per kg body weight as the waste products are removed and muscle wasting starts in the patient. To make up the muscle loss and weight loss proteins are increased in the diet.

Fats: Good fats, i.e., omega 3 fatty acids are recommended in such patients according to the RDAs.

Vitamins and minerals: Adequate amounts of vitamins and minerals are given , sometimes supplements are needed to cope up the harsh treatment of dialysis in the patient.

6.6 WATER AND ELECTROLYTE BALANCE IN KIDNEY DISORDERS

Water and electrolytes are vital to the various functions of our body and for life. The various electrolytes like sodium, potassium, calcium, magnesium, etc., in their required range manage various functions of our body from the normal maintenance of the water content of the body, production of the brain cells energy, maintain the heart rhythm, electricity of the nerve cells, etc. The balance of water and electrolytes in our body is very important and this important function is carried out by our kidneys. The kidneys play a central role in maintaining the various electrolytes as well as water balances and hence are responsible for maintaining the homeostasis in our body by maintaining the proper water, electrolyte and acid-base balance in our body. So primarily any imbalance to the functioning of our kidneys like kidney disorders will directly have an effect on the water and electrolyte balance of our body. The disorder of the kidney can be chronic or acute, and in both the cases it can cause multiple imbalances in the water and electrolyte balance. Some of the kidney disorders are also induced by some drugs also leads to the development of kidney disorders.

6.6.1 Fluid and Electrolyte Balance in Our Body

There are various minerals that are present in our body and from those minerals those that carry a charge on them are basically termed the electrolytes. The various electrolytes present in our body are:

- Sodium
- Potassium
- Calcium
- Phosphate
- Chloride
- Magnesium

These electrolytes are acquired by our body through the various foods that we eat as well as the various fluids we drink. These are of utmost importance for the normal functioning of our body. Importance of electrolytes:

- The required amount of water in our body is maintained and balanced.
- The pH of the body is maintained by balancing the acid-base balance of our body.

- Enables the movement of nutrients into various cells.
- Helps in the removal of various waste and unwanted substances out of the cells.
- Working of the nerves ensured.
- Muscle functioning maintained.
- Working of the vital organs like the heart and the brain is supported.

The levels of electrolytes in our body keeps on fluctuating. Sometimes the electrolytes can become too low while sometimes they become too high. These fluctuations depend on the changes of the water content present in our body. So, proper levels of electrolyte in our body is maintained by maintaining the required level of water in our body. This is achieved by replacing the water that is lost from our body. The amount of water that should be taken should be equal to the amount of water lost from our body through various processes like urination, respiration, sweating, etc. But in case of kidney disorders this balance gets disturbed and leads to various conditions like dehydration when the water level becomes too low and when water level becomes too high it leads to the development of the condition called overhydration.

6.6.1.1 Importance of Various Electrolytes in Our Body

6.6.1.1.1 Sodium

Most of the natural food items that we consume contain sodium. While processed foods contain a higher amount of sodium than all the other natural foods. Sodium plays some important functions in our body which are as follows:

- The regulation of the pressure of the blood
- The regulation of the volume of the blood
- Regulation of the functions of the nerves
- Regulation of the contraction of the muscles
- Regulation of the pH. of the blood by maintaining the acid-base balance
- Regulation of the amount of water that is eliminated as well as the amount of water that is retained in the body.

6.6.1.1.2 Potassium

Most of the food items that we consume contain potassium. It is also a mineral that is already present naturally in the body. It plays major roles in our body like:

- Regulation of the regular heartbeat
- Regulation of the proper working of the muscles
- Regulation of the proper fluid balance in the blood
- Regulation of the proper electrolyte balance in the blood.

6.6.1.1.3 Phosphorous

This mineral gets absorbed into the body through the small intestine whenever a food rich in phosphorous is consumed. This mineral is mainly responsible for functions like: maintenance of healthy bones as well as is important for the development of the bone. It also is responsible for the development of the connective tissues as well as the organs. It also helps in the movement of various muscles.

6.6.2 Maintenance of Water Balance by the Kidneys

To maintain proper homeostasis in the body maintaining a proper water level in the body is very important as half the weight of the body is constituted by water. And this is achieved by balancing the amount of intake of water with the amount of output of water. Since the largest output of water is through the urine produced by the kidney by adjusting the amount of urine excreted by the kidney, the amount of output of water from the body can be controlled. The amount of water output is adjusted by the kidney based on the water requirements of the body. That is, when the body is dehydrated due to lack of water, the urine is concentrated by the kidney and when the body has sufficient amount of water the urine output is increased by diluting the urine. These adjustments in the urine output are controlled by the body by the reabsorption process that is carried out by the kidneys. The ADH (antidiuretic hormone) is responsible for adjusting this reabsorption process of the kidney, which is particularly responsible for preventing the diuresis or increased urine output by directing the kidneys to increase the reabsorption of water from the tubules and hence decrease the urine output when the body is having sufficient amounts of water.

All the kidney functions that maintain a balance of the water and electrolytes in the body mainly depends on the process of filtering water and electrolytes from the blood. This is balanced by returning some of this filtered water and electrolytes into the blood as well as excreting excess amounts present in the urine. For this mainly the structural and functional unit of the kidney that is the nephron as well as the vessels present in the renal medulla region play the vital role. The permeability of the nephrons enables to achieve this process of excretion and reabsorption that is carried out by the various regions of the tubules of the nephrons. Apart from this various hormones also play a major role in this process. During the filtration process sodium is mainly reabsorbed from the filtrate into the blood by the renal tubules of the nephrons. While potassium is mainly excreted into the excrete from the blood in the collecting duct of the kidney. Mainly two hormones are involved in this process of reabsorption and secretion of these electrolytes and they are:

- **Aldosterone:** This hormone mainly increases the reabsorption of the sodium in the tubules as well as the excretion of potassium.
- **Angiotensin II:** This hormone increases the constriction of the vessels and hence increases the blood pressure. This leads to an increase in the glomerular filtration rates. This mainly increases the amount of the filtrate produced and released into the bowman's capsule. Aldosterone also increases the blood sodium levels as well as increases the secretion of potassium into the filtrate.

6.6.3 Maintenance of Calcium and Phosphate Balance by the Kidneys

The regulation of calcium and phosphate is balanced mainly by 3 main hormones and they are:

- **Parathyroid hormone** is released into the blood when the blood calcium levels falls. It inhibits the loss of calcium from the kidneys by directing the kidney to reabsorb more calcium from the tubules and hence increases the blood calcium level when it falls. It also reduces the loss of phosphate from the kidneys and hence increases blood phosphate levels.
- **Dihydroxy vitamin D:** It functions by stimulating intestinal calcium and phosphorus absorption. It stimulates bone calcium movement & then increases renal resorption of calcium.
- **Calcitonin** gets released in conditions when the calcium levels in the blood increases.

Depending upon the levels of calcium in the blood, these hormones are released into the blood.

6.6.4 Electrolyte Imbalances in Kidney Disorders

Patients with chronic and acute renal disorders are most probably found to have the tendency to develop the following conditions.

Hypervolemia: It is a medical condition in which too much of fluid is present in the blood. The other name for hypervolemia is fluid overload. In this condition the fluid gets accumulated in the intravascular compartments. The major cause for this condition of hypervolemia is presence of an increased sodium content in the body and hence extracellular water consequently increases in the body. The major cause is the imbalance in the regulation of sodium in the body which occurs as a result of certain diseases like kidney failure. The other diseases that create a similar condition are during congestive heart failure and liver disorders. The major treatment provided to solve this condition is

- to provide the patient with diuretics, that is, the substances that increase the urine output, and
- to reduce the intake of sodium, salt and fluids.

Hyperphosphatemia: Hyperphosphatemia is a medical condition in which the phosphate levels increases in the blood required. Mainly kidney disorders are the 4 major causes of this condition but sometimes even other diseases also contribute to this condition. Kidneys play a vital role in balancing the phosphate levels in our blood but in cases where the kidney functions get disturbed, the kidney becomes incapable of excreting the excess levels of phosphate from the blood and hence this condition develops. If hyperphosphatemia persists for a longer time. It may lead to conditions like bone disorders, calcification and mineral disorders, etc. The basic treatment provided for this condition in kidney disorder patients is through proper diet as well as through drugs.

Hypocalcaemia: Hypocalcaemia is also known as calcium deficiency disease. During kidney disorders kidney becomes unable to maintain a normal calcium level in the body which leads to decreased levels of calcium in the body which show symptoms like osteoporosis, thin nails and slower hair growth, etc.

Bicarbonate deficiency: In a normal healthy individual, the kidneys are primarily responsible for maintaining a constant acid-base balance in our body. This is achieved by the kidneys by excreting the acid urine as well as the organic acids that are produced as a by-product of the various metabolic functions in our body. In patients with various kidney disorders the kidneys will not be able to function properly and hence will not be able to excrete the various organic acids that are continuously produced by our body and also kidneys will also not be able to either reabsorb or even produce the required amount of bicarbonates from the glomerular filtrate. And hence a deficiency of sodium bicarbonates is produced in the body.

Hyponatremia: An abnormal decrease in the sodium level of the blood, that is 135 meq/L leads to the development of a condition which is termed hyponatremia. The determination of the sodium levels of the body is achieved by firstly determining the amount of sodium in the blood, and secondly the amount of water in the blood. In most of the cases it is not always necessary that the condition of a low sodium level is developed due to lack of sodium rather it is often due to the increased levels of the amount of water in the body which is required by the present sodium levels. The various reasons responsible for the decrease in the sodium levels of our body are:

- **Actual fall of sodium levels in the blood:** This occurs when there is a loss of the sodium from the body through various processes like sweating, diarrhoea, vomiting, etc. This condition can further develop to serious consequences which may lead to the development of conditions like seizers or even may lead to death.
- **Increase in water content of the body:** In advanced kidney failure, the patients are more likely to get into this condition–of presence of excess water in the body.
- **Syndrome of inappropriate antidiuretic hormone production**: Antidiuretic hormone produced by the hypothalamus is responsible for maintaining the required level of water by the kidney. In certain conditions when the ADH is produced in a higher amount this leads to the fall in the sodium concentration in the body.
- **Rise of kidney problems:** Kidneys are the important organs that are responsible for the process of performing one of the most important functions of the body that is excretion, filtering the impurities from the blood as well as maintaining the water and electrolytes balance in the body and are of the size of a fist and are two in number that are present under the rib cage one each on each side of the spine.

Kidney disorders develop when the kidney's structure gets affected and as a result the kidneys become unable to perform its functions. There are various conditions of the body or various diseases that affect the structure and functioning of the kidneys and thus leads to various kidney disorders. The diseases can be diabetes, high blood pressure or some other long-term conditions like the presence of some kind of chronic diseases. The various kidney disorders, in turn, lead to the development of various other diseases as well as various conditions like malnutrition, loss of bone density, as well as nerve disorders. If the diseases of the kidneys are allowed to get progressed they lead to major failure of the kidneys that may lead to complete stoppage of the functions performed by the kidneys. Some of the kidney disorders are also induced by certain drugs as well as like the anticancerous drugs. Certain anti-cancerous drugs induce nephrotoxicity.

6.6.5 Glomerulonephritis

It is a condition in which the glomerulus, the extremely small, tiny structures present inside the kidney that gets inflamed. Glomerulus plays the vital role of filtering the blood. There are various reasons for the development of this condition which includes, heredity and it occurs just after the birth. In some of the conditions, infections in the glomerulus leads to the infection. Sometimes the consumption of some drugs also leads to the development of this condition as some drugs cause side effects that lead to the infection of the glomerulus. But the glomerulonephritis in most of the cases gets cured by itself without the requirement of any complicated treatments.

6.6.6 Symptoms of Water and Electrolyte Imbalances

Mainly electrolyte imbalances that are very mild usually don't create any specific symptoms at all. Usually these types of mild electrolyte imbalances are not identified and probably go unidentified and are noticed only during some blood tests are carried out as well as during conditions when certain disorders get into their highly severe states. The various symptoms of electrolyte imbalances that are commonly observed in the patients are:

- Irregularity in the heartbeat
- Increase in the rate of heartbeat
- Feeling of tiredness
- Lack of energy
- Occurrence of seizures
- Nausea
- Vomiting
- Cramps in muscles
- Diarrhoea
- Constipation
- Cramps in abdomen
- Weakness in the muscles
- Irritability
- Feeling confused
- Headaches
- Numb feeling

The various symptoms of the lower or higher levels of sodium in our body mainly depend upon the severity of the condition. It also depends upon the rate at which this condition of hyponatremia develops. It can have both mild symptoms as well as severe symptoms. Mild symptoms include headaches while on the other hand severe symptoms include conditions like the development of abnormalities in the gait of the patients, changes in the rhythm of the heart as well as cramps, etc. One dangerous symptom caused by the decrease in the sodium level is the development of seizures. Therefore the treatment of this condition of hyponatremia is very important.

6.6.7 Management of Water and Electrolyte Imbalance

The management of this condition of water and electrolyte imbalance is done mainly by focusing on assessing and managing the fluid level of the body. Proper hydration of the patient is very important. For specific patients the fluid treatment is calculated and planned individually. Fluid intake planning is personalised depending on the specific condition of the patient. The fluid and electrolyte balance is continuously assessed and appropriate changes are introduced to this fluid plan based on the rapidly changing medical conditions of the patient with the renal disorders. For this the condition of the patient should be assessed from time to time.

Since along with the fluid the electrolyte balance in our body also gets disturbed in kidney disorders, patients with kidney disorders also suffer from disorders of sodium, potassium, calcium, phosphate, chloride, etc. These disorders can be life threatening and hence treatment should also focus on improving and balancing this electrolyte imbalance.

Treatment is also focused on maintaining a proper nutritional status of the patients.

6.6.8 Treatment of Hyponatremia

The treatment of natremia depends on the cause that leads to the decrease in the blood sodium level as well as the rate at which this condition developed. That is, in those conditions where the increase in body water levels lead to the development of low sodium levels, treatment will be focused on increasing the water excretion from the body so as to correct the decreased sodium levels or to restrict the amount of water intake by the patients. While in those cases where the actual sodium loss from the body happens the treatment of this condition will include the administration of sodium tablets or to increase the sodium intake.

But treatment of the hyponatremia should be done carefully as a sudden correction or change in sodium levels can prove to be dangerous specially in those cases where the patient was going through this condition for a long time.

6.6.9 Dietary Recommendations

Kidney patients can monitor the sodium intake by the following methods:

- Before consuming the packed foods, patients should check the food labels and should only consume foods in which the sodium contents are less.

- Serving sizes of the various foods consumed should always be carefully maintained.
- The consumption of packaged meats should be avoided by the patients and rather fresh meat should be consumed.
- Always fresh fruits as well as fresh vegetables should be preferred and the consumption of dried, pickled and canned fruits and vegetables should be completely avoided.
- Always avoid the consumption of processed foods.
- Food cooked at home is to be preferred without the addition of salt.
- Total sodium consumption is to be restricted to 400 mg per meal.

6.6.9.1 Monitoring of Potassium Intake by the Patients

The various methods that the patients should follow so as to maintain and monitor the potassium intake are as follows:

- A proper eating plan should me made so as to control the intake of the potassium.
- Foods that are high in potassium should be restricted.
- The milk and its various products that are mainly high in potassium contents should be reduced.
- Always fresh fruits as well as fresh vegetables should be consumed.
- Salt substitutes as well as seasonings that contain potassium should be avoided.
- Food labels should be carefully read before eating any food and should avoid those foods that contain potassium.
- The serving size of the food should always be considered and carefully managed.
- Always a food journal is to be managed.

6.6.9.2 Monitoring of Phosphorous Intake by the Patients

Phosphorous is found in every food that we consume. The various tips that need to be followed so as to keep the phosphorous levels in safe level are:

- Foods that are low in phosphorous content is to be consumed.
- Each time smaller portions of foods should be consumed that are mainly higher in protein content.
- Always fresh fruits as well fresh vegetables should be consumed.
- Packaged foods should be avoided mainly those containing high phosphorous contents.
- Food journal maintenance is very important.

6.6.9.3 Regulation of Fluids

Regulation of fluids is of increased importance mainly in those patients with chronic kidney diseases. In these patients normal fluid consumption is not possible and leads to accumulation of fluids in the body leading to further complications. In those patients who are put into dialysis, there is a decrease in the urine output and therefore an increased fluid intake will lead to the building up of pressure in the various major organs of our body like the heart and the lungs.

The calculations of the amount of fluids that a patient can consume is completely personalised and is calculated on the patient's urine output as well as on the patients on dialysis, the fluid intake amount is calculated based on the particular dialysis settings the patient is put on. So as to control the fluid intake, the patients should follow the following methods:

- The intake of water of a patient should be as per the doctor's or the nutritionist's advice.
- Apart from the direct fluids that are consumed, the other foods that are liquid at room temperature is also considered.
- The amount of water that is used in the cooking is also to be considered carefully.

6.7 OTHER TREATMENTS

6.7.1 Diuretics

The use of diuretics is the most common kind of therapy used for correcting electrolyte imbalance in kidney disorders. In those patients where there are excess amounts of certain electrolytes such as calcium, potassium, etc., that gets buil it up in the body these diuretic drugs are used. These drugs are administered through the mouth. These diuretics help in getting rid of this excess amount of electrolytes from the body as these drugs increase the urine output and hence the excess electrolytes get eliminated from the body through the urine.

6.7.2 Potassium Lowering Medications

Medications like sodium polystyrene sulfonate which are potassium lowering medicines that are given to those patients with the condition of hyperkalemia or increased potassium levels. Also, sodium polystyrene sulphate is administered to patients through mouth or through enema.

CASE STUDIES

1. TO PLAN A DAY'S DIET FOR A MAN, 68 YR OLD SUFFERING FROM GLOMERULONEPHRITIS

Personal Data

Age: 68 years

Gender: Male

Recommended Dietary Allowance

Energy: 1936 kcal/day

Protein: 68 g/day

Carbohydrates: 290 g/day

Fats: 43.2 g/day

Dietary Modifications

Energy: 1936 kcal/day

Protein: 55 g/day, assuming the patient is having proteinurea.

Carbohydrates: 290.4 g/day

Fats: 53.7 g/day

Food Exchange List

Food exchange	Number of exchange	Energy (Kcal)	Protein (g)	Carbohydrate (g)	Fat (g)
Milk	2	340	16	24	20
Meat	1	80	7	Neg.	6
Pulse	1	100	7	17	-
Cereal	12	840	24	180	-
Veg. A	1	20	1	3.5	-
Veg. B	1.5	60	3	10.5	-
Fat	6	270	-	-	30
Sugar	10	200	-	50	-

Exchange Distribution

Exchange	Total no.	Early morning	Break-fast	Mid-morning	Lunch	Evening snacks	Dinner
Milk	2		0.6		0.4	0.2	0.8
Meat	1		1				
Pulse	1				1		

Cereal	12	2	2	2	3	1	2
Veg. A	1				½		½
Veg. B	1.5		½		½		½
Fat	6	1	1		2		2
Sugar	10		2	2	2	2	2

Diet Chart

Meal	Food item	Amount	Menu	Energy (kcal)	Protein (g)	Carbohydrate (g)	Fat (g)
Early morning (8:00 am)	Ragi + Butter	40 g (2 in no.) + 2 tbsp	Ragi cheela	128.2 45	2.8	26.7	Neg. 10
Breakfast (10:00 am)	Milk + Sugar	150 mL 2 tbsp	Milk	91.54 40	5.6 -	7 10	4.5 -
	Egg whole	1	Boiled egg	97	7	-	7
	Vermicelli + Butter + Onion	2 katori 1 tbsp ½ katori	Onion vermicelli	199.6 45 6.89	6 - Neg.	10.4 - Neg.	Neg. 5 Neg.
Mid-morning (12 noon)	Puf. Rice	40 g	Puf. Rice	130	3	30	Neg.
	Lemon sugar water	2 tbsp sugar + 250 mL water + 1 lemon	Shikangi	40	-	10	-
Lunch (2:00 pm)	Butter milk + Sugar	100 g 2 tbsp	Sweet butter milk	60 40	3 -	2.98 10	3.99 -
	Lobia + Tomato + Onion	25 g (1 katori) 25 g 25 g	Lobia	80 4.7 6.89	5.3 Neg. Neg.	13.4 Neg. Neg.	Neg Neg. Neg.
	Wheat flour + Rice + Butter	40g (2 chapati) 1 katori 2 tbsp	Chapati	128 267 90	4.2 5.9 -	25.6 58.6 -	Neg Neg. 10

Evening snacks (5:00 pm)	Milk + Sugar	50 g 1 tbsp	Tea/coffee	30.51 20	1.86	2.33 5	1.5
	Wheat flour + Sugar	1 paratha 1 tbsp	Sweet paratha	64 20	2.1 -	12 5	Neg. -
Dinner (8:00 pm)	Wheat flour + Potato + Onion + Butter	20 g 50 g 25 g 2 tbsp	Aloo and onion paratha	64 48 6.89 90	2.1 Neg. Neg. -	12 11.3 Neg. -	Neg. Neg. Neg. 10
Bedtime (9:30 pm)	Milk + Sugar	200 2 tbsp	Sweet milk	65 40	4 -	5 10	3.2 -
Total				1942	53.8	285.6	54.2

Important Points

- Low protein intake due to proteinuria.
- High biological value proteins to be given like eggs, milk, etc.
- Low sodium and fluid intake in cases of oedema.
- Fats and carbohydrates should be the major sources for energy.
- Include butter and cream in diet as they are emulsified and easy to digest.
- Fruit intake to be restricted due to high content of potassium due to hyperkalemia.
- Potassium rich foods to be avoided like banana, mango, amla, coffee, chocolate, cocoa, nuts, etc.
- Food like rice, sugar,vegetables, sago, honey to be included.
- Intake of water to be reduced.
- In case of thirst moisten your mouth with lemon wedge/candy/chewing gum.
- Foods to be avoided:
  - ◊ Potato
  - ◊ Amaranth leaves
  - ◊ Meat
  - ◊ Chicken
  - ◊ Plums

2. TO PLAN A DAY'S DIET FOR A MAN, 41 YEARS OLD SUFFERING FROM GLOMERULONEPHRITIS

Personal Data

Age: 41 years

Gender: Male

Recommended Dietary Allowance

Energy: 1883 kcal/day

Protein: 70/day

Carbohydrates: 60%E

Fats: 15-25%E

Dietary Modifications

Energy: 1883 kcal/day

Protein: 70 g/day, assuming the person is not having proteinurea.

Carbohydrates: 282.45 g/day

Fat: 47.3 g/day

Food Exchange List

Food exchange	Number of exchange	Energy (Kcal)	Protein (g)	Carbohydrate (g)	Fat (g)
Milk	2	340	16	24	20
Meat	1	80	7	Neg.	6
Pulse	1	100	7	17	-
Cereal	13	910	26	195	-
Veg. A	1	20	1	3.5	-
Veg. B	1.5	60	3	10.5	-
Fat	6	270	-	-	30
Sugar	10	200	-	50	-

Exchange Distribution

Exchange	Total no.	Early morning	Break-fast	Mid morning	Lunch	Evening snacks	Dinner
Milk	2		0.6		0.4	0.2	0.8
Meat	1		1				
Pulse	1				1		
Cereal	13	2	2	2	3	2	2
Veg. A	1				½		½

Veg. B	1.5		½		½	½	
Fat	6	1	1		2		2
Sugar	10		2	2	2	2	2

Diet Plan

Meal	Food item	Amount	Menu	Energy (kcal)	Protein (g)	Carbohydrate (g)	Fat (g)
Early morning (8:00 am)	Ragi	40 g (2 in no.)	Ragi cheela	128.2	2.8	26.7	Neg.
	+ Butter	+ 2 tbsp		90			10
Breakfast (10:00 am)	Milk	150 mL	Coffee/ tea	91.54	5.6	7	4.5
	+ Sugar	2 tbsp		40	-	10	-
	Egg whole	1	Boiled egg	97	7	-	7
	Vermicelli	2 katori	Onion vermicelli	199.6	6	10.4	Neg.
	+ Butter	1 tbsp		45	-	-	5
	+ Onion	½ katori		6.89	Neg.	Neg.	Neg.
Mid morning (12 noon)	Wheat flour	1 paratha	Sweet paratha	64	2.1	12	Neg.
	+ Sugar	1 tbsp		20	-	5	-
	Puf. rice	40 g	Puf. rice	130	3	30	Neg.
Lunch (2:00 pm)	Curd	100 g	Sweet curd	60	2	2.98	3.99
	+ Sugar	2 tbsp		40	-	10	-
	Lobia	25 g (1 katori)	Lobia	80	5.3	13.4	Neg
	+ Tomato	25 g		4.7	Neg.	Neg.	Neg.
	+ Onion	25 g		6.89	Neg.	Neg.	Neg.
	Wheat flour	40 g (2 chapati)	Chapati	128	4.2	25.6	Neg
	+ Puff. rice	1 katori		130	3	30	Neg
	+ Butter	2 tbsp		90	-	-	10
Evening snacks (5:00 pm)	Milk	50 g	Tea/ coffee	30.51	1.86	2.33	1.5
	+ Sugar	1 tbsp		20	-	5	

	Wheat flour + Sugar	1 paratha 1 tbsp	Sweet paratha	64 20	2.1 -	12 5	Neg. -
Dinner (8:00 pm)	Wheat flour + Cauliflower + Onion + Butter	20 g 50 g 25 g 2 tbsp	Cauli-flower and onion paratha	64 48 6.89 90	2.1 Neg. Neg. -	12 11.3 Neg. -	Neg. Neg. Neg
	Curd + Sugar	100 g 2 tbsp	Sweet curd	60 40	2 -	2.98 10	3.99 -
Total				1894.4	68	285	45.98

Important Points

- No change in protein intake due to absence of proteinuria.
- High biological value proteins to be given like eggs, milk, etc.
- Low sodium and fluid intake in cases of oedema.
- Fats and carbohydrates should be the major sources for energy.
- Include butter and cream in diet as they are emulsified and easy to digest.
- Fruit intake to be restricted due to high content of potassium due to hyperkalemia.
- Potassium rich foods to be avoided like banana, mango, amla, coffee, chocolate, cocoa, nuts, etc.
- Foods like rice,sugar,vegetables, sago, honey to be included .
- Intake of water to be reduced.
- In case of thirst moisten your mouth with lemon wedge/candy/ chewing gum.
- Foods to be avoided:
    - ◊ Potato
    - ◊ Amaranth leaves
    - ◊ Meat
    - ◊ Chicken
    - ◊ Plums
    - ◊ Bakery products like breads
    - ◊ Sweet potato
    - ◊ Drumsticks
    - ◊ Spinach

3. TO PLAN A DAY'S DIET FOR A FEMALE, 61 YEARS OLD SUFFERING FROM GLOMERULONEPHRITIS

Personal Data

Age: 61 years

Gender: Female

Recommended Dietary Allowance

Energy: 1782 kcal/day

Protein: 58/day

Carbohydrates: 60%E

Fats: 15-25%E

Dietary Modifications

Energy: 1782 kcal/day

Protein: 48 g/day, assuming the person is having proteinurea.

Carbohydrates: 267.3/day

Fat: 49.5 g/day

Food Exchange List

Food exchange	Number of exchange	Energy (kcal)	Protein (g)	Carbohydrate (g)	Fat (g)
Milk	1	170	8	6	10
Meat	1	93	8	Neg.	6
Pulse	1	80	7	17	-
Cereal	13	840	24	180	-
Veg. A	1	20	1	3.5	-
Veg. B	1	40	2	10.5	-
Fat	7	315	-	-	35
Sugar	10	200	-	50	-

Exchange Distribution

Exchange	Total no.	Early morning	Break-fast	Mid morning	Lunch	Evening snacks	Dinner
Milk	1	0.2			0.4	0.2	0.2
Meat	1		1				
Pulse	1				1		
Cereal	12	2	3	2	2	2	2
Veg. A	1				½		½
Veg. B	1		½		½		
Fat	6	1	1		2		2
Sugar	10	2		2	2	2	2

Diet Plan

Meal	Food item	Amount	Menu	Energy (kcal)	Protein (g)	Carbohydrate (g)	Fat (g)
Early morning (8:00 am)	Bulgur wheat	20 g	Milk dalia	68	2	13.8	Neg.
	+ Milk	+ 150 mL		91.54	5.6	7	4.5
	+ Sugar	2 tbsp		40	-	10	-
	Potato	50 g		48	Neg.	11.3	-
Breakfast (10:00 am)	Ragi	20 (2 in no.)	Ragi cheela	64	1.4	13.35	Neg.
	+ Butter	+ 2 tbsp		90	-	-	10
	Egg whole	1	Boiled egg	97	7	-	7
	Vermicelli	2 katori	Onion vermicelli	199.6	6	10.4	Neg.
	+ Butter	1 tbsp		45	-	-	5
	+ Onion	½ katori		6.89	Neg.	Neg.	Neg.
Mid-morning (12 noon)	Wheat flour	1 paratha	Sweet paratha	64	2.1	12	Neg.
	+ Sugar	1 tbsp		20	-	5	-
	Puf. rice	40 g	Puf. rice	130	3	30	Neg.
Lunch (2:00 pm)	Curd	100 g	Sweet curd	60	2	2.98	3.99
	+ Sugar	2 tbsp		40	-	10	-
	Red gram dal	30 g (1 katori)	Lobia	99	6.51	16.5	Neg
	+ Tomato	25 g		4.7	Neg.	Neg.	Neg.
	+ Onion	25 g		6.89	Neg.	Neg.	Neg.
	Wheat flour	2	Chapati	128	4.2	25.6	Neg
	+ Butter	2 tbsp		90	-	-	10
Evening snacks (5:00 pm)	Milk	50 g	Tea/ coffee	30.51	1.86	2.33	1.5
	+ Sugar	1 tbsp		20	-	5	
	Wheat flour	1 paratha	Sweet paratha	64	2.1	12	Neg.
	+ Sugar	1 tbsp		20	-	5	-

Dinner (8:00 pm)	Wheat flour + Cauliflower + Onion + Butter	20 g 50 g 25 g 2 tbsp	Cauli-flower and onion paratha	64 48 6.89 90	2.1 Neg. Neg. -	12 11.3 Neg. -	Neg. Neg. Neg
	Curd + Sugar	100 g 2 tbsp	Sweet curd	60 40	2 -	2.98 10	3.99 -
Total				1834.1	47.87	257	45.98

Important Points

- Low protein intake due to proteinuria.
- High biological value proteins to be given like eggs, milk, etc.
- Low sodium and fluid intake in cases of oedema.
- Fats and carbohydrates should be the major sources for energy.
- Include butter and cream in diet as they are emulsified and easy to digest.
- Fruit intake to be restricted due to high content of potassium due to hyperkalemia.
- Potassium rich foods to be avoided like banana, mango, amla, coffee, chocolate, cocoa, nuts, etc.
- Foods like rice,sugar,vegetables, sago, honey to be included .
- Intake of water to be reduced.
- In case of thirst moisten your mouth with lemon wedge/candy/ chewing gum.
- Foods to be avoided:
  - ◊ Potato
  - ◊ Amaranth leaves
  - ◊ Meat
  - ◊ Chicken
  - ◊ Plums

4. TO PLAN A DAY'S DIET FOR A MAN, 38 YEARS OLD SUFFERING FROM NEPHRITIC SYNDROME

Personal Data

Age: 38 years

Gender: Male

Recommended Dietary Allowance

Energy: 2450 kcal/day
Protein: 56/day
Carbohydrates: 60%E
Fats: 15-25%E

Dietary Modifications

Energy: 2450 kcal/day
Protein: 70 g/day
Carbohydrates: 383 g/day
Fat: 54.3 g/day

Food Exchange List

Food exchange	Number of exchange	Energy (kcal)	Protein (g)	Carbohydrate (g)	Fat (g)
Milk	1	170	8	12	10
Pulse	3	300	21	51	-
Cereal	14	980	28	210	-
Veg. A	3	60	3	10.5	-
Veg. B	2	80	4	14	-
Fruit	4	180	-	40	-
Fat	7	315	-	-	35
Sugar	7	140	-	35	-

Exchange Distribution

Exchange	Total no.	Early morning	Break-fast	Mid morning	Lunch	Evening snacks	Dinner
Milk	1	0.2		0.2	0.2	0.2	0.2
Pulse	2		1		1		
Cereal	14	2	3	2	3	2	3
Veg. A	3	1			1		1
Veg. B	2	½	½		½		½
Fruit	4	1		1		1	1
Fat	7	1	2		2		2
Sugar	7	1 ½		1	1 ½	1	2

Diet Chart

Meal	Food item	Amount	Menu	Energy (kcal)	Protein (g)	Carbohydrate (g)	Fat (g)
Early morning (8:00 am)	Full cream milk	½ glass (125 mL)	Milk oats	109.7	4.7	5.85	7.5
	+ Sugar	½ tbsp		10	-	2.5	-
	+ Oats	1 bowl		90	3.3	15	-
	Apple	1 medium		43	-	10	-
	Cracked wheat	1 bowl	Sweet cracked wheat porridge	68.3	2.16	13.8	-
	+ Ghee	2 tbsp		90	-	-	10
	+ Sugar	1 tbsp		20	-	5	-
	Carrot	25 g		6.78	Neg	Neg	Neg
	+ Beet root	25 g		5.43	Neg	Neg	Neg
Breakfast (10:00 am)	Green gram	1 katori (30 g) raw wt.	Sprouts	100	7	17	Neg.
	Sago	2 katori (50 g) raw wt.	Sago	120	Neg.	30	-
	+ Onion	30		3.89	Neg	Neg	Neg
	+ Butter	5 g		45	-	-	5
	Puffed rice	1 katori (20 g)	Roasted puffed rice	20	1.5	15	-
	+ Ghee	+ 1 tbsp ghee (5 g)		45	-	-	5
Mid-morning (12 noon)	Milk	125 mL	Rice kheer	109.7	4.7	5.85	7.5
	+ Sugar	1 tbsp		20	-	5	-
	+ Rice	1 katori		267	5.9	58.9	-
	Apple	1 medium		43	-	10	-
Lunch (2:00 pm)	Curd	100 g	Sweet curd	60	2	2.98	3.99
	+ Sugar	1 ½ tbsp		35	-	7.5	-
	Bengal gram dal	I katori	Dal palak	131	6	18.68	-
	+ Spinach	60 g		14.62	3.5	6	Neg.
	+ Onion	30 g		3.89	Neg.	Neg	Neg.
	+ Ghee	5 g		45	-	-	5
	Chapatti	3		192.15	6.34	38.4	-
	+ Butter	5 g		45	-	-	5

Evening snacks (5:00 pm)	Green Gram	1 katori (30 g) raw wt.	Sprouts	100	7	17	Neg.
	Biscuit	1		54.5	Neg.	7.5	2.3
	Milk + Sugar	50 g 1 tbsp	Tea/ coffee	30.51 20	1.86 -	2.33 5	1.5
	Apricot	½ medium		50		5	
Dinner (8:00 pm)	Wheat flour + Potato + Onion + Butter	60 g 50 g 12 g 2 tbsp	Potato and onion paratha (3 paratha)	192 48 3.3 90	6 Neg. Neg. -	36 11.3 Neg. -	Neg. Neg. Neg
	Curd + Sugar + Apple	100 g 2 tbsp 1 medium	Sweet apple curd	60 40 43	2 - -	2.98 10 10	3.99 - -
Total				2471	68	383	51.78

Important Points

- Low cholesterol intake should be there.
- Low sodium due to oedema and water retention in body.
- Low sugar intake.
- There is reduction in fat intake due to hypercholesterolemia and hyperlipidemia.
- Low intake of water, approximately 500 mL – 1 L/day.
- Take pulses along with cereals to improve the quality of protein.
- Potassium rich foods like carrots, potatos, onion, spinach can be given.
- Due to chances of calcium deficiency curd and milk can also be given.
- Pulses should be taken in sufficient amount.

5. TO PLAN A DAY'S DIET FOR A WOMAN, 40 YEARS OLD SUFFERING FROM NEPHRITIC SYNDROME

Personal Data

Age: 40 years

Gender: Female

Recommended Dietary Allowance

Energy: 2625 kcal/day
Protein: 75/day
Carbohydrates: 60%
Fats: 15-25%

Dietary Modifications

Energy: 2625 kcal/day
Protein: 75 g/day
Carbohydrates: 393 g/day
Fat: 58.3 g/day

Food Exchange List

Food exchange	Number of exchange	Energy (kcal)	Protein (g)	Carbohydrate (g)	Fat (g)
Milk	1	170	8	12	10
Meat	1	80	8	Neg	6
Pulse	3	300	21	51	-
Cereal	14	980	28	210	-
Veg. A	3	60	3	10.5	-
Veg. B	2	80	4	14	-
Fruit	4	180	-	40	-
Fat	8	360	-	-	40
Sugar	7	140	-	35	-

Exchange Distribution

Exchange	Total no.	Early morning	Break-fast	Mid-morning	Lunch	Evening snacks	Dinner
Milk	1	0.2		0.2	0.2	0.2	0.2
Meat	1					1	
Pulse	3		1		1	1	
Cereal	14	2	3	2	3	2	3
Veg. A	3	1			1		1
Veg. B	2	½	½		½		½
Fruit	4	1		1		1	1
Fat	8	1	2		2	1	2
Sugar	7	1 ½		1	1 ½	1	2

Diet Chart

Meal	Food item	Amount	Menu	Energy (kcal)	Protein (g)	Carbohydrate (g)	Fat (g)
Early morning (8:00 am)	Full cream milk	½ glass (125 mL)	Milk oats	109.7	4.7	5.85	7.5
	+ Sugar	½ tbsp		10	-	2.5	-
	+ Oats	1 bowl		90	3.3	15	-
	Apple	1 medium		43	-	10	-
	Cracked wheat	1 bowl	Sweet cracked wheat porridge	68.3	2.16	13.8	-
	+ Ghee	2 tbsp		90	-	-	10
	+ Sugar	1 tbsp		20	-	5	-
	Carrot	25 g		6.78	Neg	Neg	Neg
	+ Beet root	25 g		5.43	Neg	Neg	Neg
Breakfast (10:00 am)	Green gram	1 katori (30 g) raw wt.	Sprouts	100	7	17	Neg.
	Sago	2 katori (50 g) raw wt.	Sago	120	Neg.	30	-
	+ Onion	30		3.89	Neg	Neg	Neg
	+ Butter	5 g		45	-	-	5
	Puffed rice	1 katori (20 g)	Roasted puffed rice	20	1.5	15	-
	+ Ghee	+ 1 tbsp ghee (5 g)		45	-	-	5
Mid-morning (12 noon)	Milk	125 mL	Rice kheer	109.7	4.7	5.85	7.5
	+ Sugar	1 tbsp		20	-	5	-
	+ Rice	1 katori		267	5.9	58.9	-
	Apple	1 medium		43	-	10	-

Lunch (2:00 pm)	Curd +	100 g	Sweet curd	60	2	2.98	3.99
	Sugar	1 ½ tbsp		35	-	7.5	-
	Bengal gram dal +	I katori	Dal palak	131	6	18.68	-
	Spinach +	60 g		14.62	3.5	6	Neg.
	Onion +	30 g		3.89	Neg.	Neg	Neg.
	Ghee	5 g		45	-	-	5
	Chapatti +	3		192.15	6.34	38.4	-
	Butter	5 g		45	-	-	5
Evening snacks (5:00 pm)	Green gram +	1 katori (30 g) raw wt.	Sprouts	100	7	17	Neg.
	Butter	5 g		45	-	-	5
	Egg whole +	1	Full fry egg	97	7	-	7
	Butter	5 g		45	-	-	5
	Biscuit	1		54.5	Neg.	7.5	2.3
	Milk +	50 g	Tea/coffee	30.51	1.86	2.33	1.5
	Sugar	1 tbsp		20	-	5	
	Apricot	½ medium		50		5	
Dinner (8:00 pm)	Wheat flour +	60 g	Cauliflower and onion paratha (3paratha)	192	6	36	Neg.
	Cauliflower +	50 g		48	Neg.	11.3	Neg.
	Onion +	12 g		3.3	Neg.	Neg.	Neg
	Butter	2 tbsp		90	-	-	5
	Curd +	100 g	Sweet apple curd	60	2	2.98	3.99
	Sugar +	2 tbsp		40	-	10	-
	Apple	1 medium		43	-	10	-
Total				2520	68	394.8	58.6

Important Points

- Low cholesterol intake should be there.
- Low sodium due to oedema and water retention in body.

- Low sugar intake.
- There is reduction in fat intake due to hypercholesterolemia and hyperlipidemia.
- Low intake of water, approximately 500 mL – 1 L/day.
- Take pulses along with cereals to improve the quality of protein.
- Potassium rich foods like carrots, potatos, onion, spinach can be given.
- Due to chances of calcium deficiency curd and milk can also be given.
- Pulses should be taken in sufficient amount.

6. TO PLAN A DAY'S DIET FOR A WOMAN, 59 YEARS OLD SUFFERING FROM NEPHRITIC SYNDROME

Personal Data

Age: 59 years

Gender: Female

Recommended Dietary Allowance

Energy: 2625 kcal/day

Protein: 75/day

Carbohydrates: 60%E

Fats: 15-25%E

Dietary Modifications

Energy: 2625 kcal/day

Protein: 75 g/day

Carbohydrates: 393 g/day

Fat: 58.3 g/day

Food Exchange List

Food exchange	Number of exchange	Energy (kcal)	Protein (g)	Carbohydrate (g)	Fat (g)
Milk	2	340	16	24	20
Meat	1	80	7	Neg.	6
Pulse	2	200	14	34	-
Cereal	13	910	26	195	-
Veg. A	2	40	2	7	-
Veg. B	2	80	4	14	-
Fat	6	270	-	-	30
Sugar	10	200	-	50	-

Exchange Distribution

Exchange	Total no.	Early morning	Break-fast	Mid-morning	Lunch	Evening snacks	Dinner
Milk	2		0.6		0.4	0.2	0.8
Meat	1		1				
Pulse	1				1		
Cereal	13	2	2	2	3	2	2
Veg. A	1				½		½
Veg. B	1.5		½		½	½	
Fruit	4	1		1		1	1
Fat	6	1	1		2		2
Sugar	10		2	2	2	2	2

Diet Plan

Meal	Food item	Amount	Menu	Energy (kcal)	Protein (g)	Carbohydrate (g)	Fat (g)
Early morning (8:00 am)	Ragi + Butter	40 g (2 in no.) + 2 tbsp	Ragi cheela	128.2 90	2.8	26.7	Neg. 10
	Apple	1 medium		43	-	10	-
Breakfast (10:00 am)	Milk + Sugar	150 mL 2 tbsp	Coffee/tea	91.54 40	5.6 -	7 10	4.5 -
	Egg whole	1	Boiled egg	97	7	-	7
	Vermicelli + Butter + Onion	2 katori 1 tbsp ½ katori	Onion vermicelli	199.6 45 6.89	6 - Neg.	10.4 - Neg.	Neg. 5 Neg.
Mid-morning (12 noon)	Wheat flour + Sugar	1 paratha 1 tbsp	Sweet paratha	64 20	2.1 -	12 5	Neg. -
	Puff. Rice	40 g	Puff. rice	130	3	30	Neg.
Lunch (2:00 pm)	Curd + Sugar	100 g 2 tbsp	Sweet curd	60 40	2 -	2.98 10	3.99 -
	Lobia + Tomato + Onion	25 g (1 katori) 25 g 25 g	Lobia	128 130 90	4.2 3 -	13.4 Neg. Neg.	Neg Neg. Neg.

	Wheat flour + Puff. Rice + Butter	40 g (2 chapati) 1 katori 2 tbsp	Chapati			25.6 30 -	Neg Neg 10
Evening snacks (5:00 pm)	Milk + Sugar	50 g 1 tbsp	Tea/coffee	30.51 20	1.86 -	2.33 5	1.5
	Apricot	1 medium		50		5	
	Wheat flour + Sugar	1 paratha 1 tbsp	Sweet paratha	64 20	2.1 -	12 5	Neg. -
Dinner (8:00 pm)	Wheat flour + Cauliflower + Onion + Butter	20 g 50 g 25 g 2 tbsp	Cauliflower and onion paratha	64 48 6.89 90	2.1 Neg. Neg. -	12 11.3 Neg. -	Neg. Neg. Neg
	Curd + Sugar	100 g 2 tbsp	Sweet curd	60 40	2 -	2.98 10	3.99 -
	Apple	1 medium		43	-	10	-
Total				2620	60	390	55.98

Important Points

- Low cholesterol intake should be there.
- Low sodium due to oedema and water retention in body.
- Low sugar intake.
- There is reduction in fat intake due to hypercholesterolemia and hyperlipidemia.
- Low intake of water, approximately 500 mL – 1 L/day.
- Take pulses along with cereals to improve the quality of protein.
- Potassium rich foods like carrots, potatos, onion, spinach can be given.
- Due to chances of calcium deficiency curd and milk can also be given.
- Pulses should be taken in sufficient amount.

7. TO PLAN A DAY'S DIET FOR A MAN, 63 YEARS OLD SUFFERING FROM NEPHRITIC SYNDROME

Personal Data

Age: 63 years

Gender: Male

Recommended Dietary Allowance

Energy: 2800 kcal/day

Protein: 80/day

Carbohydrates: 60%E

Fats: 15-25%E

Dietary Modifications

Energy: 2800 kcal/day

Protein: 80 g/day

Carbohydrates: 420 g/day

Fat: 62 g/day

Food Exchange List

Food exchange	Number of exchange	Energy (kcal)	Protein (g)	Carbohydrate (g)	Fat (g)
Milk	2	340	16	24	20
Meat	1	80	7	Neg.	6
Pulse	3	300	14	34	-
Cereal	14	980	28	210	-
Veg. A	3	60	3	10.5	-
Veg. B	2	80	4	14	-
Fruit	4	180	-	40	-
Fat	8	360	-	-	40
Sugar	7	140	-	35	-

Exchange Distribution

Exchange	Total no.	Early morning	Break-fast	Mid morning	Lunch	Evening snacks	Dinner
Milk	2		0.6		0.4	0.2	0.8
Meat	1		1				
Pulse	3		1		1		1

Cereal	14	2	2	2	3	2	3
Veg. A	3	1			1		1
Veg. B	2	½	½		½		½
Fruit	4	1		1		1	1
Fat	8	1	1		2	1	2
Sugar	7	1 ½		1	1 ½	1	2

Diet Plan

Meal	Food item	Amount	Menu	Energy (kcal)	Protein (g)	Carbohydrate (g)	Fat (g)
Early morning (8:00 am)	Ragi	40 g (2 in no.)	Ragi cheela	128.2	2.8	26.7	Neg.
	+ Butter	+ 1 tbsp		45			5
	Apple	1 medium		43	-	10	-
	Cucumber	1 medium	Salad	20	1	3.5	Neg.
	+ Carrot			30	2	7	Neg.
	Lemon and Honey	1 tbsp	Lemon and honey water	19	-	5	-
Breakfast (10:00 am)	Milk	150 mL	Coffee/tea	91.54	5.6	7	4.5
	+ Sugar	2 tbsp		40	-	10	-
	Egg whole	1	Boiled egg	97	7	-	7
	Vermicelli	2 katori	Onion vermicelli	199.6	6	10.4	Neg.
	+ Butter	1 tbsp		45	-	-	5
	+ Onion	½ katori		6.89	Neg.	Neg.	Neg.
Mid-morning (12 noon)	Wheat flour	1 paratha	Sweet paratha	64	2.1	12	Neg.
	+ Sugar	1 tbsp		20	-	5	-
	Puff. Rice	40 g	Puff. rice	130	3	30	Neg.
	Apple	1 medium		43	-	10	-
Lunch (2:00 pm)	Curd	100 g	Sweet curd	60	2	2.98	3.99
	+ Sugar	2 tbsp		40	-	10	-
	Lobia	25 g (1 katori)	Lobia	128	4.2	13.4	Neg
	+ Tomato	25 g		130	3	Neg.	Neg.
	+ Onion	25 g		90	-	Neg.	Neg.

	Wheat flour	40 g (2 chapati)	Chapati	128	4.2	25.6	Neg
	+						
	Puff. rice	1 katori				30	Neg
	+						
	Butter	2 tbsp				-	10
Evening snacks (5:00 pm)	Milk	50 g	Tea/coffee	30.51	1.86	2.33	1.5
	+						
	Sugar	1 tbsp		20	-	5	
	Apricot	1 medium		50		5	
	Wheat flour	1 paratha	Sweet paratha	64	2.1	12	Neg.
	+						
	Sugar	1 tbsp		20	-	5	-
Dinner (8:00 pm)	Wheat flour	20 g	Cauliflower and onion paratha	64	2.1	12	Neg.
	+						
	Cauliflower	50 g		48	Neg.	11.3	Neg.
	+						
	Onion	25 g		6.89	Neg.	Neg.	Neg
	+						
	Butter	2 tbsp		90	-	-	
	Green gram	1 katori (30 g) raw wt.	Sprouts	100	7	17	Neg.
	+						
	Butter	5 g		45	-	-	5
	Curd	100 g	Sweet curd	60	2	2.98	3.99
	+						
	Sugar	2 tbsp		40	-	10	-
	Apple	1 medium		43	-	10	-
Total				2786	80	420	60

Important Points

- Low cholesterol intake should be there.
- Low sodium due to oedema and water retention in body.
- Low sugar intake.
- There is reduction in fat intake due to hypercholesterolemia and hyperlipidemia.
- Low intake of water, approximately 500 mL – 1 L / day.
- Take pulses along with cereals to improve the quality of protein.
- Potassium rich foods like carrots, potatos, onion, spinach can be given.
- Due to chances of calcium deficiency curd and milk can also be given.
- Pulses should be taken in sufficient amount.

8. TO PLAN A DAY'S DIET FOR A WOMAN, 43 YEARS OLD SUFFERING FROM ACUTE RENAL FAILURE

Personal Data

Age: 43 years

Gender: Female

Recommended Dietary Allowance

Energy: 2006 kcal/day

Protein: 60/day

Carbohydrates: 60%E

Fats: 15-25%E

Dietary Modifications

Energy: 2100 kcal/day

Protein: 60 g/day

Carbohydrates: 315 g/day

Fat: 46 g/day

Food Exchange List

Food exchange	Number of exchange	Energy (kcal)	Protein (g)	Carbohydrate (g)	Fat (g)
Milk	1	340	8	12	10
Pulse	3	300	17	51	-
Cereal	11	770	24	165	-
Veg. A	3	60	3	10.5	-
Veg. B	2	80	4	14	-
Fruit	2	90	-	20	-
Fat	8	360	-	-	40
Sugar	8	160	-	40	-

Exchange Distribution

Exchange	Total no.	Early morning	Break-fast	Mid morning	Lunch	Evening snacks	Dinner
Milk	1		0.4		0.2	0.2	0.2
Pulse	3		1		1		1
Cereal	11	1	2	2	2	2	2
Veg. A	3	1			1		1
Veg. B	2	½	½		½		½

Fruit	1					1	
Fat	8	1	2		2	1	2
Sugar	8	1		2	2	2	1

Diet Plan

Meal	Food item	Amount	Menu	Energy (kcal)	Protein (g)	Carbohydrate (g)	Fat (g)
Early morning (8:00 am)	Ragi	20 g (1 in no.)	Ragi cheela	64	1.4	13.35	Neg.
	+	+					
	Butter	1 tbsp		45	-	-	5
	Apricot	1 medium		50		5	
	Cucumber		Salad	20	1	3.5	Neg.
	+	1 medium					
	Carrot			30	2	7	Neg.
	Lemon and Honey	1 tbsp	Lemon and honey water	19	-	5	-
Breakfast (10:00 am)	Milk	150 mL	Coffee/tea	91.54	5.6	7	4.5
	Green gram	1 katori (30 g) raw wt.	Sprouts	100	7	17	Neg.
	Egg whole	1	Boiled egg	97	7	-	7
	Vermicelli	2 katori	Onion vermicelli	199.6	6	10.4	Neg.
	+						
	Butter	2 tbsp		90	-	-	10
	+						
	Onion	½ katori		6.89	Neg.	Neg.	Neg.
Mid-morning (12 noon)	Wheat flour	2 paratha	Sweet paratha	64	2.1	12	Neg.
	+						
	Sugar	2 tbsp		40	-	10	-
	Puff. rice	40 g	Puff. rice	130	3	30	Neg.
Lunch (2:00 pm)	Curd	100 g	Sweet curd	60	2	2.98	3.99
	+						
	Sugar	2 tbsp		40	-	10	-
	Lobia	25 g (1 katori)	Lobia	80	5.3	13.4	Neg
	+						
	Tomato	25 g		4.7	Neg.	Neg.	Neg.
	+						
	Onion	25 g		6.89	Neg.	Neg.	Neg.

	Wheat flour + Butter	40 g (2 chapati) 2 tbsp	Chapati	128 90	4.2 -	25.6 -	Neg 10
Evening snacks (5:00 pm)	Milk + Sugar	50 g 1 tbsp	Tea/coffee	30.51 20	1.86 -	2.33 5	1.5
	Wheat flour + Sugar	2 paratha 1 tbsp	Sweet paratha	128 20	4.2 -	24 5	Neg. -
Dinner (8:00 pm)	Wheat flour + cauliflower + Onion + Butter	20 g 50 g 25g 2 tbsp	Cauliflower and onion paratha	64 48 6.89 90	2.1 Neg. Neg. -	12 11.3 Neg. -	Neg. Neg. Neg
	Curd	100 g	Apple curd	60	2	2.98	3.99
	Apple	1 medium		43	-	10	-
	Green Gram	1 katori (30 g) raw wt.	Steamed Sprouts	100	7	17	Neg.
Total				2070	56	318	45.98

Important Points

- Water intake to be reduced to 500 L/day
- Food to be avoided:
  - ◊ Protein concentrates
  - ◊ Eggs
  - ◊ Meat
  - ◊ Junk foods
  - ◊ Bakery products
  - ◊ Potato
- Rice, sago, vermicelli, suji, oats can be included in diet.
- Intake of pulses should be reduced

QUESTIONS

1. Define acute kidney failure. Give its etiology, symptoms, risk factors associated, prevention and management.
2. Differentiate between acute and chronic kidney failure.
3. What is nephrotic syndrome? Give management and prevention of the disease.
4. Discuss about dietary management of glomerulonephritis along with causes, symptoms and complications related to it.
5. Define dialysis. Discuss about different types and their procedures.
6. Write short notes on:
   (i) Renal calculi
   (ii) Acute kidney failure
   (iii) Chronic kidney failure
   (iv) Nephrotic syndrome
7. Differentiate between haemodialysis and peritoneal dialysis.
8. What is the importance of water and electrolyte balance in kidney diseases?
9. Plan a day's diet for a male patient of 10 years suffering from nephrotic syndrome.
10. Plan a day's diet of a 70 years old patient of chronic kidney failure undergoing haemodialysis.

7

Liver Disorders

7.1 CIRRHOSIS

Liver is composed of hepatocytes or hepatic cells and is located in the right upper quadrant of the abdomen just below the diaphragm. Hepatic cells regulate the synthesis and breakdown of small and complex molecules. Liver synthesizes proteins, detoxifies different metabolites and produces different biochemicals necessary for digestion of different components. It also helps in the metabolism of carbohydrates, proteins and lipids.

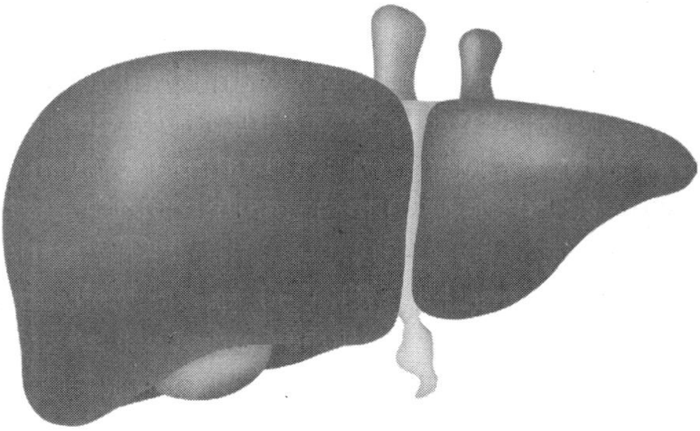

Decomposition of RBCs (red blood cells), production of hormones and regulation of body store of glycogen are its other functions; and is only found in vertebrates. Other functions of liver include production of bile, which is stored in gall bladder. When normal hepatic cells don't function properly and are replaced by scar tissue then this condition is termed cirrhosis. There are many manifestations of cirrhosis which arises either due to failure of hepatic cells or resultant portal hypertension (high blood pressure in hepatic portal vein). It occurs slowly and gradually over a period of time. Generally, it is well advanced before the appearance of clinical signs and symptoms. Initially, there are no visible symptoms of the disease but with time a person may become weak, tired, itchy, and swelling in the lower legs is generally seen.

Cirrhosis is the disease of the human liver. In cirrhosis the liver tissue is replaced by a scar tissue and fibrosis. The scar tissue prevents blood and the bile from flowing through the liver which leads to a loss of function in the liver. Cirrhosis is caused mostly by alcoholism, hepatitis B or hepatitis C. Ascites is the most common complication for cirrhosis. Cirrhosis is defined as the histological development of regenerative nodules which are surrounded by fibrous bands in response to chronic injury to the liver, which leads to portal hypertension and end stage liver disease.

7.1.1 Signs and Symptoms

Symptoms of liver cirrhosis include fever, nausea and vomiting, diarrhoea, anorexia, vague right upper quadrant pain, weight loss, loss of appetite, broken blood vessels, jaundice, ascites, redness of the palms of the hands (Palmer Erythema), oedema, spider angiomas, parotid gland enlargement, digital clubbing, muscle wasting, decreased body hair in men, menstrual irregularities in women, variceal hemorrhage.

7.1.1.1 Jaundice

A person may develop yellow skin, spider-like blood vessels on the skin and fluid buildup in the abdomen. Hepatic encephalopathy, bleeding from dilated veins in stomach or oesophagus and liver cancer are other severe complications. First signs and symptoms are not easily seen in this disease, but some people may develop initial signs like bruising or bleeding, sensitivity to medicines, acute kidney injury (also known as acute renal failure, loss of kidney function), and may even develop into hepatic encephalopathy (varying levels of consciousness due to liver failure). Enlarged or shrunken liver, gynecomastia (increase in breast gland size of men, and is non-cancerous), spider angiomata (vascular lesions of arteriole), hypogomadism (decrease in male sex hormones), palmar erthema (reddening of palms), fetor hepaticus (musty odour breath), ascites (accumulation of fluid in peritoneal cavity) and jaundice (yellowing of skin and sclera of eyes) are the direct consequences of improper functioning of hepatic cells. Cirrhosis due to portal hypertension develops oesophageal varices (enlargement of blood vessels in stomach and oesophagus), splenomegaly (increased size of spleen), Cruveilhier-Baumgarten murmur (humming sound heard on examination) and caput medusa (dilated periumbilical collateral veins). Liver is enlarged initially, but decreases in size with the progression of disease. Surface being irregular, firm consistency and discolouration (yellow colouration) is seen. Cirrhosis is characterized by the presence of either regenerating nodules of hepatocytes or fibrosis (deposition of connective cells).

Cirrhosis on the basis of size of nodules is categorized into three: micro-nodular, macro-nodular and mixed cirrhosis. Micro-nodular form is also known as Laennec's cirrhosis or portal cirrhosis; in this the nodules are less than 3 mm. On the other hand, in macro-nodular, nodules are larger than 3 mm. Nodules in mixed cirrhosis are of varying size. Cirrhosis is also classified on the basis of cause-specific abnormalities. Cardiac cirrhosis (one in which there are erythrocytes and more amount of fibrosis around tissues surrounding hepatic veins.), primary biliary cholangitis (also known as primary biliary cirrhosis, autoimmune disorder of liver leading to fibrosis around the bile duct.), alcoholic cirrhosis (due to excess of alcohol). It is diagnosed by liver biopsy. But is best predicted by ascites, spider angiomata, platelet count $<160{,}000/mm^3$, and a Bonacini cirrhosis discriminant score greater than 7. The severity of cirrhosis is generally given by Child-Pugh score. It uses bilirubin, albumin, INR and presence of ascites.

7.1.2 Background and Causes of Cirrhosis

Globally, cirrhosis leads to 2 million deaths per year; making it 11th top most cause of death. Cirrhotic liver has found its way into many families because of the extensive addiction of alcoholic beverages and increased hepatitis infection. But, the exact global estimation of the disease is still not found. From the estimates given by WHO in May 2014, 216,865 people in India died due to the deadly liver disease, which is about 2.44 per cent of the total deaths. Within the total population of India, 39.5 and 19.6 per cent males and females respectively, were having cirrhotic liver in 2012; making India stand on the position of 61st on the cirrhotic liver death rates globally. From the report of WHO, 780,000 people are affected with cirrhotic consequences of hepatitis B, irrespective of type. 170 million of the population is the carrier of cirrhosis, who are at the risk of developing full-fledged disease. 3 per cent of the total population is affected with Hepatitis C virus infections.

7.1.3 Alcohol

Alcoholic cirrhosis develops for 10-20% of individuals who drink heavily for a decade or more. Excessive chronic alcohol use can cause several different types of chronic liver disease, including alcoholic cirrhosis. Chronic alcohol use can produce fibrosis in the absence of inflammation or necrosis. Fibrosis can be central lobular, per cellular or per portal. Women are more affected to alcohol related liver disease with shorter durations and doses of chronic consumptions. Because in women lesser amount of alcohol dehydrogenase secreted in the gut which raises the proportion of body fat in women and changes the fat absorption due to menstrual cycle.

Reason behind the development of liver cirrhosis because of alcohol is formation of fibrosis because of the action of pro-inflammatory cytokines like TNF-alpha, interleukin-6 & 8, oxidative stress, lipid per oxidation and acetaldehyde. Acetaldehyde stimulates hepatic stellate cells for the collagen deposition. Other factors cause inflammation, apoptosis and ultimately occurrence of fibrotic liver cells.Further, NADPH oxidase and P-4502E1 contribute to the formation of oxidants. Formation of oxidants along with the acetaldehyde protein adducts damage the cell membrane. These factors cause inflammation, apoptosis and eventually fibrosis of the liver cells. The liver has tremendous capacity to regenerate and even when 75% of hepatocytes are dead, it continues to function as normal. Alcohol is the leading cause of cirrhosis in the US; 14 million cases of alcohol abuse were reported in the US.

Alcoholism can cause either fibrosis (in the absence of inflammation) or necrosis. From another research, it was found that alcoholic hepatitis leads to the development of cirrhosis in 20 percent of the cases.

7.1.4 Hepatitis

Liver cirrhosis is also caused by hepatitis B. People who are affected due to hepatitis B also developed cirrhosis. In US 2 million people are carriers of hepatitis B, whereas in other parts of the world hepatitis B virus (HBV) is endemic (i.e., Asia, Southeast Asia, and sub-Saharan Africa). Thus, over 300-400 million people are affected due to hepatitis B. Up to 40% patients who are affected with chronic hepatitis B virus infection develop serious complications during their lifetime. Up to 12% of patients with HBV cirrhosis die of liver failure and up to 10% perish from liver cancer. Cirrhosis is most commonly caused by alcohol, hepatitis B, hepatitis C, non-alcoholic fatty liver disease, autoimmune hepatitis and Wilson's disease. Causes of non-alcoholic fatty liver disease include overweight, diabetes, high blood fats and high blood pressure. Liver cirrhosis has many possible causes sometimes more than one cause is present in the same person.

Hepatitis C is a liver disease caused by hepatitis C virus (HCV). It is a blood-borne virus and the most common mode of infection is through unsafe injection practices, inadequate sterilization of medical equipment, and the transfusion of unscreened blood and blood products. Globally, 130-150 million people have chronic hepatitis C virus (HCV) infection. And the people who are affected to hepatitis C develop gradually liver cirrhosis. Approximately 700,000 people die each year from hepatitis C related liver disease. Hepatitis C virus (HCV) causes both acute and chronic infection. Acute HCV infection is generally asymptomatic and it is rarely associated with life threatening disease, in about 15-45% of patients the defence system spontaneously clears the virus within 6 months of infection without any treatment. 55-85% people develop chronic HCV infection. The people, who are affected with chronic HCV infection, will develop the risk of cirrhosis of liver between 15-30% within 20 years. Hepatitis C is found worldwide. The people who live in regions of Africa and Central and East Asia are more affected due to hepatitis C. hepatitis C virus is a blood borne virus. Hepatitis C virus (HCV) can also be transmitted through sexually and can be passed from an infected mother to her baby, but these modes of transmission are much less common. The hepatitis B virus causes liver inflammation and injury that can lead to cirrhosis after several years. Chronic hepatitis B virus (HBV) infection is a major global public health problem which results in 1 million deaths per year of individuals worldwide, liver failure and hapatocellular cancer (HCC).

The early phase of hepatitis B virus infection is asymptomatic with active virus replication and very little liver necro inflammation. In this phase hepatitis B antigen (HBeAg) is present; this phase is also known as immune tolerant phase. The immune tolerant phase lasts for several years before the appearance of hepatitis symptoms. In the immune tolerant phase the immune elimination of HBV takes place. During this phase the levels of HBV DNA are decreased and the sero conversion from HBeAg to HBe antibody (anti-HBe) takes place complications like jaundice, ascites, hepatic encephalopathy (HE). Other causes of cirrhosis include autoimmune hepatitis and non-alcoholic fatty liver. Patient who is suffering from autoimmune hepatitis will not be able to take the immunosuppressive therapy with glucocorticoids or azathioprine. In this situation, liver biopsy does not show a significant inflammatory infiltrate. Diagnosis in this case requires positive autoimmune markers such as anti-nuclear antibody (ANA) or anti-smooth muscle antibody (ASMA). Patient, who is suffering from autoimmune hepatitis with cirrhosis and active inflammation accompanied by elevated liver enzymes, is able to take the immunosuppressive therapy. People who are affected with non-steato hepatitis also develop cirrhosis.

Alcoholic cirrhosis caused 40% of the total deaths in US. 80% of the total cases of hepatitis C virus developed into chronic cirrhosis. 170 million people of the total population of Egypt are affected because of the hepatitis C. Both macro and micro-nodular cirrhosis are seen in the patients who develop cirrhosis as a consequence of hepatitis C viral infection. Along with hepatitis C infection, hepatitis B infection also contributes to the development of cirrhotic liver. 40 per cent people with hepatitis B infection develop complications of liver cirrhosis, 10 percent develop liver cancer, while 12 per cent die because of the liver failure. The rate of survival for the

HBV patient is negligible, with a life expectancy of maximum 5 years. About 62%, 98% and 80% population of China, sub-Saharan Africa and Pacific Islands are subjected to the viral hepatitis B infection. Chronic hepatitis B affects an estimated population of 350 million, among which 75 per cent is native to Asia and 12 per cent resides in Africa. Most common reasons behind the high rate of prevalence are alcohol, hepatitis C, hepatitis B, autoimmune hepatitis, non-alcoholic fatty liver and Wilson's disease. Non-alcoholic fatty liver is a result of obesity, hypercholesterolemia (high blood cholesterol levels, diabetes and hypertension. Generally, it is observed that two or more than two complications are present there to cause cirrhosis. Hard core alcohol drinkers develop alcoholic cirrhosis over a decade or so; the rate of alcoholic cirrhosis is 10-20 per cent.

Complications like portal hypertension, ascites, coagulation disorders, hepatic encephalopathy and hepato-renal syndrome are seen with last stage cirrhosis or hepatic failure. Initially, steatosis or fatty liver develops because of the excessive alcoholism. If alcohol intake is reduced and dietary modifications are done, then the fatty liver can be cured. From a study conducted on the alcohol intake by both the men and women was conducted, and its side-effects were studied. From the results, it was concluded that, intake of 75-100 mL/day and 25 mL/day alcohol for 20 years or more by, men and women respectively, increases the chances of getting cirrhosis by 7-47%. From another study conducted in Russia, it was found that with 1 litre increase in the overall alcohol consumption, there is an increase of liver cirrhotic mortality rate by 7.0% and 6.2% in men and women respectively. From the analysis of results, the death rates in men and women were found to be 61.4% and 56.4% respectively One of the other leading causes of cirrhosis is hepatitis C virus, with death rate of 700,000 per year. 15-30% cases of hepatitis C infection upgrade themselves in cirrhosis over a span of 20 years. Hepatitis B virus also progresses to cirrhosis, with a global death rate of 1 million per year. Progression of hepatitis B infection into cirrhosis can be explained by the duration of the immune tolerant phase of hepatitis B. More the duration of this phase, more are the chances of getting cirrhotic liver. Immune tolerant phase is the presence of HBeAg (hepatitis B antigen). This phase generally lasts for several years; in this phase, reduction in the levels of HBV DNA takes place, and conversion to HBe antibody takes place. Ascites, jaundice and hepatic encephalopathy are the common complications. Another reason for the development of this liver disorder is Wilson's disease. Wilson's disease is a rare autosomal recessive disorder, affecting 1 in 30,000 individuals. In this disease, there is copper buildup in different organs especially liver and brain. Process of excretion of excess copper in bile is impaired. Symptoms generally occur during childhood and teenage. If untreated, scarring of the liver tissue takes place and finally leading to the development of cirrhosis.Cirrhosis just like other diseases runs in genes, with a family history the chances of getting the disease is increased by 12%.

7.1.5 Wilson's Disease

Wilson's disease is a condition where too much copper builds up in the body, mainly in the liver and brain. Wilson's disease is a rare inherited disorder that affects about 1 in 30,000 people. In this disease a particular gene on chromosome 13 does not work. The gene normally controls the way of liver cells to get rid of excess copper. Normally, the liver cells pass out excess copper into the bile. If this process does not work properly then the copper builds up in liver cells. When the copper storage capacity is exceeded, the copper flows into the bloodstream and gets deposited in other parts of the body, mainly in the brain. Symptoms of Wilson's disease start developing between the age of 6 and 20, most commonly in the teenage years. Symptoms of liver problems develop first. The toxic effect on liver cells causes the inflammation of the liver. And if the disease is left untreated the damaged liver cells starts developing scarring of the liver which causes liver cirrhosis. The deposition of copper in the brain can cause symptoms like depression, difficulty with speech, headache, mood swings, seizures, dementia, severe rigidity, inability to concentrate, muscular weakness, etc. Copper may develop in the layer at the front of the eye (called the cornea). This causes a characteristic feature called Keyser-Fleischer rings, a brownish pigmentation of the cornea. Liver cirrhosis is a chronic condition that is not possible to heal. Wilson's disease can be diagnosed by various tests like blood test, urine test. Blood test is done to measure caeruloplasmin. Caeruloplasmin is a protein that binds copper in the bloodstream. The level of this protein is low in people who are affected with Wilson's disease. This test is done to measure the copper levels and the test of liver function. Urine test is done to measure the amount of copper in the urine. The amount is typically higher than normal. Liver biopsy is done to diagnose the cirrhosis of the liver. In liver biopsy a small sample (biopsy) of the liver is taken to look under the microscope. This shows the toxicity of copper in the liver and the extent of any scarring of the liver cirrhosis (Aggarwal A, Bhatt M, 2013). The diagnosis of alcoholic cirrhosis is liver biopsy, which needs to be maintained for at least 6 months to determine residual, non-reversible disease. In patients who are suffering from cirrhosis and who continue to drink, there is a <50% 5 year survival. In these cases liver transplantation is the only option.

Treatment of the patients with cirrhosis due to Wilson's disease includes the use of medicines like penicillamine, trientine, zinc, etc. Penicillamine is a medicine which removes the copper from the body. Due to the penicillamine the excess of copper from the body passes out in the urine. When the excess of copper from the urine is cleared from the body, then the dose is reduced and maintained for a year. Trientine is an alternative to penicillamine. It is a chelating agent and removes copper from the body. Zinc absorbs the copper from food by blocking the gut. Therefore, it does not remove excess copper from the body but it can prevent any further buildup of copper. It is recommended for the people who are diagnosed at early stage of the disease and have no symptoms. People who did not follow the treatment with medication will develop the late stage of liver cirrhosis, after which the liver transplantation is the only option. Although there is no cure for cirrhosis of the liver, there are treatments available that can stop or delay its progress, minimize the damage to liver cells and reduce complications.

7.1.6 Dietary Management

Though there is no cure for the deadly disease, but with dietary modifications and lifestyle changes, life expectancy can be increased. Complications like malnutrition, ascites, glucose intolerance, hepatorenal syndrome and hepatic encephalopathy occurs. The ill effects can be reduced by dietary management.

Energy: A close check on all the nutrients should be kept. The energy intake of the person is increased by 120-140%. If the complications are severe, energy intake is increased up to 150-175%. Per day calorie requirement is around 25-35 kcal per kg body weight per day. Energy requirement for patients who is affected from liver cirrhosis is about 120% to 140%. 150-175% of increased energy is recommended for the patient who is suffering from ascites, infection or malabsorption. 25 to 35 calories per kilogram body weight is recommended to the liver cirrhotic patients. Oral nutritional supplement or tube feeding is effective for the malnourished patients.

Carbohydrates: Carbohydrates should be the main source of energy. 1 gm each of carbohydrate, protein and fat provide 4, 4 and 9 kcal of energy respectively. Carbohydrate-rich diet is prescribed. Foods rich in carbohydrates like fruits, sugar, sweets, milk, vegetables, bread and potatoes should be given. Carbohydrate intake should be around 350 gm or more depending upon the condition. More of carbohydrates are given for meeting the energy demands as well as protein sparing action. Diet rich in fibre is advised; fibre not more than 35 gm should be given as it gives the feeling of satiety and patient refuses to eat. Carbohydrates are the main source of energy for the body. 1 gm of carbohydrates provides the body with 4 kcal foods that are rich in carbohydrates include sugar, sweets, fruit, bread, flour, potatoes, milk and vegetables. High carbohydrate diet is recommended to provide energy in the liver cirrhotic patients.

Proteins: Protein intake should not be more than 0.8 gm per kg body weight. From research, it has been found that mortality rate decreases with the increase in protein intake. The protein intake in hepatitis or cirrhosis is between the ranges of 0.8-1 gm per kg body weight. While, in case of sepsis, ascites, or alcoholic hepatitis, the required intake of protein is 1.5 gm per kg body weight. In alcoholic hepatitis or decompensate disease such as sepsis, infection, ascites, at least 1.5 gm of protein per kg/day should be recommended.

Fats: Implication of high fat intake, saturated fats and PUFA to the patient is done. Fat should contribute about 25-40% of the total calories. More of unsaturated fats from sources like avocado, olive oil, nuts, and vegetable oil. Coconut oil is better tolerated. Omega-3 fatty acids are given. In cirrhosis plasma-free fatty acids, glycerol and ketone bodies are increased in the fasting state. A range of 25% to 40% calories as fat should be given to the cirrhotic patients. High intake of total fat, saturated fat, and polyunsaturated fat is implicated to the patients

Vitamins and minerals: Vitamin and mineral deficiencies are very common in cirrhosis. Proper supplementation should be done. Fat soluble vitamins should not be given in excess, because of toxicity. Vitamins like A, C, D, E, K, thiamine, niacin, B12, riboflavin, folate and pyridoxine should be administered. Because of the oedema and ascites, sodium intake is restricted. Sodium not more than 2000 mg should be given. Other minerals like selenium and magnesium should also be administered. Proper check of fluid intake is done because of the presence of ascites. Feeding can either be oral or tube feeding. Small and frequent meals should be given. Foods included are sugar, potato, bread, vegetables, fruits, milk, sweets, avocados, berries, coconut, figs, green peas, turnips, beans, nuts and seeds. Foods to be avoided include high sodium food, packed food, canned soups, non-vegetarian food, snacks, alcohol and fried food. Careful monitoring should be done in maintaining the electrolyte and fluid balance. High fibre diet is recommended for the liver cirrhotic patients. High fibre foods include avocados, pears, berries, coconut, figs, artichokes, green peas, okra, turnips, beans and legumes, flaxseeds, chia seeds, etc.

7.1.7 Role of Herbs

Apart from diet, herbs also help in reducing the complications of the disease and help in early recovery. One such herb is *Silybum marianum*.

7.1.7.1 *Silybum marianum*

Silybum marianum is being used extensively for its pharmacological benefits in the treatment of various diseases like liver disorders, supportive treatment in cases of mushroom poisoning, cancer prevention and treatment, and is also known as milk thistle. It belongs to family of Asteraceae. Commonly it is also called from the names like cardusmarianus, blessed milk thistle, mary thistle, Mediterranean milk thistle and scotch thistle.

From a study, it has been found that milk thistle helps in the treatment of fatty liver, hepatitis, cirrhosis, radiation toxicity and ischemic injury. It helps because of antioxidant, anti-lipid peroxidative, anti-inflammatory, immunomodulatory, anti-fibrotic and liver regeneration properties. All these hepato-protective properties come from the mixture of flavonolignans, silibinin, silychristin and silydianin; combined to form silymarin.

Silymarin supports the production of hepatic glutathione and helps against cellular damage. From a review, it was found that large doses of the herb have therapeutic activity. It helps in the treatment of cirrhosis, has hepato-protective, anticarcinogenic, antioxidant and immunomodulatory properties. No side-effects of the herbs are reported. Though headache, heart burn and upset stomach are the complications reported because of the laxative effect of the herb.

The most common and difficult to handle myth about the liver disease is that there is complete restriction of dietary fat and protein intake in diet which is in contrast to the actual dietary advices for the patients. Hence, we should always recommend the patients to take high protein and fat rich diet with less amount of salt and fluid.

CASE STUDIES

1. TO PLAN A DAY'S DIET FOR A MAN, 40 YEARS OLD SUFFERING FROM CIRRHOSIS AND OBESITY

Nutrition plays a vital role in the management of patients with cirrohosis and obesity. Diet is an important part of the treatment plan, along with medications. The diet must provide enough calories to ensure that muscles are not wasted alpng with decreasing the fat stores. This becomes a challenge as most patients have very poor appetite. Depending upon the condition, restriction is to be done.

General Instructions

- Weight should be brought around expected ideal weight.
- Regular exercise should be integral part of daily routine.

- Eat plenty of vegetable protein like beans.
- Take 400 mg to 800 mg of vitamin E.
- Fat intake should not exceed 20 gm per day.
- High fibre diet should be consumed.
- Eat lots of fruits and vegetables but remember the salt limit.

Foods Allowed

- High fibre foods like whole cereals, whole pulses, sprouts and fruits.
- Low fat substitutes like skimmed milk, curd.
- Foods rich in soluble fibre like curry leaves, methi leaves.

Foods to be Avoided

- eliminate alcohol
- refined cereals like suji, maida
- eliminate all high fructose corn syrup
- eliminate most sodium — the goal 1500 mg of salt.
- eliminate all added dietary sugar
- whole milk and its products
- deep fried foods
- bakery products as they contain baking soda

To make your food palatable use spices like cardamom, cinemon, lemon juice, etc.

Dietary Allowances

Energy: 1400 kcal
CHO: 250 gm
Protein: 55 gm
Fat: 25 gm

Food Exchange List

Servings	No. of servings	Energy (kcal)	Cho (gm)	Proteins (gm)	Fats (gm)
Cereals	5	500	100	18	2
Pulses	2	200	50	12	2
Meats	1	150	--	17	7
Vegetables	4	130	40	4	1
Fruits	4	160	40	--	--
Milk and products	2	140	20	6	4
Fats and oils	2	90	--	--	10
Total		1370	250	57	26

Servings	Early morning	Breakfast	Mid-morning	Lunch	Evening snack	Dinner	Bed time
Cereals	2			1		2	
Pulses				1		1	
Meats				1			
Vegetables		1		2		2	
Fruits		2	2				
Milk and products		1					1
Fats and oils				1		1	
Sugars							

Timing	Menu	Amount (G)	Energy (kcal)	Cho (G)	Protein (G)	Fats (G)
Early morning	Jeera water	200 mL	--	--	--	--
Breakfast	Blueberry milk shake + oats and besan cheela (2 pc)	120 g + 200 mL + 60 g	390	70	11	6
Mid-morning	Fruit	100 g	40	10		
Lunch	Salad + 1 chapati + vegetable + lean chicken curry	100 g + 30 g + 100 g + 50 g	370	85	29	7
Evening snacks	Tea + roasted makhana	150 mL + 35 g	100	20	2.5	
Dinner	2 chapati + dal + vegetables	50 g + 35 g + 100 g	390	75	12	5
Bedtime	Milk (with pinch of turmeric)	250 mL	90	10	3	6

2. TO PLAN A DAY'S DIET FOR A MAN, 55 YEARS OLD SUFFERING FROM HEPATITIS AND ASCITES

Nutrition plays a vital role in the management of patients with Hepatitis and ascitis. Diet is an important part of the treatment plan, along with medications. The diet must provide enough calories to ensure proper functioning and repair of body and organ tissues. This becomes a challenge as most patients have very poor appetite. Depending upon the condition, restriction is to be done.

General Instructions

- Weight should be maintained along expected ideal weight.
- Regular light exercise should be integral part of daily routine.
- Water intake is restricted depending on the stage of ascites, generally between (1.5-2 L/day).

- Fat intake should not exceed 20 gm per day.
- Moderate protein diet should be consumed.
- Slight lift in carbohydrate content in the diet.
- Salt intake is generally restricted to 2 g/day.

Foods Allowed

- Green leafy vegetables (broccoli, cauliflower), kale, beans, fruits in moderation
- Freshly made vegetable juices, curd
- Foods rich in whole grains
- Lean meats and fish

Foods to be Avoided

- refined cereals like suji, maida
- whole milk and its products
- deep fried foods
- bakery products as they contain baking soda, maida
- Wheat products (rich in gluten)
- Packed fruit juices

To make your food palatable use spices like cardamom, cinnamon, lemon juice, etc.

Dietary Allowances

Energy: 1600 kcal

CHO: 300 gm

Protein: 70 gm

Fat: 20 gm

Food Exchange List

Servings	Servings	Energy (kcal)	Cho (gm)	Proteins (gm)	Fats (gm)
Cereals	6	600	120	13	1
Pulses	3	300	70	18	--
Fish and meat products	2	230	--	35	6
Vegetables	4	120	40	4	--
Fruits	4	160	40	--	--
Nuts	1	81	2	3	4
Fats and oils	2	90	--	--	10
Total		1581	272	73	21

Servings	Early morning	Breakfast	Mid morning	Lunch	Evening snack	Dinner	Bed time
Cereals		1		2	1	2	
Pulses			1	1		1	
Fish and meat products				1		1	
Vegetables		1		2	1		
Fruits		1	2			1	
Nuts							1
Fats and oils				1		1	
Sugars							

Diet Chart

Timing	Menu	Amount (g)	Energy (kcal)	Cho (g)	Protein (g)	Fats (g)
Early morning	Black tea	150 mL	80	--	--	--
Breakfast	Oats khichri (70% vegies and 30% oats) + fruit	30 g + 100 g + 100 g	210	50	4	--
Mid-morning	Sprouts and fruit salad	30 g + 160 g	140	33	6	
Lunch	Brown rice + Fish curry + vegetable	25 g + 40 g + 100 g	410	80	27	12
Evening snacks	Tea + Quinoa vegetable chat	150 mL + 25 g + 100 g	210	30	3	
Dinner	Steamed Chicken Biryani (less oil) + Nav ratna dal +fruit	60 g + 50 g + 30 g 80 g	430	76	23	9
Bedtime	4 almonds	30 g	81	2	3	4

QUESTIONS

1. Discuss about different liver disorders, along with their etiology and management.
2. Define liver cirrhosis. Give its causes, symptoms and dietary management.
3. Define hepatitis. Discuss about different types of hepatitis.
4. What is acute viral hepatitis? Discuss about its causes, symptoms and dietary management.
5. What is alcoholic hepatitis?

6. Discuss about the symptoms, causes and management of Wilson's disease.
7. Plan a day's diet for a male patient of 45 years suffering from alcoholic hepatitis.
8. Plan a day's diet for female patient of 38 years suffering from liver cirrhosis.
9. Diffrentiate between acute viral hepatitis and alcoholic hepatitis.
10. Write short notes on:
    (i) Liver cirrhosis
    (ii) Hepatitis B
    (iii) Alcoholic hepatitis
    (iv) Wilson's disease

8

Inborn Errors of Metabolism

8.1 PHENYLKETONURIA

Inborn errors actually mean birth defects in the newborn. The explanation for IEM is mutations in which the gene of the person is a code for an enzyme resultant in the synthesis of defective enzyme activity in the body. This enzyme activity can affect reciprocally to the effects of the traditional function of a metabolic pathway.

Phenylketonuria is a genetic disorder that results in reduced metabolism through the amino acid as phenylalanine. Protein is a very essential nutrient for our human body. In the diet, high protein is found in the dairy products, pulses and legumes, and meat products. It has many functions, which help to maintain the body like repairing cells and tissues, growth and many more. When protein is taken or eaten then it breaks down with the help of enzymes present in the body and makes the amino acid. Phenylketonuria is the inherited metabolic disorder of phenylalanine metabolism. When the phenylalanine increases and flows in the bloodstream in the human body then it affects the functioning of the body.

Phenylketonuria causes to changes on the pattern of behavior, intellectual disability, mental disorders and seizures. It can also cause a musty smell and lighter skin. It is an autosomal recessive genetic condition which means the deficiency in the enzyme phenylalanine hydroxylase (PHA). The enzyme is very essential for the body to metabolize the amino acid (protein) phenylalanine (Phe). When the enzyme phenylalanine hydroxylase is absent then conversion of phenylalanine to make tyrosine (amino acid) does not form in the human abody. Then phenylalanine hydroxylase is lacking then the phenylalanine accumulates and converts into phenylpyruvate (another name of phenylpyruvate is phenyl ketone). This was detected in the test of urine. The normal range in blood of phenylalanine level is about 1 mg/dL in the human body.

8.1.1 Stages of Phenylketonuria

Phenylalanine and special supplements are used to treat the phenylketonuria as they are low foods. Newborn babies are recommended to be fed by the special technique and little quantity of breast milk. From the help of the diagnostic Phe level mutation testing which is performed in the medical field can categorise the different stages of PKU and explain the amount of phenylalanine that can be tolerated by the patient. The condition of PKU patient can be understood by mild to the severe while seeing the signs and symptoms of patient.

First stage: Infants suffering classic PKU disorder that can be shown after a few months. Without checking or not taking treatment of PKU, then these children develop problem like a permanent intellectual disability, delayed development, behavioural problems, seizures and psychiatric disorders. The test is done in laboratory that shows the phenylalanine concentration in blood. It is more at 20 mg/dL (>1200 µmol/L) in the babies.

Second stage: The second stage is "moderate or mild PKU". The Phe levels rises then the proper treatment is required. It is more than 6 mg/dL but it is lower than 20 mg/dL (360-1200 µmol/L).

Third stage: The third stage is "Hyperphenylalanemia" (HyperPhe). This term is used to that patient in which phenylanine concentration increased more than the normal level. Nevertheless, it can be handled by the dietary management because it is still less enough to control. Moreover, in the third stage the Phe level in blood is less than 6 mg/dL (<360 µmol/L).

8.1.2 Variations of PKU in Accordance with Severity

They are of two types:

1. **Classical PKU:** Classic PKU is the most severe kind of disorder in which the enzyme is converted into phenylalanine and is severely reduced which lowers the levels of phenylalanine and causes damage.
2. The deficiency of PAH causes patterns of diseases, which includes phenylketonuria and mild hyperphenylalaninemia, thalassemia accumulation of levels are still high than in general people having normal pH of phenylalanine. People who face "hyper phe" suffer from pulmonary arterial hypertension that are prone to handle a big quantity of phenylalanine as compared to those having classical PKU, but a person faces the problems for blood levels which are high by Phe and they are with typical PAH.

- In mild or moderate forms of PKU some functions of enzyme are retained, so phenylalanine levels are not as high and they result in the smaller risk of brain damages.

8.1.3 Metabolic Pathway

Pathophysiology of phenylketonuria is caused by phenylalanine hydroxylase enzyme, a functional enzyme that is absent. Amino acid phenylalanine is converted into amino acid by enzyme phenylalanine hydroxylase. Phenylalanine accumulates in case where the phenylalanine hydroxylase enzyme is absent. Excessiveness of phenylalanine can be broken down into phenylketones through small pathways that is a transamutespaturay with some of glutamates. Phenylalanine, phenylpyrumate and phenethylanine are included into metabolites. The eminent stages of phenylalnine present in the blood and investigated by the phenylketons in the discharge of a patient then it is diagnostic and patients are checked through newborn screen.

8.1.4 Development of Phenylketonuria

Genes are transferred from the parents. We have two inherited genes–one from female and another from the male body. Genes help in the designing of characteristics of baby like eye and hair colour, height in the teenage time and the gender. In the PKU condition the gene does not work properly. The condition of recessive inherited affects both the males and females equally.

When the baby has both the carriers of recessive gene in the condition of PKU then the chances of increase in the baby body. And it has:

- 25% chances of getting PKU disorder in baby (inheriting two defective genes).
- 50% increase in the chances of being a carrier means child has defective gene, which does not show any symptom of PKU (inheriting one PKU gene and one normal gene).
- 25% is the chance of patient (baby) have the inheriting two normal genes.

The mild forms of PKU in the newborn can, however, go undetected if the mother is discharged very soon or if newborn baby is unable to consume any protein. However, the suffering child who is diagnosed and treated appropriately at birth is less likely to show the symptoms. Long-term care focuses on adhesion to dietary therapy, monitoring of blood Phe and Tyr levels and assessing for the potential cognitive impairment.

Flowchart representing biosynthetic pathway of phenylketonuria

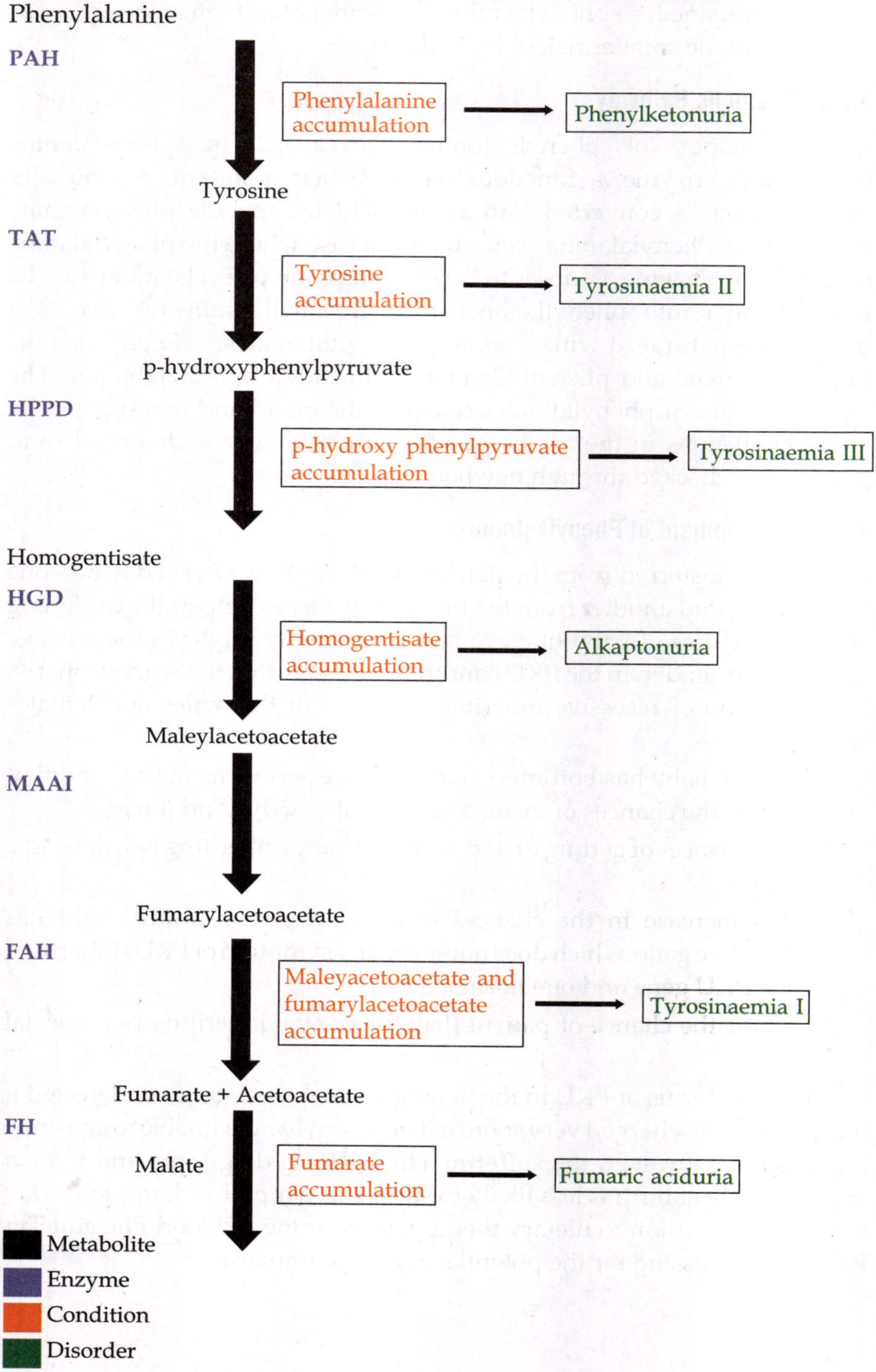

8.1.5 Screening

In order to test phenylketonuria a blood sample is taken from a 2-week old baby. PKU is generally incorporated in the screening tracts for the newborn in many places over the world having various methods to conduct this and find their results. The few drops of blood are taken as a sample from the baby by the nurses or lab technicians to check the heel or the band in your baby arm.

Many in the newborn in advanced countries do early screening of PKU as soon as the baby is boned. Doctor takes needle for lancet to take blood from baby's arm to test the positive or negative for disorder. Screening tests are suggested by the doctor if he has an idea that he or she may be the patient of this disease. The screening is done when the baby is 1-2 day in age and still present in the hospital with the mother.

If it is confirmed about that the baby is suffering from PKU:

- Then the child has to undergo additional test to check about the PKU, which includes the cloting test and faeces discharge test
- Genetic testing is performed for you and your baby to identify the gene mutations.

8.1.6 Symptoms of Phenylketonuria in Infants

The problem of PKU starts showing at the age of 6 months, the signs and symptoms can be seen on the body and how he or she responds to the environment. The body shows symptoms like the jerky movements in arm and leg of baby, eyes and skin lighter due to melanin cannot be synthesized in the body, and is responsible for the lighter skin and hair problems. Moreover, there are other indications also like the small head size of baby, musty body smell seizures, and skin rashes all over the body. And when the baby takes longer time to sit, crawl or walk as compared to other children, show less interest in surroundings like in playing and delay in mental and social skills development,intellectual disabilities and behaviour problems, like being hyperactive baby.

The detailed symptoms which are included in this disorder are following:

- A musty order in urine and skin due to too much presence of phenylalanine in the body.
- The neurological problems always include seizures in joints and rashes in upper body layer
- Small size of head (microcephaly)
- Hyperactivity

- Late development
- Psychiatric disorders
- Behavioural problems and changes, emotional problems and social problems
- Intellectual disability

8.1.7 Pregnancy and PKU

The women suffering from PKU have high risk of another form of disease that is known as maternal PKU. In case the female does not take appropriate diet when a mother is just to a conceiving situation, the level of red clots of phenylalanine are higher and can cause miscarriage or can harm a foetus.

- A women who faces this problem she may face the difficulties during the pregnancy.
- Babies from mothers with higher phenylalanine levels do not often inherit PKU. Women is at a high risk when she faces some difficulties in the cloting levels. The complications may include the following points:
- Low birth weight
- Heart problems and other heart defects
- Development which has been late to be performed
- Problem of size of mini head
- Developmental changes through brain and difficulties
- Disabilities related to intelligence
- Facial abnormalities

8.1.8 Sources of PKU

Abnormal inherited mutations are sources of the phenylketonuria. Some deficiencies which increases the levels of amino acids. There is a risk in making up of phenylalanine which occurs by the consumption of foods which contain more protein like milk, paneer or non-veg food products, and even cereals like bread and pasta or eat different kinds of manmade sweet items. It prepares the acids in deserts which harms the brain cells.

Many difficulties and abnormalities can be seen in the initial period of pregnancy and some kind of brain problems and damages are found.

- Sensational difficulties are found.
- Developmental and social difficulties, emotional problems in the older children and in youngster.
- Some fitness and strength development difficulties.

8.1.9 Treatment or Management of Phenylketonuria

8.1.9.1 Dietary Management

The diet of phenylketonuria is very complicated because it has restriction of phenylalanine. In addition, the options of food are less. There are many barriers regarding to the PKU diet which affect the patient's health, and cause the other harmful effects on the human body. These barriers are explained in below:

- Poor access of treatment of PKU diet. People do not consult the dietician about the food that should be avoided or eaten by the person or child or pregnant women.
- Social functioning of the poor.
- Illiteracy and person have the problem in learning new thing.
- The stability of patient in the living arrangement as if the person is not living with his family or may be family have problem between them.
- Patient does not have any information regarding to dietary habits of phenylketonuria.
- The family of patient is not educated enough.
- During the period of PKU treatment it takes times to manage all this.
- Difficulties in navigating medical services.
- Infant or person dislikes low protein food on the daily basis
- Family culture can affects on PKU diet.
- When the patient does not accept her condition then there is negative impact on the treatment whether the medicine or dietary habit.

8.1.9.2 Nutritional Care Objective for the Patient

- Phenylalanine-free formula or medical care taken.
- Low phenylalanine food should be consume.
- Take the supplements of tyrosine under the guidance of doctor and dietician.
- The detail of formula should be told to the family and child.
- There should be adequate amount of nutritional intake from food.
- Regular monitoring of growth.
- Education on label reading and food choices.

8.1.10 Diet

Ideally the ranges are between the range of 1 20 and 360 umol per litre or consistently 2-6 mg per dL and target to achieve during at least the initial decade to permit the development of brain. The perfect age for people suffering from phenylketonuria may adopt the diet safely and the diet is subjected to few debates. The perfect age is 8 and 10 for the maintenance of diet.

The restricting and eliminating diets are:

- Soya bean
- White part of eggs
- Shrimps
- Chicken breasts
- Spirulina
- Watercress
- Fish
- Nuts
- Crayfish
- Lobster
- Tuna legumes
- Low fat cottage cheese

Foods which contain more starch like potatoes and corn can be taken in less amounts, but the amount of Phe should be in limit. Milk and its products should not be taken. Take other food products instead of bread slices and its products, you may take some cereals based foods Lower-proteins substitutes can be used, which contain a required amount of Phe. Large quantity of vegetable and fruit can be eaten. To provide all the subsequent benefits of breast milk they may still breastfed the quantity of breast feed should be observed and supply for the nutrients which are missing and is required for the growth. In many of diet eatables or soft drinks in which sweetener aspartame is presented are recommended to avoid, as it is fused into phenylalanine.

The amount of Phe varies person to person in their dietary schedule but all cannot tolerate it. The effects of dietary Phe can be determined with the regular blood tests by intake the blood Phe levels.

Some other foods to be avoided

- Due to some restriction you should not take more protein containing foods following;
- Chicken
- Beef
- Pork

- Fish
- Cheese

8.1.10.1 Phenylalanine- Free Formulas for Phenyketonuria Patient

Phenylalanine-free formula are those formulas, which are blends of amino acid that provide nutrients without the presence of amino acid phenylalanine. These formulas also contain other nutrients such as carbohydrates, fat, vitamins and minerals to help meet the person daily nutrition requirement need. PKU formulas also help in other ways also as person does not feel hungry, repair and build impaired cells during the sickness, help in the concentration in work and stay focused all day, build the muscle of the body. Supplement should be Phe-free formula is given with the breast milk during the infancy cow milk can also be given. Non-essential amino acid can be given to the growing child . PKU formulas are easy to be consumed by the child or adult. To improve the effect of treatment low protein food products is necessary. 90 per cent of protein and the 80 per cent of energy comes from the mixtures of the phenylalanine-free formula. Nowadays these formulas come in different flavours.

There are different types of PKU formulas in the market as explained below:

- **Shake-like formulas:** Shake like formulas are made by the powder and get mixed with water and shake for a few minutes, then the drink is made. Shake-like formulas are the drinks, which give all the nutrients with phenylalanine-free protein. These drinks contain high amount of calorie that is daily requirement according to the RDA.
- **Low volume formulas:** As the person grows and gets older then the requirements of protein increases according to the age and weight of the person. To fulfil requirements of protein is taken from the formula. However, the person may not need as many calories from formula because of the eating low protein food. So low volume formulas have fewer calories, mixed with water, and consumed by the person.
- **Ready-to-drink formulas:** Ready-to-drink formulas is a good choice. These formulas of Phe come in both the shake-like formula and the less-to-drink formula can be decided to complete the needs.
- **The tablet:** If the person does not want or lie to change formula drink, he or she can take tablets. The patient can take multiple tablets of phenylanine free to complete the daily requirement of the body.

8.1.10.2 Low Protein Diet

If the baby is suffering from PKU then the low protein food should be started from the birth in form of a formula, milk is given along with the breast milk. Food products, which contain low amount or moderate amount of phenylalanine, should be consumed. Prescribed foods and supplements are suggested by the dietician for the different age groups and pregnant woman for daily requirement of energy for developing the body and mind. When the baby starts growing after the six months different types of food groups can be introduced after short intervals. The pureed fruit or vegetables can be given to the baby after 6 months. In addition, other foods like finger foods can be given to the baby in 7 to 8 months.

People suffering from PKU get maximum of the protein from medical formula or Phe-free formula. Other proteins help in the growth of the baby and functioning of the body organs. The food should be eaten along with the formula having the low protein. Foods that can be consumed are the vegetables and fruit and other cereal products which are low in proteins like pasta, rice and breads. Fats can be taken in the form of vegetable oil and person can consume sugar in the appropriate amount in PKU.

8.1.10.3 Pregnancy Diet

In the mother's body, when foetus starts growing then it is seen that phenylalanine acceptance in the mother's body increases. The reason behind this is the requirement of foetus for building of body tissues with the phenylalanine, an amino acid. During pregnancy it is necessary to watch the phenylalanine levels in the blood. When the phenylalanine level is lower than the 2 mg/dL in the blood then the mother can consume the foods containing phenylalanine. During pregnancy, formulas are very essential for the mother's body because they are the main sources of protein to be absorbed. The formulas are explained above.

8.1.10.4 Controlling Phenylalanine

As we know that higher concentration of phenylalanine is toxic for body and therefore the requirements of the developing foetus change in the each trimester of pregnancy. Phenylalanine and tyrosine in the blood levels in the women should be carefully checked during the whole pregnancy period.

- It is important to prescribe the tyrosine supplements to the pregnant lady if the levels are low.
- Take phenylalanine formula every day as it covers the calorie and other nutrient requirement for the human body on the daily basis.

- Consumption of low protein diet. The low protein food like bread can be given in the form of sandwich and other example are like pasta in that we can add vegetables that are low in Phe and the crackers quarter-hour before the person taking medical formula.
- Formula drink should be consumed in small amounts.
- Eat small meals at regular intervals.
- Phenylalanine intake should be tracked during the pregnancy. The levels of phenylalanine can start to lower in the 2nd and 3rd trimesters that can help in the growth and development of foetus.

Common difficulties during pregnancy which are to be taken care of:

- Women should eat small amounts foods that are prescribed by dietician.
- Women should drink more water or beverages. Moreover, drink water in between the meals.
- Women should avoid the fried foods and highly spicy foods.
- Seasonal vegetables should be included in diet.
- Women should try to consume fruits and vegetables with their skin because raw vegetables help in the constipation.
- Women should eat small food before making the meals.
- While eating the meals she should sit in straight posture and chew the food carefully and slowly.
- Women should go for walk after the eating the meal.
- After eating, she should avoid lying down on the bed because it can be cause heartburn.
- If the women is suffering from constipation then she should take high fibre cereals. Low protein diet can be taken in the morning with prune juice.
- During pregnancy, women should exercise or practise yoga.

8.1.10.5 Adulthood

In adulthood, person suffering from phenylketonuria has a very tough lifestyle. Because he or she has many restrictions regarding food. When the patient starts realizing that how things are different from others in eating pattern can harmfully increase the level phenylketonuria in the blood.

The is one way that encourage in this is S.A.M. Just keep in mind that S.A.M. is the mode that can be support for the tough time during the diet and pursuing the healthy lifestyle throughout the life.

In S.A.M, the first letter 'S' is for Strong. It means livelihood for those who trust in the dealing with the PKU disorder and maintaining the PKU diet.

The second letter 'A' is for Attitude. For those people who have an positive attitude and eat the low protein diet.

The third letter 'M' is for Manageability, for those persons, who can balance their life with the diet of PKU.

In adulthood, person should have the all the information regarding to the medical formulas:

- Person should drink a glass of Phe formula. It can be taken with the meal or before the meal on the each day.
- While the person going to work place or college or going for some other work, he or she should drink a glass formula shake before leaving the house.
- Ask the dietician about the other beverage substitutions in the daily life.
- Manage the formula of intake the whole day. The body also absorbs all the essential nutrients.
- Person should always carry the bottle of mouthwash so that person can clean his mouth after drinking the formula.

8.1.10.6 Infant/Childhood Diet

After the birth of a child there is less time to find out that child is suffering from PKU. If the report states that baby has PKU then breast milk is not given to the children. By giving the formula to the baby helps the level of phenylalanine to be managed in the blood quickly. The grouping of bottle-feeding and the mother breast feeding both the methods are manageable by the babies easily. Breast milk contains all the essential nutrients that are needed for the babies to grow and stay healthy. The baby has regular source of nutrients from the breast milk. Additionally, the clinical team prescribes the PKU infant formula to the parent.

Formulating the formula (standard infant formula or PKU infant formula)

- First, the person should clean the pan and boil fresh water for infant formula. Leave it for 30 minutes to cool down.
- Clean the surfaces of bottle and wash hands thoroughly.
- In the sterile bottle of baby, pour the cold water in the appropriate amount.
- Then, in the water add the number of scoops as prescribed by the dietician or doctor with the help of scoop provided with the formula. (1 scoop each is 30 mL/1 oz)
- Shake the bottle very well.

- Quickly cool the bottle in the running tap water.
- Check the temperature of the bottle that it can be consumed by baby.

Children take time to adjust to the flavour of food and texture items.

Food that can be given in between 6 to 12 months: The types of food that can be given to the baby can be cooked very well and mashed so that it can be easily swallowed or strained. Baby rice cereal can be given in mashed form, fruit and vegetable puree can be given that are low in phenylalanine and should be prepared at home. Vegetables that can pureed are carrots, squash and beets. Pulped form of fruits, are apricots, pears, peaches, and apples.

During the 10-12 months, bread with low protein, can be made for baby. Other low protein food products such as pasta spirals, crackers, etc., can be given.

Keep track and measure correctly: Accurate measures of food items should be taken with proper tools. The calculations should be done properly of what is consumed everyday by you, meals and snacks consumed should be in accurate portions on your daily basis schedule. The list of foods which can be consumed by a child should be maintained.

Buy some low amount of protein foods: If you want to consume the different type of food items in your diet then you can buy some of the other products that do not contain high amount of protein , rice, flour and bread which you can easily find through speciality industries. Now by having a survey at different places you may find some different variety of foods.

Recommendations on the dietary management of phenylketonuria

1. Screening test should be done so that treatment and checkup can be initiated by minimizing the delay, indeed days of age.
2. Blood phenylalanine concentration should be taken with an average that may be in early morning when the concentration is at peak level. Daily monitoring can be done.
3. The intake of phenylalanine can be adjusted rendering to the blood phenylalanine concentration, by taking care of the maintaining the consistency of milligrams quantity taken whole with the kilograms seriously. It may be applicable or remotely adaptable with the clotting of acids consistency.
4. The standard protocol should be managed for the illness which ensures good substitutions of energy and protein.
5. The goal is handle acid levels by checking frequently. The above deadline is 480 umol/L instead of 360 umol/L.

6. Adults and adolescents who face PKU they require continuing support facilities in the particular timings. Biochemical monitoring services and facilities should be provided through medications.
7. The people who conceive during phenylalanine concentrations have dangerous problems.

8.2 GALACTOSEMIA

Galactosemia signifies 'galactose in the blood' and it is the disability of the body to breakdown the sugar called galactose. The dairy products contain galactose and in galactosemia undigested form is present in blood.

Breast milk is the full source of nutrients to a baby. The immunoglobulins, all vitamins and minerals and antibodies are provided to them which keep them healthy and away from diseases. But there are infants born with galactosemia which is a metabolic disorder and this shows the inability of the digestive system to breakdown galactose, a sugar in the milk. This disorder is fatal and can prove to be life threatening to babies.

Galactosemia is a genetic disorder and it is passed on through the parents. In this condition the genes that produce enzymes to break galactose to glucose are absent. The genes are unable to pass the information to secrete enzymes that breaks the galactose. This results in accumulation of galactose in the blood.

There are three types of galactosemia and their causes, signs and side effects and seriousness are given as under.

8.2.1 Classic and Clinical Variant Galactosemia

Classic and clinical variant galactosemia is a rare genetic metabolic disorder.

The patient has harmful mutations copy of GALT Genes and their blood shows no residue of GALT activity. In the vast majority of cases, the GALT mutations in classic and clinical variant galactosemia are inherited so that both parents of an affected child are carriers. Exceptions are always there. In this disorder the person having galactosemia is not able to fully metabolize the galactose into glucose. Endogenous galactose is also made by human body. Other molecules derived from galactose, such as galactose-1-phosphate (Gal-1P), galactitol, and galactonate, may also build up in the cells and tissues of patients with galactosemia. Galactose is built up in the body as well so if high levels of galactose accumulate in the body due to high intake of milk then the infant can suffer from jaundice, vomiting, and diarrhoea, to liver disease and failure to thrive, and eventually to *E. coli* sepsis, which can be fatal.

It is also known as classic galactosemia. It refers to a disorder arising as a result of profound deficiency of galactose-1-phosphate uridyltransferase (GALT) enzyme. Classic galactosemia is an autosomal recessive disorder. It is inherited when both the parents are carriers and the child gets both the recessive genes for the disorder from each parent. People with only one recessive gene become carriers; they themselves are not affected with the enzyme deficiency, but can pass on the disorder to future generations. It arises due to compound heterozygous or homozygous deletion or mutation in the GALT gene. Mutation leading to 95 per cent decrease in the enzyme activity is very common. Mutations which reduced GALT activity rather than ceasing it lead to milder variant of the disorder. 1 in 40,000 to 1 in 60,000 live births in western countries is affected with type I galactosemia.

Manifestation of classic galactosemia is observed by poor feeding behaviour, *Escherichia coli* related sepsis in untreated infants, bleeding problems and failure of neonates to thrive. In this type, infants exhibit rapid symptoms of indigestion after the ingestion of lactose containing milk either through breast-feeding or formula feeding. Symptoms of indigestion include diarrhoea and vomiting. Because of the rapid and overlapping symptoms of galactose intolerance and lactose intolerance, infants are sometimes termed lactose intolerant. Despite sharing common physical signs and symptoms (diarrhoea and vomiting), there is a profound clinical distinction between the two, galactosemia and lactose intolerance.

Infants with classic galactosemia who consume meals containing galactose or lactose may suffer from hypoglycaemia, elevated blood galactose, hyperbilirubinemia, hyperchloremic metabolic acidosis, hypergalactosemia, hyperaminoaciduria, urinary galactitol excretion and impaired liver function, which may lead to liver cirrhosis if left untreated.

Nearly 230 different mutations in the gene encoding GALT enzyme have been identified. These mutations result in three main forms of type I galactosemia. Forms of galactosemia type-I are as: classic, clinical variant and biochemical variant.

The most common mutation detected in Caucasians takes place in the allele Q188R. In this mutation glutamine (Q) is substituted by arginine (R) at 188 amino acid, which lies in close proximity of the active site of the enzyme. Very little or no activity of GALT in the erythrocytes of the homozygotes for allele Q188R can be seen. The majority of homozygotes show no activity of the GALT enzyme activity, some exhibit a very low level of GALT activity of not more than 20 per cent.

The most commonly detected mutation in the European population is K285N, S135L and N314D. As a result of mutation in K285N, 0 per cent and

50 per cent GALT activity is seen in homozygous and heterozygous individuals, respectively.

The N314D mutation in the GALT gene results in two different biochemical variants of classic galactosemia. D_1 variant (the Los Angeles variant) occurs as a result of mutation solely in N314D. While D_2 variant (the Duarte variant) occurs as a result of both mutation in the coding region of (N314D) GALT gene as well as deletion of GTCA (-119 to -116) in the promoter region of the gene. The GTCA nucleotide is responsible for positive regulatory domain in the GALT promoter, loss of which causes impairment of the regulatory action. A Duarte variant infant arises rarely through the inheritance of a D_2 allele from one parent and a pathogenic GALT mutation from the other parent. Duarte variant form of classic galactosemia patients has 14-25 per cent of the erythrocyte GALT activity when compared to normal individual. D_2 variant infants are generally asymptomatic even when exposed to lactose containing food (breast milk or formula milk). Jaundice or hyperbilirubinemia resolves on its own after the complete removal of lactose in the diet.

Prenatal detection of galactosemia involves measurement of erythrocyte levels of galactose-1-phosphate as well as erythrocyte GALT activity. A person is considered galactosemic if erythrocyte levels of galactose-1-phosphate are elevated and levels of GALT activity reduced or absent.

8.2.2 Duarte Variant Galactosemia

The Durate variant galactosemia is called DG and it's another common form of galactosemia that is results from mutations in GALT genes.In Duarte variant of galactosemia one GALT copy is severe and second one is mildly impaired and it shows characteristic sequence change and named "Duarte" which is the D or D2.

There is additionally a variation of exemplary galactosemia called DUARTE VARIANT GALACTOSEMIA in which the individual has the change in the GALE quality yet has just halfway lack of the protein.

The children are affected with this type and its total genetics with one of the parent suffering as a carrier of severe GALT gene with Duarte variant. Initially, with infants there are no symptoms present of this disease and we do not have to restrict the diet with milk or lactose. The infant does not show any symptoms of liver ailments. The children suffering from Duarte variant galactosemia are at risk of long term growth hinderances. A study has shown that girls suffering from this disorder may experience premature ovarian insufficiency.

Another study found that there was no significant difference in the development of the children specially in the first year of life with Duarte variant galactosemia. Duarte variant galactosemia is doubtfully detected in the newborn and a normal screening test for galactosemia is found. So it is difficult to diagnose a Duarte variant galactosemia.

8.2.3 Galactokinase Deficiency (Type 2)

Second form or type II galactosemia arises as a result of mutation in the enzyme gene galactokinase (GALK1), leading to the development of deficiency of the enzyme. Infants who continue to feed on milk based diets despite being suffering from type II galactosemia, accumulate abnormally high levels of galactose in tissues and blood, as seen in infants with classic galactosemia. Patients with type II galactosemia also suffer with cataracts, but the condition is resolved by making dietary modifications and ruling out lactose completely from diet. Patients with GALK deficiency do not experience long term complications if galactose restricted diets are followed; which is contrary to the classic galactosemia. Biochemically and clinically this difference, between classic and type II galactosemia, is quite significant. This difference among the two provides compelling evidence supporting the fact that accumulation of galactose does not take place in type II disorder, but galactose-1-phosphate (Gal-1-P), or even some other metabolic derivative of Gal-1-P. This accumulation of Gal-1-P or its derivative is considered the primary culprit behind the disease. Type II disorder is rare with a chance factor of <1 in 100,000 live births. It is not severe disorder because of the lack of conclusive evidence in favour of long term complications.

The transformation of GALK 1gene and is shown by insufficiency of galactokinase 1. Seldom, this sort causes pseudotumourcerebri (a condition which emulates the manifestations of a huge mind tumor when no cerebrum tumour is available). However the treatment is available for galactokinase deficiency (Type 2)

8.2.4 Galactose Epimerase Deficiency (Type 3)

It is brought about by the changes in GALE quality and described by the insufficiency of protein called UDP-galactose-4-epimerase. Manifestations and seriousness of this sort relies upon whether the insufficiency is kept to specific kinds of platelets or is available in all tissues. A few people with this sort has no sign and side effects, while others have side effects like sort 1, for example, exemplary galactosemia.

Newborn children with this structure may have jaundice, which settle when changed to a low galactose recipe. A few examinations have demonstrated that individuals with this sort have higher danger of neurodevelopment issues. Legacy of galactosemia is an autosomal passive. The determination might be suspected dependent on the side effects or the consequences of the infant screening tests and can be affirmed by estimating compound movement and hereditary testing. Contingent upon the kind of galactosemia, treatment may include expelling galactose sugar from the eating regimen (when suspected), calcium supplementation, and individualized consideration of any extra manifestations.

It is the form of galactosemia arising as a result because of mutation in enzyme gene UDP-galactose-4-epimerase (GALE), which leads to the deficiency of the enzyme. Two different types of GALE deficiencies have been identified. Deficiency affecting RBCs (red blood cells) and WBCs (white blood cells) is the most common recurring deficiency. It is relatively more benign than the other one. The other form of GALE deficiency is characterized by severe enzyme impairment. It affects multiple tissues and organs; and has symptoms very similar to classic form (GALT deficiency). It is very rare; only 8 cases have been reported till date. This is placed on second position after classic type in case of severity. Initially, it can be controlled with dietary interventions, but over a prolonged period of time, diet loses its effectiveness because of arising long term complications.

8.2.5 Type IV Galactosemia

In 2018, several new cases of galactosemia were reported. After assessment it was found that the complication was because of deficiency of enzyme GALM, thus giving type IV its place in the run.

Both type II and type III are rarer when compared to type I galactosemia. Enzyme inactivating mutations is one of the leading causes of the accumulation of abnormally high levels of galactose in the tissue and blood. This accumulated galactose enters polyol pathway of carbohydrate metabolism. In polyol pathway, galactose is reduced to galactitol with the help of catalyst aldose reductase. The thus formed galactitol is excreted in the urine. In some cases, oxidation of galactose into galactonate, assisted by enzyme galactose dehydrogenase, is also observed. Galactonate is considered less harmful than galactitol.

If the person continues to consume galactose in diet, all the above-mentioned galactosemias can lead to life threatening conditions like blindness, liver failure and even brain damage. Blindness is caused as a result of conversion of free circulating galactose into galactitol (a sugar alcohol derivative) facilitated by an energy dependent enzyme, namely, aldose reductase. The enzyme aldose reductase is present in the lens of eyes and in the neural tissue. Osmotic swelling is seen in the lens if the concentration of galactitol is high, this increased concentration gives rise to cataracts and other symptoms related to eyes leading to blindness. However, under normal conditions when the level of free circulating galactose is less, conversion of galactose to galactitol by aldose reductase does not cause any harmful physiological impact on the body.

8.2.6 Galactose Metabolism

The primary wellspring of galactose sugar is lactose present in milk and dairy items. After its ingestion, lactose is hydrolyzed in the intestinal lumen by the lactase into glucose and galactose. Galactose is moved over the enterocyte brush fringe layer by the sodium/glucose dynamic co-transporter SGLT1, and through encouraged dissemination by the GLUT2 transporter over the enterocyte basolateral film. After entering the circulatory system it is conveyed by the entry blood to the liver, the significant site for galactose digestion where it is disguised by the low liking high limit GLUT2.

8.2.7 Galactose Accumulation in the Body

8.2.7.1 Galactosemia

Metabolism: Milk and dairy products are the primary sources of galactose in diet. Galactose is present in the form of lactose (milk sugar). During digestion of milk, lactose is catabolised into two monosaccharide units, namely, glucose and galactose. Galactose contributes to 20 per cent of the total energy in newborn babies. Synthesis of glyoconjugates is also done with the help of galactose. Glucose is the primary carbohydrate which is absorbed and used by the body. So as to be used by the body, galactose undergoes the process of glycolysis, resulting in its conversion to glucose-1-phosphate (G1P). The conversion of glucose to G1P occurs through a series of steps, and is referred as the Leloir pathway (named after the scientist who determined the process of galactose utilization, Luis Federico Leloir). Any deviation of galactose from Leloir pathway arising due tȯ any reason leads to galactosemia.

Galactose exists in two different stereo-isomeric forms, namely, alpha-D-galactose (α-form) and beta-D-galactose (β-form). The α-form is metabolized in the Leloir pathway. For β-form to be utilized in the body, it is first converted into α-form. Conversion of β-form to α-form galactose is facilitated by the enzyme galactose mutarotase. This enzyme mutarotase is encoded by GALM gene (also known as aldose-1-epimerase).

Steps involved in the Leloir pathway: The Leloir pathway is a multistep reaction leading to the metabolism of galactose. In the first step of the pathway, α-D-galactose is phosphorylated into galactose-1-phosphate with the activity of enzyme galactokinase. The galactokinase enzyme is encoded by the gene GALK1. Further, galactose-1-phosphate is epimerized into glucose-1-phosphate (G1P) with the transfer of UDP. UDP is transferred from UDP-glucose facilitated by galactose-1-phosphate uridyltransferase enzyme (GALT). Action of GALT results in the generation of UDP-galactose and G1P. The UDP-glucose formed as a result of GALT is further epimerized to UDP-glucose with the action of UDP-galactose-4 epimerase (GALE). Then the exchange of UDP portion takes place generating glucose-1-phosphate. This G1P is then converted into glucose-6-phosphate (G6P) by the action of enzyme phosphoglucose mutase.

Coding of enzymes: Galactokinase protein is encoded by the GALK1 gene located on 17q25.1 chromosome. The GALK1 gene contains 8 exons, which encodes for 392 amino acid proteins; it also spans 7.3 kilo base pair (kbp).

Galactose-1-phosphate uridyltransferase enzyme is encoded by the GALT gene located on 9p13.3 chromosome. The GALT gene contains 11 exons, which generate two alternatively spliced mRNAs that encodes for two distinct isoforms of the enzyme, GALT-1 and GALT-2. GALT isoform-1 is a protein composed of 379 amino acids, while GALT isoform-2 is composed of 270 amino acids.

UDP-galactose-4 epimerase enzyme is encoded by GALE gene located on 1p36.11 chromosome. It is composed of 13 exons, which generate three mRNAs spliced alternatively. All three mRNAs encode the same 348 amino acids. GALE catalyses two epimerization reactions which are distinct but analogous in nature. Epimerization of both UDP-galactose to UDP-glucose and UDP-N-acetylgalactosamine to UDP-N-acetylglucosamine is done by GALE.

Under normal conditions, galactose is metabolised to glucose with the help of different, specific, organic catalysts or enzymes. In galactosemia, the catalyst which converts galactose-1-phosphate to glucose-1-phosphate becomes inactive and further conversion ceases. Due to this metabolic block in conversion of galactose, accumulation of galactose-1-phosphate in the body tissues takes place. Accumulated galactose-1-phosphate is believed to be the culprit behind liver damage and cataracts. Galactose is present in urine and blood samples in detectable quantities of person suffering from galactosemia. Due to less conversion of galactose to glucose, low levels of blood sugar are very common in the patients of galactosemia. High galactose level, low blood sugar level or both are the possible causes of mental retardation observed in galactosemic children. According to estimates, approximately 18,000 infants are galactosemic because of hereditary transfer of galactose intolerance.

There are other minor pathways of galactose metabolism in humans as well which do not involve all three enzymes (GALK1, GALT and GALE) used in completion of the Leloir pathway. With the sequential activities of GALK, UGP2 (UDP-glucose pyrophosphorylase-2) and GALE, conversion of galactose into UDP-glucose can take place. In case of galactosemia resulting from GALT and GALK1 deficiencies, galactose can be reduced to galactitol by the action of NADPH-dependent aldose reductase. And then finally oxidation of galactose to galactonate is done with the assistance of galactose dehydrogenase. In non-galactosemic people, these alternative pathways metabolise only trace amount of galactose in the body.

8.2.8 Metabolic Pathway of Galactose

8.2.8.1 Reduction to Galactitol

In galactosemic patients, the gathering of galactose turns into the substrate for compounds that catalyze the polyol pathway for sugars digestion. The primary response of this pathway is the decrease of aldoses, sorts of sugars including galactose to sugar liquor. Aldose reductase is the compound liable for the essential phase of the response. Hence, aldose reductase diminishes the galactose sugar to its liquor sugar structure, for example, galactitol. Galactitol, be that as it may, doesn't go about as a substrate in the subsequent stage of the pathway for the chemical polyol dehydrogenase.

In this way the alcoholic type of the sugar amasses in the body tissue and is discharged in the pee of the galactosemic patients. Amassing of galactitol has unfriendly impact on the galactosemic patients particularly with the great galactosemia (GALT inadequacy or Galactose-1-phosphate uridylytransferase lack), galactokinase insufficiency and epimerase lack with the glucose sugar.

Oxidation to galactonate: Gathered galactose can likewise experience an elective response: oxidation to galactonate. The component of galactonate arrangement is as yet indistinct. Nonetheless, the ongoing examinations recommend that the chemical galactose dehydrogenase is liable for the transformation of the galactose sugar to galactonolactone, which then unexpectedly or enzymatically changes to galactonate. When created, the galactonate enters the pentose phosphate pathway. Consequently, oxidation to galactonate fills in as a substitute pathway for utilizing galactose sugar. This oxidation renders galactonate which is less destructive than the alcoholic type of the galactose sugar, for example, galactitol.

Metabolic pathway of Galactose

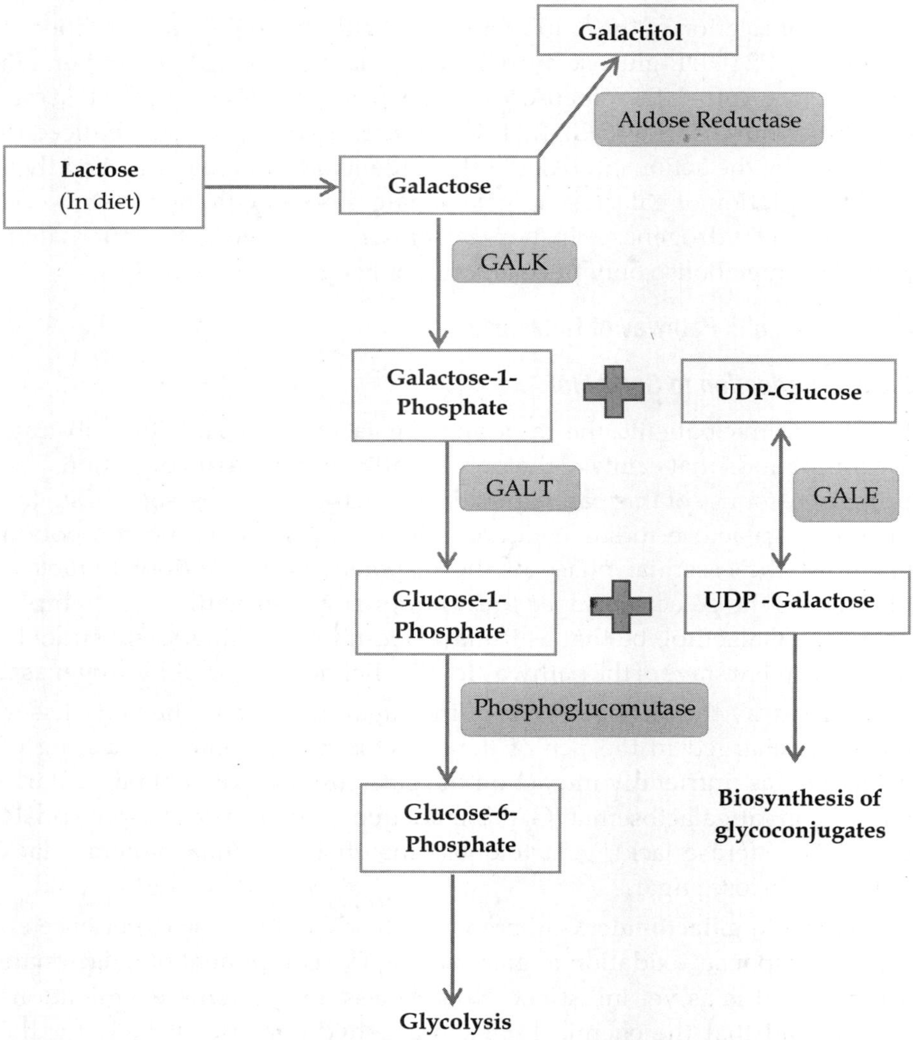

Diagnosis: Detection of galactosemia can be done even in prenatal period. Prenatal diagnosis is done by collecting the amniotic fluid sample and checking its culture for the deficiency of GALT. For perinatal detection of galactosemia, blood sample of the infant is collected and sample is checked for galactose and galactose-1-phosphate levels.

Treatment: Treatment of all the four types of galactosemia entails avoiding galactose containing food. Dietary modifications begin in infants, both human milk and cow's milk are replaced by soy-based milk products or protein hydrolysate formulas. Human and cow milks contain lactose, which, in turn, is made up of galactose, while soy milk and protein hydrolysate formulas are devoid of galactose in any form. If the lactose and galactose free diet is instituted in early infancy and maintained for at least 3 years of age, the chances of developing cataracts, mental retardation and even liver damage can be diminished. With prolonged modification in diet, galactose tolerance may increase in some individuals. Though life threatening conditions can be avoided with dietary modifications, the affected individual is still at the high risk of getting speech problems, cognitive impairment and developmental delay (verbal dyspraxia and dysarthria). Most of the females affected with classic galactosemia develop hyper-gonadotrophic hypo-gonadism or premature follicular atresia (premature ovarian failure) resulting in ovarian insufficiency infertility. Individuals should be provided with early intervention for speech and developmental delay. Females should be regularly screened for premature ovarian failure.

A person may exhibit biochemical signs, like elevated erythrocyte levels of galactose-1-phosphate and urinary excretion of galactitol, of GALT deficiency even when on a galactose-free diet. Due to the above-mentioned persistent clinical complications, the individual is advised to undergo routine tests and check-ups for the accumulation of erythrocyte Gal-1-P, elevated urinary excretion of galactose, liver function tests, formation of cataracts and tests for speech and cognitive development. Calcium supplementation is advised for the galactosemia individuals.

The main treatment for galactosemia is wiping out lactose and galactose from the eating regimen. Indeed, even with early detection, analysis and confined eating regimen in any case, a few people with galactosemia experience long haul inconveniences, for example, discourse troubles, learning challenges, neurological hindrance such as tremors, etc. Side effects have not been related with Duarte galactosemia. Galactosemia is frequently mixed up with lactose prejudice, however the previous is an increasingly genuine ailment. Lactose is acquired or procured with lack of the lactase hormones and experience stomach torment in the wake of ingesting the dairy items, and doesn't has long haul impact. Conversely, the galatosemic isolate who expends galactose can make changeless harm their bodies.

8.2.9 A Case Study

Aim: ID and practical examination of three unmistakable transformations in the Human Galactose 1-phosphate Uridyltransferase quality related with galactosemia in a solitary family.

The researcher recognized three changes related with transferase - lack galactosemia in a three age family remembering influenced individuals for two ages and have demonstrated every one of the three - age transformations in a yeast articulation framework.

A succession of family, biochemical, and atomic investigations of the Galactose 1-phosphate Uridyltransferase (GALT) proteins and hereditary locus in both influenced and bearer individual uncovered three unmistakable base substitutions right now, (Q188R and S135L) that had been accounted for already and one (V155A) that was novel.

Biochemical investigations of red platelet lysates from the applicable family proposed that every one of these transformations was related with sensational weakness of GALT movement in these cells.

While this perception was predictable with the past discoveries concerning the Q188R change communicated both in people and in a yeast framework model it was inconsistent, demonstrating that in their COS cell articulation framework the S135L substitution, carried on as ordinary impartial polymorphism.

To address this obvious Catch 22, just as to explore the practical criticalness of the recently distinguished V151A substitutions, each of the three changes were reproduced by site coordinated mutagenesis in any case wild sort GALT grouping and were communicated both separately and in the fitting allelic mixes in a GALT inadequate strain of the yeast *S. cerevissae*.

The yeast of these yeast demonstrating contemplates were completely reliable with the patient information, prompting the end that at any rate inside the setting of the cell types examined, in the homozygous state Q188R is a transformation that eliminates GALT action, S135L and V155A are both change that debilitate GALT movement to <6% of the wild sorts esteems.

8.2.10 Dietary Options

To follow a low-galactose diet, keep away from a lactose - free nourishments, including 1. Milk 2. Spread 3. Cheddar 4. Frozen yogurt 5. Dairy items.

You can supplant a significant number of these items with sans dairy options, similar to almond or soy milk or coconut milk. A few patients with Duarte galactosemia may at present go for best - taking care of in any case. While the Habitats for Illness Control and Anticipation (CDC) best milk as the most ideal path for babies to get supplements, they don't prescribe breast feeding a baby with galactosemia. Rather, you'll have to utilize a sans lactose equation. Get some information about recipe alternatives.

8.3 MAPLE SYRUP URINE DISEASE

Branched chain ketoaciduria, BCKDH deficiency, branched chain alpha ketoacid dehydrogenase deficiency, BCKD flaw and ketoacids decarboxylase flaw are some of the other terms that can be used for Maple syrup urine disease. Faulty decarboxylation process which affects the branched chain amino acids (BCAAS). For the development of Maple syrup urine disease the main requirement is two copies of defected genes thus, it is also known as autosomal recessive disorder.

An irreversible oxidative decarboxylation reaction occurs in the from branched chain to oxocids in the mitochondria of the cell which is aided by the branched chain keto acid dehydrogenase complex. A bio ester- branched chain acyl co is the product procured out of this reaction. There is a bunch of enzymes, particular for each branched chain amino acid that helps in metabolism of these thio esters from which they were derived. Branched chain kiel acid dehydrogenase complex defects are the main reason behind the maple syrup urine disease. Several organic ria's branch chain keto acid dehydrogenases are caused by enzymes in the pathway.

The infant or newborn appears to be normal at the time of birth but as soon as the child reaches to the age of 4 - 5 days of birth, the child starts, showing poor food intake, vomiting, lack of energy and periodic hypertonia that involves uncontrollable muscle spasms, stiffening of muscle. A sweet and malty odour from urine can be noticed at the end of 1st week after birth. If it is not treated or if there is a non-fulfillment to treat this adverse condition proceeds to acidosis, neurological decay, coma and seizure that leads finally to death.

Early intervention and careful biochemical control in infants and children who are affected by the maple serum urine disease, also taking into account the severity of the enzyme defect, can help more fruitfully in the treatment. In children who are normal or have low range difference can be seen in pattern of appropriate growth and intellectual development. Early diagnosis (up to 7 days of age) and metabolic control for a long period of time can help in maintaining normal intellectual development in the child.

E2 forms the core of the enzyme complex and is the reason behind the acyl callay products formation. Dye hydro light immediate dehydrogenase is a part of the flavour protein-e3 subunits. During the catalytic cycle they reduce and oxidize to e2 subunits for regulating the reactions of the branched chain keto acid dehydrogenase complex activity, which is mediated through an association of kinase and a phosphatase which are sensitive to the levels of brains change to oxoacids and the branched chain amino acids respectively.

Other names of maple syrup urine disease:

- Branched chain ketonuria
- BCKDC deficiency.
- Branched chain ketoaciduria.
- Branched chain alpha keto acid dehydrogenase.

8.3.1 Pathology of Maple Syrup Urine Disease

The normal maintenance of plasma leucine concentration should be at between 2 and 5 mg/dL (150 to 380 µmol/L) is recommended. The concentration higher than 10 mg/dl (760 µmol/L) is integrated with disease like alpha ketoacidemia and neurologic indication.

8.3.2 General Characteristics of Maple Syrup Urine Disease

Estimated to have prevalence of around 1 and 185,000 around the world with most incidences in the population of Mennonite, maple syrup urine disease is recessively autosomal in nature. Any defect in the complex subunits of the three branched chain keto-acid dehydrogenase results in the building up of the two oxoacids to up.

8.3.3 Classification of Maple Syrup Urine Disease

1. **Classic maple syrup urine disease:** Coma and death are the most common results of the classic maple syrup urine disease, which is the most severe type as it cannot be recognised easily due to absence of strong symptoms. Children who survive classic maple syrup disease tend to have other cognitive and intellectual disabilities in later life.
2. **Intermittent maple syrup urine disease:** Overall, a normal neurological development is seen in children suffering from intermittent maple syrup urine disease. The disease only progresses when the patients tends to undergo high level of protein breakdown in the body which can be seen in case of any infection, vomiting, fasting, fever, etc., leading to saturated activity of branched chain keto acid dehydrogenase.
3. **Thiamine responsive maple syrup urine disease:** The e2 subunits of the branched chain keto acids dehydrogenase complex is defected in this type of maple syrup urine disorder. It lowers the enzyme's ability to hold on the obligate cofactors of diaminepyrophosphate. Though it is absent during the time when the child is a neonate, but in the later life symptoms same as those of intermediate maple syrup urine disease, start showing up. Supplementing the patient

with thiamine can help in overcoming the decreased thiamine pyrophosphate affinity, thus improving the residual activity as branched chain keto acids dehydrogenase complex.

4. **Intermediated maple syrup urine disease:** It is a lll deficient maple syrup urine disease. Branched chain keto acid dehydrogenase complex is a part of short chain oxalic acid.

8.3.4 Causes/Etiology

1. Gene defect is the main reason behind maple syrup urine disease (MSUD). Patients with MSUD are unable to break amino acids (leucine, isoleucine and valine), leading to the building of these in the blood.
2. Physical stress conditions such as fever, infections and poor appetite for long period of time can cause damage to the brain in severe cases of maple syrup urine disease.
3. Maple syrup urine disease are also of milder versions that arise and are easily curable. But still they can lead to intellectual disability and high leucine levels due to repetitive physical stress.

8.3.5 Manifestation/Symptoms

Poor appetite or difficulty in feeding, irritability, weight loss, convulsions, coma, vomiting, maple odour from the urine of the patient. Symptoms are mostly related to an odour of maple syrup in the urine, metabolic acidosis, hypertonia, loss of motor reflex, severe damage to the brain damage, etc.

Lab findings: High levels of branched chain amino acids (isoleucine, leucine, and valine) in serum and urine.

Role of genes: Faulty genes is the main cause for the Maple syrup urine disease. Gene are the carriers of the information which is hereditary in nature. These genes then help in the process of the body formation like eye colour, hair colour, blood group, etc., by transferring traits from both the parents into the offspring as he/she inherits one set from each parent. The genes are rearranged in pairs and then the process of replication starts, i.e., transferring information in each of the cells. The child who is born with MSUD has faulty genes which he or she inherited from parents. The height and blood test to check nutrient and amino acid level of the child with MSUD is taken into account during clinic visits. Changes in the growth pattern and the diet should be studied and then modifications in the diet should be done as per the dietary habits and need of the child. There are diets mixes and formulas available in the market which can almost fulfil the needs of amino acids especially for consumption of the people suffering from maple syrup urine disorder. In order to ensure that these mixes also provide enough branched chain amino acids to the infant for proper growth and development, these mixes come with small amounts of cow milk or standard infant formula. There is also a need to maintain the biochemical balance in infants, which can be obtained by providing supplements of L-valine or L-isoleucine. The main aim for successful treatment of MSUD is diet management, that can be attained by preventing catabolism and maintenance of plasma BCAA range by providing enough minerals and vitamins through the diet and reduction of BCAA (branched chain amino acids).

8.3.6 Dietary Management

- Branched chain amino acids intake should be avoided.
- Plasma amino acid should be monitored on regular intervals.
- Keeping a check on concentration of plasma leucine.

The treatment of acute stage maple syrup urine disease requires two methods, peritoneal dialysis and hydration. When plasma lucine concentration sufficiently decrease in the body then branched chain amino acids are involved into the diet. The resultant neurologic damage and precise mechanism for complete decarboxylase reaction is not clearly known. Not even the reason why lucine metabolism is more unusual than that of other two branched chain amino acids understood. The degree of impaired strength after some time of improvement is most likely to be relatable to the degree of abnormality of lucine concentration and this impaired strength after some time of improvement is sometimes related to any infection. Acute infection causes life frightening medical emergencies. Branched chain amino acids have to be excluded from the diet straight away if the plasma lucine concentration increases quickly during illness and intravenous therapy ought to be begin.

Possible complications

- Coma
- Death
- Neurological damage

The clinical features and manifestation

The clinical features of maple syrup urine disease are variable but the classic form is characterized by these symptoms such as psychomotor retardation, cerebral degradation, hypoglycaemia and seizures. Adolescent children with this disease may have attention defect hyperactivity disorder and anxiety and development delay. Failure to thrive and feeding difficulties are commonly seen.

Aggressive treatment of acute metabolic decompensation

- Rapidly lower leucine concentrations.
- Infusion of glucose: inhibits protein catabolism and promotes protein synthesis.
- Stop protein intake for 24- 48 hours.

Foods to be limited in the diet

- Meat
- Fish
- Cheese
- Egg
- Pulses
- Nuts

Food groups that are included in the diet

- Fruits and vegetables.
- Bread and cereals (low protein special bread, flour and pasta).
- Meat, chicken, fish.
- Milk and dairy with special supplementation.
- Fats and sugars

8.3.7 Dietary Management

- Branched chain amino acids intake should be avoided.
- Plasma amino acid should be monitored on regular intervals.
- Keeping a check on concentration of plasma leucine.

S. No.	Food items	Examples
1.	Vegetables	Globe artichoke, Broad beans, Avocado, Mustard greens, Bean sprouts, Button squash, Corn, Mushrooms Pumpkin, Peas, Green beans, Sweet potato, Spinach, Brussels sprouts, Cauliflower, Broccoli Red cabbage,Asparagus, Potato, etc.
2.	Grain, Flour, Pasta, Biscuits, Bread, and Cereals	Baking mixes, Low protein flour, Rice and Breakfast Cereals, Corn flour, Custard powder, Sago, Tapioca, Arrowroot, Yeast, Vermicelli, Baking powder/soda, Tartar cream, Food colours and essences, etc.
3.	Oils and Fats	Margarine, Cooking fat, Ghee, Whipped cream, Butter, etc., with a content of less than 0.3 g protein per serving.

4.	Sugar	Jam, Maple syrup, Honey, Jelly, Vegetable Gum (except gelatine), Marmalade and Golden syrup, etc.
5.	Stocks, Spices and Condiments	Salt, pepper, Herbs, Spices powder and pastes, Salad dressing, Sauces such as Tomato, Barbecue and Worcestershire, Mustard, etc, Chutney, Pickles, Readymade food items, stock cubes and stock, etc. **Note:** Avoid using stock made from meat/bones or vinegar.

8.3.8 Diet Plan for 2 Years Old Patient of Maple Syrup Urine Disease

- Leucine tolerance recommendation-: 450 mg/day
- Formula Mix/Medical foods/day can be made by combination of – Ketonex-2 = 100 g, isomil powder = 38 gm and water= 28 oz. It gives 570 kcal energy, 34.2 gm protein and 388 mg of leucine.
- Diet plan to fulfil around 50 mg leucine through food

Food	Amount	Amount of leucine content present
Breakfast:		
Formula mix	6 oz	
Canned peaches	60 gm	9 mg
Kix cereals	1 tablespoon	5 mg
Lunch:		
Formula mix	6oz	
Cooked carrots	20 gm	9 mg
Canned apricots	20 gm	9 mg
Jelly	20 gm	----
Bread (low protein)	1 piece	4 mg
Evening time:		
Formula mix	6 oz	
Apple	4 slices	4 mg
Crackers (low protein)	5 pieces	3 mg
Dinner:		
Formula mix	6 oz	
Pasta (low protein)	½ cup	5 mg
Cooked green bean	9 gm	7 mg
Butter or margarine		---
Total		55 mg

- Leucine tolerance recommendation: 550 mg/day
- Formula Mix/ Medical foods/day can be made by combination of Ketonex-2 = 100 gm, isomil powder = 38 gm and water = 28 oz. It gives 570 kcal energy, 34.2 gm protein and 388 mg of leucine.

Diet plan to fulfil around 50 mg leucine through food

Food	Amount	Amount of leucine content present
Breakfast:		
Formula Mix	6 oz	35 mg
Rice Krispies	6 oz	7 mg
Non-dairy Creamer	2 tablespoon	
Lunch:		
Formula Mix	6oz	
Grapes	50 gms	7 mg
Vegetable soup	2 tablespoon+ ¼ cup water	30 mg
Cookies (low protein)	3 pieces	3 mg
Cracker (low protein)	5 pieces	3 mg
Evening time:		
Formula mix	6 oz	
Jelly	1 teaspoon 4 slices	---
Rice cakes	1 small (1 gm)	7 mg
Dinner:		
Formula mix	6 oz	
Diced potato	30 gm	33 mg
Sauted zucchini	45 gm	24 mg
No-dairy margarine	1 teaspoon	---
Total		149 mg

8.3.9 Prevention

Couples with a history of maple syrup urine disease in the family should opt for genetic counselling when planning children. Many states have now made it mandatory for all the newborns to undergo blood tests for detection of maple syrup urine disease.

If the screening test of the newborn comes out that the newborn may be or is infected, an immediate blood test for amino acid is recommended to confirm the presence of maple syrup urine disease.

8.3.10 Complications

- Sensory disturbances, unconsciousness or convulsions
- Swelling in the brain
- Inability to see (blindness)
- Muscle tightness (uncontrolled)
- Uneven flow of blood into the brain.
- Difficulty in focussing
- Neurological damage

Hospital therapy's primary goals

Lowering the concentration of plasma leucine.	› 750 μmol/L/day
Maintaining plasma concentrations	400-600 μmol/L
Maintaining the concentration of serum sodium	138-145 mEq/L
Maximum avoidance of osmolality changes	› 5 mosm/L/day or 0.25 mosm/L/60 minutes
Maintenance of optimal urine output	2-4 mL/kg/hour

Aims of laboratory monitoring maintaining

Concentration of plasma leucine	Between 150-300 μmol/L
Concentration of plasma isoleucine	Concentration of plasma leucine
Concentration of plasma valine	Twofold concentration of leucine concentration

8.4 GLYCOGEN STORAGE DISEASE

Glycogen storage disease (GSD) is not a common disorder and it is related to the glucose metabolism in the body which is abnormal in this condition. Glucose is the source of energy in the body and is stored in the body in form of glycogen at the muscles and liver. The glycogen needs to be broken down to glucose to be utilized in the body by certain enzymes. But when one of the enzymes that is absent to convert glycogen to glucose the disease glycogen storage disease (GSD) is born.

GSD is a hereditary disorder and is passed to the children from parents usually. It is usually detected in infants or children.

8.4.1 Types of GSD

8.4.1.1 The Most Common Types of GSD are Type I , III and IV.

Type I or von Gierke disease: This kind is found in babies of 3-4 months old who have hypoglycaemia and enlarged liver that causes pot belly in babies. The enzyme is absent to convert glycogen to glucose and glycogen store builds up constantly in the liver.

Type III, Cori disease, or Forbes disease: The incomplete breakdown of glycogen to glucose results in their collection in the liver and muscles. The symptoms include in people most commonly are swollen belly, delayed growth and weakened muscles.

Type IV or Andersen disease: Now this is Type IV form and in this condition people form abnormal glycogen which attacks the immune system. This results in liver cirrhosis and scarring of organs such as muscles and heart.

8.4.2 Aetiology of GSD

It is a heredity disorder and the chances are more if both parents suffer from it. The both parents have abnormal gene mutation and it is passed to their generation. In most cases parents don't show any symptoms of the disease.

8.4.2.1 Symptoms of the Disease

The muscles and liver show the maximum symptoms. Most of the symptoms are as follows:

1. Hampered growth
2. Intolerance to hot environment
3. Easily wounded
4. Hypoglycaemia
5. Swollen stomach
6. Muscle pain and cramping

The glycogen storage disease is found mostly in children and the main symptoms are enlarged liver and weakness of muscles. The blood test can show the enzyme amount present in the child's body.

8.4.3 Management and Treatment of GSD

For types I, III, and IV, a special diet is prescribed to control symptoms. Drug therapy is also needed with the dietary prescription. The physical activities of children are also reduced to avoid exertion as weakness of muscles is already there. Enzyme replacement therapy is also implemented.

8.4.3.1 Complications

Glycogen build-up in the liver and muscles causes pain and discomfort. The other problems that exist are benign tumour of liver. In Type III and fibrosis, necrosis of liver cells which results in cirrhosis. Further it results in liver failure.

The children with GSD are called children with special needs and special diets with drug therapy is followed. There is no treatment for this disease.

8.4.4 Dietary Management in GSD

8.4.4.1 Type I & II GSD

The enzyme that converts galactose and fructose to glucose is not present. The glucose is immediately absorbed in the body. But fructose or galactose is not absorbed in the body and is converted to glycogen in the body which is the last thing needed in this disease. Therefore, patients with GSD Type

I or II should not consume foods that contain fructose and galactose as the goal is to try to limit the amount of non-usable sugars at all times.

There fore simple sugars are to be given and large amounts of fructose and galactose should be avoided. It is important to keep the amount of fructose plus galactose to less than 2.5 gm per meal.

Foods to be avoided completely are dairy products as they have lactose sugars. Unsweetened or plain soymilk is being recommended to such patients.

Vegetables can be given liberally as they contain very less sugars.

If fruits are to given should be only 20 gm per meal and not to be combined with meals. As the glycaemic load of the meal should not be increased.

Meat and meat products can be given but with no sauces or chutneys. All the snacks which are sweet / fried / complex carbohydrates should be avoided completely.

All types of sweetened beverages such as tea/coffee/ soft drinks/ fruit juices/shakes should be avoided completely.

8.5 CYSTIC FIBROSIS

8.5.1 Introduction

This disease affects the secretory glands (which produce sweat and mucus). It can pass down through generations to another. The salt and water balance of the body is disturbed in this disease The disease is caused due to some mutation of the gene – CFTR, which belongs to the chromosome 7. The cystic fibrosis generally affects the three main body organs, namely, the lungs, respiratory tract and the gastrointestinal tract including the pancreas along with the organs that help in precipitation. The lungs are lined by a thick bodily fluid in relation to the cystic fibrosis that can be removed by undergoing physiotherapy that helps in unsticking the fluid and turning it into sputum for removal. The thick bodily fluid sticks to pancreas and hinders the flow of stomach related chemicals originating from it, making it difficult for the patient to process nutrition from food high in fat and protein.

8.5.2 Causes/Aetiology

Cystic fibrosis (CF) is a hereditary disorder in nature. Patients of cystic fibrosis have one duplicate from the mother and one from the father of the flawed CF quality. Both the parents must have a duplicate of the imperfect gene. Person who has just one damaged duplicate CF quality are known as transporters, but they do not have the disorder. Every time two transporters have an offspring, the odds are that:

1 out of every 4 offspring will have cystic fibrosis.

1 out of every 2 offspring will a transporter but will not have cystic fibrosis.

1 out of every 4 offspring will not be a transporter and will not have cystic fibrosis.

There is always a slight differences in the quality of the Cystic fibrosis known as transformation. There are almost more than 1700 known transformations of this disorder. As most of the tests look for the changes caused in cystic fibrosis, the test results help to distinguish whether the individual is a transporter or not.

8.5.3 Diagnosis

If screening test shows the presence of the cystic fibrosis, additional tests are required to confirm the disorder:

- A sweat test, a person with cystic fibre will have a high amount of salt in the sweat.
- A genetic test, generally carried out in old children and adults who have by chance missed there newborn test. It is done by taking samples from the blood or saliva.

In heredity condition genetic test may be used to identify whether a person is a "carrier" of cystic fibrosis or not. This test may be important for people that desire to have babies but think they might contain defected gene. Mixing up of two individuals with cystic fibrosis can lead to even worse conditions, including weak and fracture-prone bones or osteoporosis. Prescribing bisphosphonates can help for sometime,diabetes- insulin and a controlled eating pattern might also help in controlling the levels of glucose, nasal polyps and sinus diseases. Anti-infecting agents, steroids, antihistamines and sinus flushes can help. Women with cysctic fibrosis have the chances of becoming a mother while there is no chance for man.

CF makes the body produce anomalous thick and clingy bodily fluid in the lungs and different organs. This bodily fluid stops the aviation routes and gives a reproducing ground to perilous lung contaminations. It can likewise obstruct the channel from the pancreas to the small digestive system, in this way diminishing or killing an individual's capacity to process nourishment. CF delivers various indications, for example, salty-tasting skin, repetitive pneumonia, inability to flourish, and incessant wheezing or hacking. CF is a hereditary malady acquired from the two guardians, similarly as one acquires hair shading or eye shading.

People who have CF have special healthcare needs including:

- extraordinary weight control plans to guarantee legitimate nourishment and development;
- prescriptions to check the impacts of the illness, including proteins to help digest nourishment; and
- chest exercise based recuperation to help release and oust the thick and clingy bodily fluid from the aviation routes.

The vast majority who have CF can have ordinary existence separated from these hesitate medicines. Most kids who have CF grow up to go to class, have companions, and participate in normal games and pastimes. Numerous grown-ups who have CF wed and have families.

Guardians of kids who have CF should raise them with similar desires that they apply to other youngsters. Having CF ought not prevent anybody from turning into a contributing citizen.

8.5.4 Nutritional Management

Energy: The energy requirement of people with CF is more as compared to the person without it which is 1 and half to 2 times more. So, basically a high calorie diet is required to fight lung infections.

Carbs: Starchy foods are to be provided as they are good energy providers.

Protein: People with cystic fibrosis need more energy for breathing as well as to fight infections but these people have a protein and fat digestion problem due to which the nutrients aren't absorbed by the body and they lack many of nutrients. The lack of protein as well as fat is the reason for muscle wasting. It is truly necessary to preserve muscle mass because it helps maintain lung function and leads to less bone loss. The recommended value for the chronic disease is 1.5 g/kg body weight.

Fat: It is recommended that 40% of the calories should come from fats as fat is the richest source of energy and is a good source of essential fatty acids and fat-soluble vitamins. Have more of unsaturated fats as they are a more healthier option.

QUESTIONS

1. What are inborn errors of metabolism? Give examples.
2. Name and define two types of inborn errors of amino acid metabolism.
3. Define inborn error of carbohydrate metabolism. Give examples
4. What is phenylketonuria? Give causes, pathophysiology and dietary management.

5. Discuss the pathophysiology of maple syrup urine disease. Also give its causes and management.
6. Galactosemia is which type of inborn error of metabolism? Discuss briefly.
7. What is cystic fibrosis? Describe briefly.
8. Discuss the causes, symptoms and management of glycogen storage disease.
9. Differentiate between galactosemia and glycogen storage disease.
10. Differentiate between phenylketonuria and maple syrup urine disease.
11. Plan a day's diet for a patient suffering from glycogen storage disease.

9

Hormonal Disorders

9.1 POLYCYSTIC OVARIAN SYNDROME (PCOS)

9.1.1 Introduction

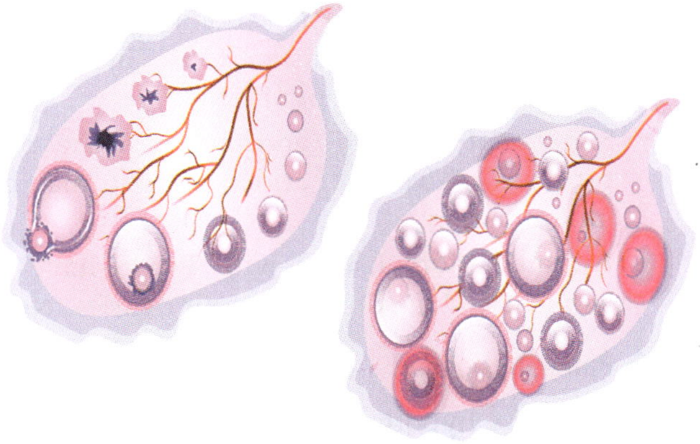

PCOS is a condition with multiple disorders. It has symptoms such as high levels of androgen, inconsistent menstrual cycle and abnormal growth of eggs in ovaries or change on ovary size. Hyperandrogenism, is an indication for PCOS which can lead to development of small types of ovarian cysts and changes in the ovulation and menstrual pattern.

New researches have shown that is becoming common in women in or below the age of 18-44 years of age. Analysis of PCOS has become a common test for women seeking doctors recommendations in conditions like disturbed menstrual cycle, obesity, inflammation of the skin, excessive hair growth and infertility issues. Patients suffering from PCOS are at a higher risk of developing high levels of cholesterol, Cardiovascular diseases, diabetes mellitus, malignant growths, etc.

9.1.2 Causes/Aetiology

PCOS is often depicted as a disease that is effected by mutation of a few genes with variations in the hereditary and natural components of the disease is biochemical, heterogeneous or clinical in nature. As the hereditary causes of PCOS are still unclear, a history of this disease in the family is somewhat seen as normal and prevalent.

Other factors behind this disease and their role in exaggerating it can come from poor or improper dietary habits, physical inactivity, lifestyle disturbances as stressful lives or sleep disorders. Alcoholism can result in PCOS. The problem of PCOS can be reversed by making alteration or small but helpful changes in the lifestyle like taking balanced and healthy diet, increasing physical activities and changing the lifestyle.

Specialists still can't seem to locate the specific reason for PCOS. Be that as it may, a few components may assume a job in whether you create PCOS. These include:

- Heredity: In the event that you have relatives with PCOS or a background marked by diabetes, you're bound to face PCOS.
- An excess of insulin: At the point when you have a lot of this hormone, your cells become resistant to it. This can cause extended androgen creation and trouble ovulating.
- Significant levels of androgen: At the point when your ovaries produce an excess of androgen, you may create hirutism and skin inflammation.
- Augmentation: Ladies with PCOS have a kind of poor quality worsening that stimulates your ovaries to deliver androgens.

9.1.3 Pathophysiology

Damage to the hypothalamus and pituitary gland can also occur which leads to irregular production and functioning of the hormones. One of the major hormones that is affected is insulin and improper functioning of the ovaries are some of the reasons of developing PCOS. But, it was earlier discussed that the exact reason behind PCOS is still unknown, it is often seen in connection with obesity and improper insulin actions. The connection of PCOS with insulin can be seen in the way that since insulin helps in the management of the ovarian function. During the times of excessive secretion of insulin, ovaries are stimulated and start producing androgens which leads to absence of ovulation.

9.1.4 Clinical indications of PCOS

High levels of gonadotropin discharging hormone (GnRH) and leuteinizing hormone (LH), leads to increased secretion of androgens. Although there are no alterations in the level of follicular stimulating hormone (FSH), but, follicular seizure can be treated by increasing the levels of (endogenous) FSH or by inserting FSH exogenously.

It is seen that PCOS is more common in younger generation who have a family history and are at the verge of hitting their puberty. Around 25% of PCOS patients have a high level of prolactin.

Medicines that are advised for curing the disorder are given with the main objective of lowering the level of insulin which will aid in decreasing the production of androgen by the ovaries, ultimately leading to expansion of sex hormone binding globulin (SHBG). This raise, in the levels of SHBG helps in coping with the causes of this disorder. Some studies have reported that when compared to an ordinary patient, a patient of PCOS has shown to have high levels of hormones like progesterone, testosterone and 17-hydroprogesterone.

Since PCOS is a disorder caused due to hormonal imbalance, some of the unexplained side effects of PCOS include: receding hairline or baldness of the type that is commonly seen in men and unwanted hair growth on face, chest and back called hirsutism which is seen in females suffering from the disorders.

9.1.5 Sign Symptoms and Complications

The indications of a female suffering from the disease have the symptoms that can be seen with naked eye:

- Male pattern baldness from your scalp and additionally hair development (hirsutism) in unforeseen spots
- Slick skin and skin break out issues
- Infertility (ovulation issues)
- Weight gain, particularly around your abdomen
- Menstrual issues
- Sadness or potentially state of mind swings

9.1.5.1 Well-being Complications Related to PCOS

Polycystic ovary disorder can bring about a large group of medical problems and difficulties. Weight gain and insulin resistance can likewise exacerbate the side effects. PCOS difficulties include:

- Gestational diabetes or hypertension during pregnancy
- Infertility
- Unnatural birth cycle or untimely birth
- Type 2 diabetes or prediabetes
- Sleep apnea
- Depression , anxiety and dietary issues
- Endometrial malignancy
- Metabolic disorders

9.1.6 Diagnosis

The following are the different standards for the identification of PCOS:

- Rotterdam criteria (2004)

  The suffering patient will be having at least two of the three conditions:

  (i) Hyperandrogenism or excessive androgen (clinical or biochemical)

  (ii) Absent or uneven ovulation pattern (oligo-ovulation)

  (iii) Presence of more than a dozen of follicles in each ovary (polycystic ovaries).

- Identification of PCOS can be done on presence of minimum two of the following parameters- chronic irregular or absent ovulation cycle with a length of more than 35 days excessive production of androgens (hyperandrogenism) and presence of multiple cysts on the ovaries (polycystic ovaries). Androgen Excess and PCOS Society (AES) & American Association of Clinical Endocrinologists (AACE) (2015).

- Important hormones for evaluating PCOS:
  1. Sex hormone binding globulin (SHBG)
  2. Follicle stimulating hormone (FSH)
  3. Testosterone
  4. Lutenizing hormone
  5. Estrogens
  6. Human chorionic gonadotropin (HCG)
  7. Androstenedione
  8. Anti-Müllerian hormone

  Following are the conditions with similar manifestations as of PCOS and in order to clear confusion these tests can be carried out.

S. No.	Condition	Test
1.	Improper functioning of thyroid gland	Thyroid stimulating hormone (TSH)
2.	Cushing syndrome	Cortisol
3.	Hyperprolactinemia	Serum prolactin
4.	Congenital hyperplasia	17-hydroxyprogesterone
5.	Acromegaly	Serum free insulin like growth factor-1 (IGF-1
6.	Adrenal tumor	Dehydroepiandrosterone sulphate (DHEAS)

- Other blood tests include:
    1. Lipid profile, that includes test of high density lipoproteins (HDL), low density lipoproteins (LDL), total cholesterol and triglycerides for understanding the chances of developing dyslipidemia or even CVD.
    2. HbA1c, for detection of diabetes and increased levels of glucose in blood.
    3. Insulin, to keep a check on the levels of insulin.
- Imaging tests: CT scan or MRI of the pelvic region, ultrasonography of the ovaries are the most commonly used imaging tests conducted for the diagnosis of PCOS.

9.1.7 Dietary Management

9.1.7.1 Vitamin D

Vitamin D deficiency has been long associated as one of the reasons behind the onset and progress of type 2 diabetes mellitus. Females who suffer from the problem of PCOS are more prone to develop deficiency of vitamin D. Although there is a bundle of studies which have shown that decreased level of vitamin D is related to increased incidences of metabolic diseases. In a study related to patients of diabetes mellitus has shown that low levels of vitamin D are inversely proportional to the insulin resistance degree.

Some of vitamin D rich foods include vitamin D fortified milk, cereals, fatty fish and eggs. Although 80-90% of the total requirement of vitamin D can be met with exposing ourselves to the sun, but sometimes use of sunscreens or geographic locations can hinder it.

9.1.7.2 Inositol

A part of the B vitamin group: Inositols (myo and d-chiro inositol), are one of the constituent of membrane of the cell. Apart from body producing inositol for itself, beans, grains, and nuts are some rich sources of inositol. Inositol supplements show no gastrointestinal side effects and also helps to better the levels of insulin and decreased intensive hungering.

Inositol is normally recommended as 4 gm/day

D-chiro-inositol has been found to improve the activity of the hormone insulin in patients of PCOS, which can be associated with its quality of improving the ovulation process.It also improves the level of cholesterol, triglycerides and the blood pressure and even serve as capable form for decreasing hyperandrogenism.

The recommended dose of myo-inositol for the disease of poly cystic ovary syndrome is about 1500-4000 mg/day. There are researches supporting the fact that doses a little higher than the recommended have shown to have even a better result. Also taking myo and DCI in combination of 40:1 ratio (4000 mg myo with 100 mg D-chiro-inositol) is also effective in the treatment of PCOS.

Women with PCOS have one of a kind concerns dissimilar to some other ailment because of the crossing point of conceptive and metabolic hormones. With PCOS, there is a characteristic insulin resistance found in most of women. This builds the hazard for diabetes and coronary illness. Diet and way of life changes are the essential treatment approaches for PCOS.

Carbohydrates: Simple carbs and refined carbs are sugars converted to small glucose particles. This implies the body doesn't need to make a effort to separate them. They enter the circulatory system quickly causing a fast ascent in glucose, which triggers a fast increment in insulin. Eating basic sugars aggravates PCOS by raising insulin levels and adding to weight gain.

Whole-grain carbohydrates can improve insulin uptake by facilitation back the upcoming of glucose and prevention of insulin spikes. Insulin levels likewise improve by expending supplements found in entire grains, for example, chromium, magnesium and selenium. In these supplements along with dietary fibre, phytochemicals and cancer prevention agents are also present. Whole grains help with weight as they are very filling. Instances of grains incorporate wheat, corn, oats, spelt, millet, dark coloured rice, kamut and quinoa.

Fruits also contain fructose. They additionally give significant nutrients, minerals and fibre and lower the insulin and cholesterol levels in the body. Fruits eaten with the skin on them (apples, blueberries, strawberries), in general, have a lower glycaemic list than organic products eaten without the skin (pineapple, watermelon).

Vegetables have high fibre content and are rich in nutrients. Nourishment is provided by broccoli, zucchini, spinach, green beans, and peppers which are non-starchy vegetables. Vegetables also comprise lentils, beans and peas. Vegetables are low in glycemic index and also do not raise blood glucose levels and are plant based proteins which are plentiful in fibre, folate, iron and other significant nutrients and minerals that improve insulin uptake in the body.

Milk is rich in calcium and protein, and is viewed as a sugar product because of its high lactose content. There is proof that milk, specifically non-fat, can add to increasing androgen and insulin levels. Consequently, it is prescribed that milk admission be restricted to two or less servings daily.

Protein nourishments are available from animal sources such as meat, poultry, pork, fish, fish, eggs and dairy. Plant-based proteins are vegetables, nuts and soy. Proteins don't require a lot of insulin to breakdown and don't raise insulin levels like starches. Eating protein with dinners can give fullness and balance the raised glucose levels because of insulin resistance.

Fat keeps us fulfilled for longer duration of times. Omega-3 fats are mandatory for women with PCOS. They help improve state of mind, cholesterol, insulin, uptake and even provide with better hair and skin maintenance. Great wellsprings of omega-3s incorporate fish, pecans, and egg yolks.

9.1.8 Case Study

Aim: To plan a day's diet for an acute polycystic ovarian disease (PCOD) female 32 years old, experiencing infertility, nausea, anxiety and also weight gain. Present weight is 85 kg with height 5.2".

General instructions:

- Weight should be brought around expected ideal weight
- Regular exercise should be integral part of daily routine
- Drink plenty of water
- Fat intake should not exceed 30 gm per day
- High fibre diet should be consumed

Foods allowed:

- High fibre foods like whole cereals, whole pulses, sprouts and fruits
- Low fat substitutes like skimmed milk, curd
- Foods rich in soluble fibre like curry leaves, methi leaves
- Foods rich in antioxidants and vitamins (A & C)

Foods to be avoided:

- Refined cereals like suji, maida
- Whole milk and its products
- Deep fried foods
- Bakery products as they contain baking soda

To make your food palatable use spices like cardamom, cinnamon, lemon juice, etc.

9.1.9 Dietary Allowances

Energy : 1700 kcal

Carbs = 70/100 × 1700
= 1190/4
= **298 g**

Protein = 17/100 × 1700
= 289/4
= **72 g**

Fats = 13/100 × 1700
= 221/9
= **25 g**

Food Exchange List

Servings	No. of servings	Energy (kcal)	Cho (g)	Proteins (g)	Fats (g)
Cereals	5	500	100	19	2
Pulses	3	300	75	21	1
Meats and eggs	2	290	--	24	3
Vegetables	4	130	40	4	1
Fruits	4	160	40	--	--
Milk and products	2	140	20	6	3
Fats and oils	4	180	--	--	20
Total		1690	295	74	30

Food Exchange Distribution

Servings	Early morning	Breakfast	Mid morning	Lunch	Evening snack	Dinner	Bed time
Cereals		1		2		2	
Pulses		1			1	1	
Meats and eggs		1		1			
Vegetables				2		2	
Fruits		2	2				
Milk and its products		1				1	
Fats and oils		1		2		1	

Diet Chart

Timing	Menu	Ingredients	Amount (g)	Energy (kcal)	Cho (g)	Protein (g)	Fats (g)
Early Morning	Aloe Vera water		200 mL	--	--	--	--
Breakfast	Strawberry Smoothie (yogurt) Oats besan cheela (1 pc) Soya, Egg white roll	Strawberry, curd Raw oats, Besan, Oil Whole wheat flour, Egg White, Mini soya chunks, Oil	120 g + 150 g 10 g + 30 g + 5 g 30 g + 15 g + 30 g + 5 g	510	78	29	12
Mid-morning	Fruit	Apple	120 g	90	20		
Lunch	Salad 2 Chapati Vegetable Fish (Salmon) grilled	Cucumber Whole wheat flour Brocoli, Carrot, Bell-peppers, Oil Salmon, Oil	100 g 60 g 100 g + 5g 80 g + 5 g	490	89	23	11
Evening snacks	Green Tea Roasted Chana		150 mL 35 g	120	20	3	
Dinner	2 chapati Dal vegetables Sweet Curd	Whole wheat flour Moong dal Spinach, potato, Oil Misti doi	50 g 35 g 120 g + 5 g 100 g	470	92	15	6
Total				**1680**	**299**	**70**	**29**

9.2 THYROID DISORDERS

9.2.1 Hypothyroidism and Hyperthyroidism

Hypothyroidism is the condition in which thyroid gland is underactive. The thyroid gland is unable to produce enough thyroid hormone to meet the daily requirement of the body. Thyroid gland is a butterfly shaped gland present in the front of the neck. The thyroid is situated just below the "Adams apple" or larynx. It is a small gland which weighs less than an ounce and it has two halves or lobes which are present on the sides of windpipe which forms a narrow tissue called isthmus.

One of the functions of thyroid gland is to take iodine and convert it into thyroid hormones that are thyroxine (T4) and triiodothyronine (T3).

Thyroid have specialised cells that can absorb Iodine and they have the ability to combine iodine and tyrosine to make T3 & T4. T3 & T4 are responsible to control metabolism all over the body. The T3 & T4 are transported from thyroid gland to the whole body through bloodstream. The role of the thyroid gland is to control the ways the body utilizes the energy and is very important to maintain the basal metabolic rate of the body. Thyroid hormones regulate metabolism and the energy expenditure is controlled by the thyroid gland. They convert the oxygen and calories to energy. The gland is responsible for production of 80% of T4 and 20% of T3 but the strength of T3 is four times more than the T4. The opposite of this disorder the overactive working of thyroid gland that results in Hyperthyroidism. When the amount of T3 & T4 hormones drops the pituitary gland secretes thyroid stimulating hormone which stimulates the gland to produce the T3 & T4 in ample amounts. And when again T3 & T4 are in required amount in the blood released by thyroid gland, the pituitary gland stops the release of thyroid stimulating hormone. Now this whole signal is sent by hypothalamus by secreting TSH releasing hormone (TRH) to the pituitary gland to secrete thyroid stimulating hormone, i.e., TSH.

The metabolism is an important parameter that has to be properly controlled because the whole functioning of body is dependent on the energy expenditure. The production of thyroid hormones is regulated by thyroid-stimulating hormone (TSH), which is made by the pituitary gland. These regulate metabolism, and they also affect the functions such as development of brain, respiration, cardiac functions, body temperature, skin dryness, menstrual cycle and weight maintenance.

9.2.2 Symptoms of Hypothyroidism

The symptoms include lethargy, obesity, slow basal metabolic rate, cold intolerance, heart rate irregularities, joint pains and aches, cramps, water retention, weakness, sleep disturbances, hair fall, brittle and thin nails constipation, loss of libido, depression and dry skin.

9.2.3 Management of Hypothyroidism

Medication is started as soon as patient is diagnosed with hypothyroidism. The synthetic thyroxine is identical to T4 hormone. It is taken on empty stomach and the dosage depends upon the levels of TSH, T3 and T4. The food is recommended after 40-45 minutes of ingesting the thyroxine hormone so that it can be better absorbed. Even tea, coffee and drinks should be avoided to get this hormone properly absorbed in the body.

9.2.4 Iodine and Nutritional Management

Iodine is an important mineral required for the function of thyroid hormone. The deficiency of iodine leads to a disorder called goitre. The best way to manage the thyroid by diet is to take iodized salt in the diet. Otherwise the people can take iodine supplements also. The foods rich in iodine are fish (such as cod and tuna), seaweed, dairy products, shrimp, and other seafoods.

The foods to be completely avoided are cruciferous vegetables, soy and soy products as they contain goitrogens.

Energy: Normal energy is required according to the RDAs. The only cut down on energy is required if the individual is gaining weight and the need to increase the BMR and weight reduction is needed.

Protein: The proteins need to be increased to increase the muscle mass in the body so that basal metabolic rate can be boosted up. The proteins can be increased to 1.2 to 1.5 gm/ kg body weight per day in an adult. Already it is told that the seafood contains high amounts of iodine so it is important for functioning of thyroid gland. So the dairy products, fish, eggs and sea weeds are rich in proteins as well.

Fats: The fats need to be restricted and low fat diet is recommended but omega 3 fatty acids are to be included which helps in weight control and are good for heart. The fats can be given 40 gm per day with invisible and visible fats combined together. The good fats should be included in the diet. The flax seeds are very good example of omega 3 fatty acids and can be given in vegan diets to reduce weight, increase HDL and smooth working of cardiac muscles.

Vitamins and minerals: Ample amounts of vitamins and minerals are required for the proper absorption of iodine in the body. So adequate amounts should be included in the diet.

9.2.5 Hyperthyroidism

The other disorder related to the thyroid gland is hyperthyroidism. The thyroid gland secretes tetraiodothyronine (T4) and Triiodothyronine (T3) in large amounts in this disorder and it becomes overactive. The finction of these hormones is to regulate the energy consumed by the body.

9.2.5.1 Aetiology

The main causes of this disorder are many but one of the condition is Grave's disease which is an autoimmune disorder. This disorder causes the Thyroid gland to secrete more amount of hormones. In Grave's disease the antibodies of the body stimulate the thyroid gland to produce the increased amount of hormones. The Grave's disorder runs more in women as compared to men.

- Genetics is the another reason for development of the Grave's disease.
- Excess iodine which is the composition of T4 & T3
- Tumor of thyroid or pituitary gland
- Inflammation or damage to thyroid gland also stimulates T4 and T3 production in excess.

9.2.5.2 Symptoms

In this disease the T4 & T3 are secreted in excess so the energy control is disturbed and the body consumes more energy. The body comes in hypermetabolic state. The patient suffers form increased heart rate, hypertension and shivering hands. The sweat glands are activated and also there is low resistance to heat. Due to increased metabolic rate an unusual weight reduction starts. The menstrual cycle is irregular and have impact on reproductive system. Goitre can develop and also the bulging out of eyes depicts the presence of Grave's disease.

There are other symptoms of increased hunger, nervousness, anxiety, sleep disorders, hair fall, brittle hair, nausea and many more. Immediate medical attention is required if the patient lies unconscious or faces difficulty in breathing and vertigo occurs. The bradycardia or tachycardia can result in stroke or heart attack in this condition.

9.2.5.3 Management of Hyperthyroidism

Medication: Antithyroid medications, such as methimazole (tapazole), is given so that over production of hormones can be stopped.

9.2.6 Dietary Management

The diet would be exactly opposite as given in hypothyroidism.

Energy: The calorie intake is increased due to hypermetabolism but healthy fats should be incorporated.

Proteins: Animal proteins and dairy products should be given, The protein requirement also increases due to muscle wasting and weight loss.

Fats: Try to inculcate the omega three fatty acids in the diet so that heart remains healthy.

9.2.6.1 Low Intake of Iodine

The mineral iodine plays a key role in making thyroid hormones. A low-iodine diet helps to reduce thyroid hormones. So take non-iodized salt, egg whites, fresh fruits and unsalted nuts. Anything with added salt is stopped such as chips, processed food, ketchups or packed snacks.

All the cabbage family or cruciferous family is allowed to hinder iodine absorption. Soy products are allowed as they have good fats also.

9.2.6.2 Vitamins and Minerals

Several nutrients are essential for thyroid health and to balance thyroid hormone production.

9.2.6.3 Iron and Selenium

Plenty of iron is recommended so include foods like green leafy veggies, nuts and oilseeds, red meats, poultry, mutton, Chia seeds, mushrooms, rice, tea are allowed.

9.2.6.4 Calcium and Vitamin D

Bones are the majorly at risk in hyperthyroidism. It causes brittle and weak bones as calcium and vitamin D are not absorbed properly. So include green leafy veggies, almond milk, white beans, kale, calcium & vitamin D fortified cereals in daily diet.

QUESTIONS

1. Define polycystic ovarian disease. Discuss its causes, symptoms and related complications along with management.
2. Differentiate between polycystic ovary syndrome (PCOS) and polycystic ovarian disease (PCOD).
3. How can lifestyle modifications help in treatment of PCOS and PCOD?
4. Plan a diet for a woman in mid-30s suffering from PCOD.
5. Describe different types of disorders of thyroid gland.
6. Differentiate between hypothyroidism and hyperthyroidism in terms of causes, symptoms and dietary management.
7. What is goitre? Give its causes, symptoms, management and prevention.
8. Plan a day's diet for a female patient of age 35 years suffering from polycystic ovarian disease.
9. Plan a day's diet for a female patient of age 40 suffering from hypothyroidism and type II diabetes mellitus.
10. Write brief notes on:
    (i) PCOD
    (ii) Hyperthyroidism
    (iii) Goiter
    (iv) Hypothyroidism

10

Cancers

10.1 TYPES AND DIETARY MANAGEMENT

10.1.1 Definition

Cancer is one of the major reasons for deaths on the planet. The development of this disease is fast and sometimes undetectable. The cells start to behave differently, developing, duplicating and spreading uncontrollably. Cancer growth resembles a battle in the body where a number of cells quit working and perform functions to benefit the body. Cancers are the uncontrolled growth of cells that are in distorted form or abnormal form that spreads in any part of the body. There are around 200 types of cancers. Some causative agents in the body which cause cancers. These agents are categorized as chemical or toxic compounds or Ionizing radiations and human genetics.

10.1.2 Development of Cancers

Our body is made of numerous cells and a cell is the basic unit of life. The cycle of cells in the body is when cells become mature, they die and new cells emerge. But sometimes the new cells that develop into the cancerous cells. The normal cells starts mutating into the abnormal cells and these cells do get exhausted and die. These new cancerous cells further grow into other tissues and then harm the body. The development of cancers in the body has a number of steps. The new cancerous cells formed in the body release growth factors and digestive enzymes. These cells continue to multiply, divide further and this way impact the working of tissues of the body. In some cases the tumours die and it takes several years to reach the size of detection. It is not applicable to all kinds of cancers.

10.1.3 Stages of Tumour Development

The growth of the tumorous cells in the body is a stepwise progression. The tumours in form of solids are called sarcomas or carcinomas. The blood cell tumours also undergo same procedure and the cells freely float around the body and not specified to a location.

Hyperplasia: In this stage the cell division starts in an uncontrollable manner and the localised division of cells occurs in one region of the tissue. The cells may appear as normal but the number is not always normal.

Dysplasia: The genetic changes start in the body and proliferation of cells is enormous. The appearance of the cells is abnormal and also the tissue has an abnormal structure as well.

Carcinoma in situ: The abnormal cells further spread and make the cells and tissue appearance more abnormal. The cells till now spread to larger areas of the body. The cells are no longer useful and do not fulfil their functions. For example, if stomach has such tumour or erosions then the digestive process is affected. Cells of this type are said to be de-differentiated or anaplastic. There is no doubt that such type of cancers which are localised can be removed by surgery easily and also their spread to other tissues also stops. Because these types do not invade the surrounding tissues.

Cancer (malignant tumours): These type of tumours have the ability to attack the surrounding tissue and these take malignant form. These types of cancers are metastatic and the tumours are most dangerous to lives of people. The abnormal cells developed in this type of cancer travel to different parts of the body. Some tumours do not progress and invasion does not start in distant tissues. Such tumours are benign. Large benign tumours can put pressure on organs. In the case of brain tumours, the limited space within the skull means that a large growth in the brain cavity can be fatal.

Tumours can be benign (non-cancerous) or malignant (cancerous). Benign tumour can often be removed and it has less chances of re-occurrence whereas malignant tumours can invade nearby tissues and spread to other parts of the body.

10.2 AETIOLOGY OF CANCER

Cancer is basically the result of changes that we people have made in the chemical environment, i.e., what we eat, drink and breathe. Today's diet is filled with chemicals and lacks nutrients. The processed foods, preservatives and many agents that are being added in the food are major causes of cancers. Most of the cancers are linked with lifestyle factors like diet, smoking and drinking alcohol. Genes are also one of the reasons for cancers but development of a suitable environment is also required for the progression of cancer. Pollution, infection, drugs, food additives, ultraviolet rays are also some of the factors which are responsible for cancers.

A carcinogen is defined as any substance, radionuclide, or radiation that promotes the formation of cancer or carcinogenesis. This may be due to the ability to damage the genome or to the disruption of cellular metabolic processes.

Talking about carcinogens , it is the substance that induces cancer by damaging the DNA. It is supported by the help of free radicals and these free radicals develop from smoking and so a diet rich in antioxidants, i.e., fruits and vegetables acts as a protector against free radicals.

One of the other reasons of cancer is poor methylation which results in high homocysteine and this further leads to an increased damage to DNA. The deficiency of vitamin B class xan be the reason. These carcinogens are categorized into three groups, i.e., physical, chemical and biological carcinogens.

Physical carcinogens: These are ionizing and the ultraviolet radiation.

Chemical carcinogens: These are the chemicals which show the carcinogenic effect They cause a problem to the regular genes. These chemicals are from the industries or can be a tobacco smoke or even aflatoxin (a food contaminant) and arsenic (a water contaminant).

Biological carcinogens: Such as infection caused by viruses, bacteria or parasites. Ageing is also one of the causes for the development of cancer. The risk of cancer increases with age. Next cause is stress which weakens our immune system and also leads to our behavioural changes due to which intake of food is decreased and there is loss of nutrients in the body due to which a person becomes more vulnerable to the cancer producing effects. Alcohol or tobacco intake are the major risk factors of cancer.

There are certain factors that can enhance the carcinogenic process and some that can inhibit the carcinogenic effect. The factors that enhance the carcinogens are given in the aetiology of cancers. The factors which inhibit carcinogenes are as under.

10.2.1 Antioxidant Activity

Some factors like UV rays, toxic drugs, carcinogens (physical, chemical and biological) and over indulgence are responsible for the increase in the number of free radicals in the body. These free radicals are basically the oxygen molecules which are highly reactive, that have lost there electron while circulating through the blood stream. So, these molecules try to become chemically stable and that to by snatching electrons from other molecules and hence, this process causes much damage to the body leading to cancers, stroke, heart disease, etc.

10.2.2 Role of Dietary Factors

There was a study done by National Cancer Institute, according to which they stated that β-Carotene given to smokers was of no benefit. It could harm a person and if given to a non-smoker or the person who has already quit smoking then it turns out to have decreased chances of lung cancer. It is because giving antioxidant to a smoker and ignoring the principle of synergy could make the matter worse. But there were many other studies that giving β-Carotene supplements with other antioxidants or given naturally with the diet shows the reduction of cancer risk. Even among smokers, a high dietary intake of β-Carotene is not linked with increased risk.

It is said that cancer patients live longer on vitamin C. A review of Vitamin C research concluded that evidence of a protective effect for cancers. As we know vitamin C is an antioxidant and has the capability to destroy the free radicals it is also capable of destroying a number of other carcinogens (cancer causing agents) such as nitrosamines. These can occur when chemicals called nitrates combine with amines. Vitamin C may be especially effective against cancers of the digestive tract because of its ability to disarm these carcinogens as well as its proven immune boosting properties.

Vitamin E is also a powerful anticancer agent especially in combination with selenium.

10.3 DIETARY MANAGEMENT

Energy: Patient should consume adequate energy to keep up their nourishment stores and to maintain the weight which is assessed through body mass index. An adult patient who has a good nutritional status needs 2000 to 2500 kcal/day for maintenance and recover from the disease. As far as malnourished patients is concerned, they require more calories, that is, 2500 to 3500 kcal/day.

Protein: Extra protein is required by the body to fix and reconstruct tissue influenced by disease treatment and to keep up a healthy immune system. An intake of 1.5–2 g/kg body weight of protein/day is required for maintenance and complete anabolism. In case the patient is malnourished an intake of 2–2.5 g/kg body weight of protein/day is recommended.

Fat: There is loss of adipose tissue so 15-20 per cent of the fat of total energy requirement should be provided.

Vitamins and minerals: Vitamins and minerals help protein and energy digestion through their coenzyme in explicit cell enzyme pathways and furthermore assume significant role in building and keeping up strong tissue.

Fluids: There are certain GI losses because of fever, infection, diarrhoea, vomiting and so adequate fluid is essential to cover up the losses.

10.4 TYPES OF CANCERS

10.4.1 Oesophageal Cancer

Oesophageal cancer refers to the cancer of the food pipe known as the oesophagus that connects the throat to the stomach. Weight loss and difficulty in swallowing the food are the most common symptoms in this type of cancer with symptoms of pain during swallowing, croaky voice, lymph nodes around the collar bones get enlarged, cough (dry), and vomit containing traces of blood.

Types of oesophageal cancer include

1. **Squamous cell carcinoma:** The one which begins from the oesophageal cells.
2. **Adeno-carcinoma:** The one which begins from the tissue (glandular) of the oesophageal cells lining.

Since there are no signs of the oesophageal cancer in the early stages, in most of the cases it is detected in advanced stages as it grows slowly and is hard to detect in early stages.

Manifestations:

- Discomfort and struggle while swallowing
- Pain or discomfort in upper and mid chest (heartburn)
- Vomit containing traces of blood
- Black coloured or stools with blood
- Inexplicable exhaustion and tiredness
- Asphyxiation while gulping food
- Feeling of uneasiness mostly during consuming food, particularly in the upper abdomen

Risk factors: Smoking tobacco, alcohol consumption, acid reflux, chewing betel nuts,

Prognosis: 5 years survival on an average.

The sickness is diagnosed by diagnostic assay done by (a fibre-optic camera).

Treatment focuses on removing the cancer through surgery. Chemotherapy and radiation may also be used.

Dietary modifications: RT Feeding 200 mL 2nd hourly.

C/O vomiting, swelling of gums due to medications , loss of appetite

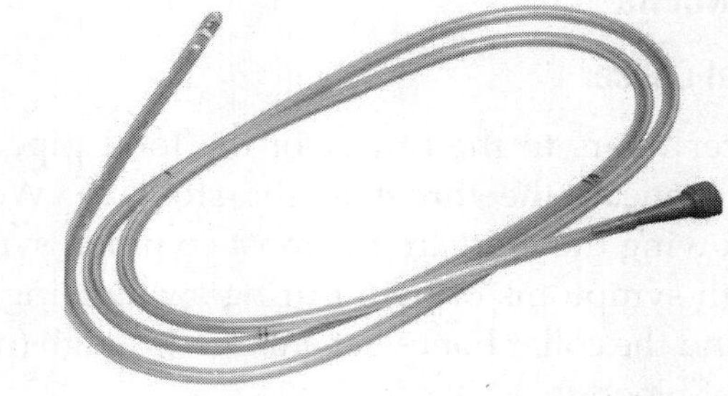

RT Feeding (Ryle's Tube)

Ryle's tube feeding, commonly known as RT feeding or naso-gastric feeding is generally opted when the patient is critically ill or is incapable of eating or swallowing food or even water. A tube called naso-gastric tube through the nostril of the patient into the stomach through the oesophagus, and this process is called naso-gastric (NG) intubation.

After inserting the tube, i.e., naso-gastric intubation, food and medicines can be provided to the patient through this tube. It is also used to remove excess/undigested food, liquid or other harmful contents from the abdomen through the process called aspiration.

Ryle's tube is a soft PVC tube which is twist resistant and comes in different sizes with a funnel that has colour coding and end connector for effortless recognition of sizes.

10.4.1.1 Example of Feed

R T FEED 200 mL

Meal	Menu	Ingredient	Amount	Energy (kcal)	Protein (g)	CHO (g)	Fat (g)	Dietary fibre (g)
Service 1 (6 am)	Milk-Bread Feed	Milk	200 mL	60 kcal	5.2 g	9.2 g	0.16 g	-
		Ataa	2 slice	350 kcal	3.9 g	28.5 g	0.6 g	1.7 g
Service 2 (8 am)	Rice-Moong dal Feed	Rice	50 g	175 kcal	4 g	35.85 g	-	1.5 g
		Moong dal	50 g	168 kcal	26 g	18.5 g	0.5 g	6.5 g
		Water						
Service 3 (10 am)	Veg. Stock Feed	Suji	10 g	34.4 kcal	1.1 g	7 g	0.1 g	1 g
		Green gram dal	20 g	66 kcal	4.6 g	12 g	-	0.72
		Carrot	20 g	8 kcal	1.2 g	1.24 g	-	0.25 g
		Pumpkin	20 g	3 kcal	0.02 g	0.45 g	-	0.20 g
		Colocasia	20 g	7.12 kcal	0.4 g	1.23	-	1 g
		Tinda	20 g	2.6 kcal	1 g	0.45 g	0.26 g	0.42 g
Service 4 (12 noon)	Buttermilk Feed	Curd	100 g	75 kcal	3.7 g	5 g	4.5 g	-
		Water	100 mL	-	-	-	-	-

Service 5 (2 pm)	Khichri Feed	Black chana Rice Oil	10 g 10 g 1.5 g	33 kcal 35 kcal 13.8 kcal	2.3 g 0.8 g -	6 g 7.17 g -	- - 1.5 g	0.36 g 0.3 g -
Service 6 (4 pm)	Milk-Biscuits Feed	Milk Ataa + Bournvita	200 mL 2 slice	60 kcal 350 kcal	5.2 g 3.9 g	9.2 g 28.5 g	0.16 g 0.6 g	- 1.7 g
Service 7 (6 pm)	Veg. Broth	Daliya Nutrella Carrot Peas Potato Tinda	10 g 20 g 20 g 20 g 20 g 20 g	34.4 kcal 66 kcal 8 kcal 3 kcal 7.12 kcal 2.6 kcal	1.1 g 4.6 g 1.2 g 0.02 g 0.4 g 1 g	7 g 12 g 1.24 g 0.45 g 1.23 0.45 g	0.1 g - - - - 0.26 g	1 g 0.72 0.25 g 0.20 g 1 g 0.42 g
Service 8 (8 pm)	Poha Feed	Poha	150 g	516 kcal	16.5 g	105 g	1.5 g	15 g
Service 9 (10 pm)	Milk-Chapati Feed	Milk Ataa	200 mL 2	60 kcal 350 kcal	5.2 g 3.9 g	9.2 g 28.5 g	0.16 g 0.6 g	- 1.7 g
Total				1095.5 kcal	37 g	167.5 g	47 g	9.49 g

General Dietary Tips (Tube is being inserted)

Type of diet: RT feed

- Drink lots of water.
- Clean the tube properly and keep the nozzle closed when not in use.
- Boil the vegetables and pulses properly and mash them in the grinder then strain it properly.
- Don't give too hot or too cold fluids through tube.
- Whey water can also be given to the patient.
- 8 scoops of protein powder as recommended by doctor to be given 3 times a day mixed well in the feed.
- Do not restrict the fats completely.
- Well strained vegetable soup can be given.
- Do not change the diet without consultation.

10.4.2 Hibernoma

In 1914, Gery explained about a certain type of fat growth showing strong similarities to the torpid glands of sure mammals and termed it "hibernoma". Originating from the residual cells of the brown fat, hibernomas are uncommon non-malignant lipomatous tumours.

Vertebrate adipose tumour, adipose tumour of embryonic fat or adipose tumours of immature fat are the different terms used for the lesion. A benign tumour in the fat tissues can be an adipose tumour. These lesion with a size of not more than 5 cm usually occur somewhat below the skin, are pain-free, soft and mobile. They can mostly be seen on abdomen, upper back and shoulders. Family history, obesity, and not enough exercise are some of the predisposing factors of the disease.

The prevalence of this cancer is found to be more in males when compared to females. The most commonly affected parts by the hibernoma are mostly in the areas of connective and muscle tissues near the pinnacle and neck areas such as shoulder, scapular and neck, followed by thigh, back, chest, abdomen, and arms. Steroid hormones are also produced as seen in some cases.

10.4.2.1 NPO (Nil per Oral)

NPO order is generally given before performing an operation, the patient is refrained from intake of any food or fluid item for a period of time to avoid the food, liquid or any other content of the stomach to breathe in into the airway (pulmonary aspiration).

The process of NPO or fasting is performed basically 2-6 hours before the operation as per the fasting guidelines, with the purpose of emptying the stomach as much as possible as even an aspiration of about 30–40 mL can prove damaging and even fatal in some cases during an operation. Conditions like filled stomach, lack of anaesthesia, obesity, changed gastrointestinal mobility, pregnancy; emergency surgeries, etc., are some of the risk factors that can also lead to aspiration. Abstaining from food for a longer period lowers the incidence of damage from aspiration.

Typically, the NPO orders are given before 6 and 12 hours prior to the surgery, but can be increased in case if there is administration of medicines which is long acting or oral post-medications were given. Severe diseases have a longer NPO period with exceptions for introducing small amount of water at regular interval if no intravenous fluid is given. It is suggested that in non-diabetic patients NPO periods can be continued for up to several days with proper ingestion of IV fluids, but in case of diabetics a shorter NPO period is advised with ingestion of insulin, IV fluids and dextrose, but a time period of more than 12 hours is still opposed.

Before the surgery there should be a restriction on consuming any solid food item for a minimum of 8 hours and all the fluid including clear fluid (that includes water, tea, coffee, pulped juices, carbonated drinks, etc.) should be restricted before 2 hours of the procedure. Drinking water 2 hours before the surgery may result in changed gastric pH to the higher side with small gastric volumes than those who have taken the liquid 4 hours before. The kind of liquid drunk is more important than the amount of liquid.

10.4.2.2 Dietary Tips

Type of diet: Soft diet

- Drink lots of water.
- Avoid eating red meat.
- Include 2 eggs daily in your diet.
- Eat lots of green vegetables in cooked form.
- Avoid eating raw foods as the immunity of the patient is currently compromise and there are high chances infections therefore prefer properly washed and cooked food only for at least 3 months.
- Can include oats cheela/ragi cheela/suji cheela in place of biscuits.
- Give small but frequent meals.
- Prefer fruits over fruit juices.
- Can change the diet from soft to normal after 3-4 days.
- In order to keep away from early satiety, drink fluids before and after meals rather than drinking while having the meals.
- Include calorie rich beverages such as milk shakes, protein shakes, etc., to the diet to fulfil the requirement of daily calories.
- Increase use of milk and milk products such as yogurt but avoid using dairy products which are not pasteurized such as soft cheese to avoid any chances of infections.
- Include foods with high calorie contents such as poultry, nuts, lean meat, etc., in the diet.

10.4.3 Acute Myeloid Leukaemia (AML)

10.4.3.1 Leukaemias

Leukaemia is a type of cancer which basically initiates from the cells and then develops into blood cells of different types. It a neoplastic fatal disorder that initiates from the white blood cells but in some cases the origin can be from the somatic cells also. The type of leukaemia is categorized depending on the following parameters:

- Progression of the disease is fast or slow (acute or chronic)
- Origin from the cells (myeloid or lymphoid)

10.4.3.2 Bone Marrow

Certain bones of the body have a soft inner part that is made up of cells which produce blood (blood stem cells), fat cells and tissues supporting them. The blood stem cells are responsible for the production of new blood cells. In this process, the produced cells are either a type of white blood cell (lymphocytes) or other type of cells which form the blood (myeloid cells). Other blood forming cells or myeloid cells transform into RBCs, WBCs (other than lymphocytes), and leucocytes. During acute myeloid leukaemia, abnormalities in the myeloid cells are seen.

Acute myeloid leukaemia (AML): Starting from the bone marrow which is the main location for the production of new blood cells, it quickly progresses into the blood. Sometimes it even escalates into different body parts such as the brain and spinal cord (central nervous system), lymph nodes, liver, spleen, etc. AML develops from cells that would turn into white blood cells, i.e., the myeloid cells, these cells grow rapidly in numbers and become cancerous thus the name myeloid leukaemia and since it's growing rapidly it is named acute myeloid leukaemia (AML), sometimes it can also be seen in other type of cells that form blood also. Repetitive infections, feeling of tiredness, high body temperature, and easily injuring the body are some of the primary symptoms of this disease. It can be due to the inadequate amount of red blood cells and leucocytes and presence of excessive immature white blood cells most of which are myeloblasts also referred to as "blast cells". Acute granulocytic leukaemia, acute myelogenous leukaemia, acute myelocytic leukaemia and acute non-lymphocytic leukaemia are some of the other names by which acute myeloid lukemia is also known.

Principle of diet-liquid diet

- Intake of plenty of water and fluid, for example, fruit juices, nectars, juice with fruit pulps, tea, coffee, etc.
- Consumption of solid food should be avoided.
- Include a lot of fluid items in the diet, food items like ice cream, custard and pudding, frozen yogurt, etc., that turn into liquid at room temperature can also be included in the diet.
- Fluid items like sugar, honey syrup, soup, broth.
- Liquid supplements like Boost, Protein powder (8 scoops/day), Resource, and other liquid supplements.
- Regular follow-up.

10.4.4 Oral Cancer (Tongue Cancer)

Oral cancer is basically the cancer of the mouth or throat tissues. It is the part of a larger body of classifications of head and neck cancers. This type of a cancer mainly develops in the squamous cells found in your mouth, tongue and lips.

One of the biggest risk factors for oral cancer is consuming tobacco which includes smoking cigarettes, cigars, and pipes, as well as chewing tobacco.

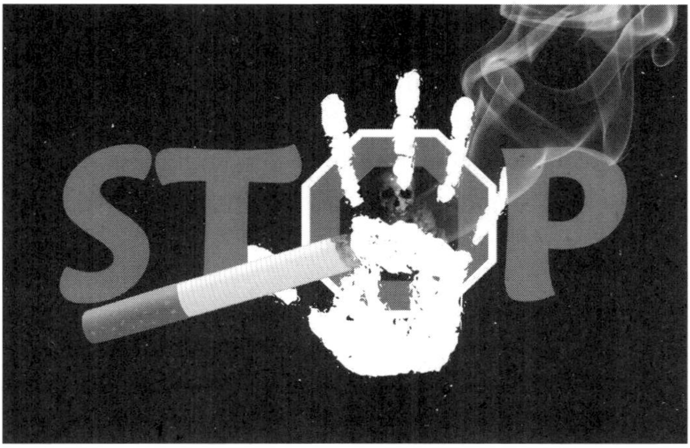

Other reasons

- Human papillomavirus (HPV) infection
- Chronic facial sun exposure
- Previous diagnosis of oral cancer
- Family history
- Weakened immune system
- Poor nutrition
- Genetic syndromes

10.4.4.1 Glossectomy Surgery

A glossectomy is the removal of part of or all of the tongue. It can be used to treat cancers of the tongue, some oral cavity (inside the mouth) and throat cancers. The functions of tongueinclude tasting, swallowing, breathing, licking and speaking.

The types of glossectomy include

Partial Glossectomy: Removal of part of the tongue. Can also include removal one side of the tongue, which may be called hemiglossectomy.

Hemiglossectomy: Removal of one side of the tongue, leaving the other side intact.

Total glossectomy: Removal of the whole tongue. This results in an inability to swallow without getting food/liquids into the lungs (called aspiration). Because of this, a laryngectomy may also be done. Laryngectomy (removal of the larynx or voice box) helps prevent aspiration, but also results in loss of your voice. Glossectomy also requires reconstructive surgery.

Type of Diet: RT Feed

- Drink lots of water.
- Clean the tube properly and keep the nozzle closed when not in use
- Boil the vegetables and pulses properly and mash them in the grinder then strain if properly.
- Don't give too hot or too cold fluids through tube.
- Whey water can also be given to the patient.
- 8 scoops of protein powder to be given 3 times a day mixed well in the feed.
- Do not restrict the fats completely.
- Well strained vegetable soup can be given.

10.4.5 Ovarian Cancer

Ovarian cancer is a broad term which is used for any kind of cancer that has its origin in the ovaries of a female. Normal physiology shows the presence of two ovaries in female reproductive system, one on each side.

In most of the cases ovarian cancer remains undetected until it starts affecting the area of pelvis and abdomen. Since this type of cancer remains undetected for a long period it is more difficult to treat and in most many proved to be lethal. But if this cancer is detected in its early stage, i.e., during the early stage gonad cancer, it can be treated with more success as the cancer is only restricted to the ovaries at that time.

10.4.5.1 Manifestations/Symptoms

Generally, there are no signs or symptoms are seen during the early stages of ovarian cancer. As the disease advances to higher stages of gonad cancer, there are some non-precise signs which can often be confused for additional common benign conditions.

- Distended or swollen abdomen
- Quick feeling of satiety
- Weight reduction
- Feeling of discomfort in the pelvis
- Altered bowel habits/constipation
- Dysuria (feeling of need of urinating frequently)

10.4.5.2 Aetiology/Causes

Till now there are no proper guidelines for what are the reasons behind the cause of this type of cancer, although a list of reasons that can negatively aid to this condition have been identified by the doctors.

Generally, cancer initiates when there is some mutation in the polymer of the cells, leading to improper growth and multiplication of the cells, producing a mass bunch of tumour consisting of abnormal cells. Slowly these abnormal cells take over the health cells and then attack the adjacent tissues and starts metastasizing within the body.

10.4.5.3 Risk Factors

Age and gender: Although it can occur at any age, but, old people and women under the age group of 50-60 years are at a higher risk of developing the cancer.

Gene inheritance: Mutated genes inherited by parents have shown to grow the chances of ovarian cancer (low incidences) in some cases. Breast cancer gene 1 (BRCA1) and breast cancer gene 2 (BRCA2) are the two genes that are jointly responsible for the incidence of ovarian cancer .

Family history: A person is more likely to develop cancer if she has a close family history of ovarian cancer.

Hormone replacement therapy: People with a history of large dose and long term use of hormonal therapies such as estrogen hormone replacement therapy, are more susceptible to this kind of cancer.

Early menarche and late menopause

Type of diet: Soft diet

- Drink lots of water.
- Avoid eating red meat.
- Include 2 eggs daily in your diet.
- Eat lots of green vegetables in cooked form.
- Avoid eating raw foods as the immunity of the patient is currently compromise and there are high chances infections therefore prefer properly washed and cooked food only for atleast 3 months.
- Can include oats cheela/ ragi cheela/ suji cheela in place of biscuits.
- Give small but frequent meals.
- Prefer fruits over fruit juices.
- Can change the diet from soft to normal after 3-4 days.
- Follow up after 3 weeks, 10:00 am.
- Avoid greasy, fried and strongly spiced foods.

- Plan to eat your biggest meal at the time when you tend to be the most hungry.
- In order to keep away from early satiety, drink fluids before and after meals rather than drinking while having the meals.
- Include calorie rich beverages such as milk shakes, protein shakes, etc., to the diet to fulfil the requirement of daily calories.
- Increase use of milk and milk products such as yogurt but avoid using dairy products which are not pasteurized such as soft cheese to avoid any chances of infection.

10.4.6 Rectosigmoid and Rectum Cancer

The last part of the large colon that is about 15-20 cms, that leads to the end of the digestive tract is called the rectum The main origin of rectal cancer is basically from the colon or the rectum, also known as colon cancer or colorectal cancer. But, since the progress and treatment of both the cancers (colon and rectum) are different, they are approached differently.

In general, the cancers arising from the rectum and sigmoid colon called rectal and recto-sigmoid cancer, shows more signs for their diagnosis than compared to other type of cancer. Symptoms include bleeding, altered bowel habits, unexplained constipation or reduced stool amount, urgent and inadequate bowel emptying. As the disease progresses there are episodes of pain in the buttocks. All these signs ultimately starts affecting the colorectal areas.

The symptoms of the cancer are generally vague during the initial stages. The symptoms are more visible only after the disease has reached its second stage or sometimes even beyond. A test called colonoscopy is generally recommended for screening the colon and rectal cancer. In many hospitals, colonoscopy a part of the routine checkups for patients above the age of 50 years or for those with the family history of any kind of cancer.

10.4.6.1 Manifestations/Symptoms

- Altered bowel activity.
  - ◊ Difficulty in passing stool (constipation).
  - ◊ Loose and watery stool (diarrhoea).
  - ◊ Hematochezia (passage of blood in stool due to bleeding in the rectum).
  - ◊ Pain and swelling in the abdomen.
  - ◊ Unexplained reduction in weight.
  - ◊ Appetite loss which is unexplained.

◊ Feeling of vomiting (nausea).
◊ Anaemia.
◊ Jaundice.
◊ Feeling of tiredness.

Type of diet: RT feed

- Drink lots of water.
- Clean the tube properly and keep the nozzle closed when not in use
- Boil the vegetables and pulses properly and mash them in the grinder then strain it properly.
- Don't give too hot or too cold fluids through tube.
- Whey water can also be given to the patient.
- 8 scoops of protein powder to be given 3 times a day mixed well in the feed.
- Do not restrict the fats completely.
- Well strained vegetable soup can be given.

After the completion of surgery or chemotherapy or if the condition of patient allows start with liquid diet and follow the instructions as under.

10.4.6.2 Principle of Liquid Diet

- Intake of plenty of water and fluid, for example fruit juices, nectars, juice with fruit pulps, tea, coffee, etc.
- Consumption of solid food should be avoided.
- Include a lot of fluid items in the diet, food items like ice cream, custard and pudding, frozen yogurt etc., that turn into liquid at room temperature can also be included in the diet.
- Fluid items like Sugar, honey syrup, soup, broth.
- Liquid supplements like protein powder (8 scoops/ day), Resource, and other liquid supplements.
- Regular follow up.

CASE STUDIES

1. TO PLAN A DAY'S DIET FOR A PATIENT OF 35 YEARS OLD SUFFERING FROM BREAST CANCER UNDERGOING CHEMOTHERAPY. THE OTHER SIDE EFFECTS ARE MUCOSITIS, VOMITING AND NAUSEA

Nutritional Requirement

Energy: 30-35 kcal/kg body wt = 35 × 55 =1925 kcal

Protein: 1.5-2 gm/kg body wt = 82.5 gm

CHO: 50-55% of total energy = 264 gm
Fats: 30% of total energy = 64 gm

Menu

Meal timing	Menu
Early morning	Milk -200 mL Almonds-20 g
Breakfast	Oats porridge • Oats-80 g • Onion-30 g • Tomato-30 g • Capsicum-30 g • Carrot –30 g • Oil/butter-5 g Pineapple juice – 50 mL
Mid-morning	Fruits (chopped) • Plum-50 gm • Melon-50 g • Apple-50
Lunch	Roti -2 nos. • Whole wheat flour-60 g Brown rice -50 g Boiled Dal -1 katori • Lentil -30 g • Onion -30 g Mix veg-1 katori • Broccoli-30 g • Carrot -30 • Oil -5 g Lean Chicken -100 g • Oil-5 g
Evening snack	Quinoa upma • Quinoa-30 g • Tomato-30 g • Onion-30 g • Capsicum-30 g • Oil-5 g
Dinner	Brown rice-50 g Roti-2 nos. • Whole wheat flour-60 g Sabji-1 katori • Turnip -30 g • Tomato-30 g • Onion-30 g • Oil -10 g

Nutritive Value

Ingredients	Amount	Energy	Protein	CHO	Fat
Milk	100 mL	70	3	5	3
Almond	20 g	65.5	2.08	8.05	5.89
Oats	80 g	308	9.2	55.2	5.6
Onion	30 g	15	0.36	3.33	3.03
Tomato	30 g	12	0.54	2.16	0.12
Capsicum	30 g	7.2	0.39	0.19	0.09
Carrots	30 g	14.4	0.27	3.18	0.06
Oil	5 g	45	-	-	5
Pineapple	50 g	23	0.2	5.4	0.05
Plum	50 g	26	0.35	5.55	0.25
Melon	50 g	8	0.1	1.665	0.1
Apple	50 g	29.5	0.1	6.7	0.25
Whole wheat flour	60 g	204.6	7.26	4.164	1.02
Brown rice	50 g	174.5	4.45	38.7	0.3
Lentil	30 g	102.9	7.53	17.7	0.21
Onion	30 g	15	0.36	3.33	0.03
Oil	5 g	45	-	-	5
Broccoli	30 g	9.3	0.75	1.8	0.12
Carrot	30 g	14.4	0.27	3.18	0.06
Oil	5 g	45	-	-	5
Chicken	100 g	109	25.9	-	0.6
Quinoa	30 g	36	1.32	6.39	0.57
Tomato	30 g	12	0.54	2.16	0.12
Onion	30 g	15	0.36	3.33	0.03
Capsicum	30 g	7.2	0.39	0.19	0.09
Oil	5 g	45	-	-	5
Brown rice	50 g	174.5	4.45	38.7	0.3
Whole wheat flour	60 g	204.6	7.26	41.64	1.02
Turnip	30 g	8.7	0.15	1.86	0.06
Tomato	30 g	12	0.54	2.16	0.12
Onion	30 g	15	0.36	3.33	0.03
Oil	10	90	-	-	10
Total		1963 kcal	81.43 g	265 g	54 g

Energy : 1963 kcal, Protein: 81.43 g CHO: 265 g Fat: 54 g

2. TO PLAN A DAY'S DIET FOR A FEMALE AGE 35 YEARS OLD SUFFERING FROM CERVIX CANCER, PATIENT HAVE SEVERE CACHEXIA AND HAIRFALL

Nutritional Requirement

Energy: 30-35 kcal/kg/IBW = 1925 kcal

Protein: 1.5-2 gm/kg/IBW = 82.5 gm

CHO: 50-55% = 264 gm

Fats: 30% of total energy = 64 gm

Menu

Meal Time	Menu
Breakfast	Veg sandwich • Cabbage-100 g • Onion-30 g • Cheese -60 g • Bread slices-60 g • Tomato-30 g Egg white-50 g
Mid-morning	Fruits (chopped) • Papaya – 100 g • Avocado – 50 g • Apple-50 g • Honey -2 tsp
Lunch	Rice – 100 g Fish curry – 1 katori • Potato – 30 g • Onion-30 g • Pumpkin-30 g • Ridge gourd-70 g • Rohu -50 g • Oil – 1 tsp
Evening Snack	Samai kheer • Samai-40 g • Skimmed milk-100 mL
Dinner	Paneer Khichidi – 1 bowl • Rice – 100 g • Masoor dal – 25 g • Onion-20 g • Paneer – 40 g • Spinach – 25 g • Mint leaves – 10 g • Oil – 1 tsp

Nutritive Value

Ingredients	Amount	Energy	Protein	CHO	Fats
Cabbage	100 g	27	1.8	4.6	0.1
Onion	80 g	40	0.96	8.88	0.08
Cheese	60 g	208	8.04	3.78	13.8
Bread slices	60 g	147	4.68	31.14	0.42
Tomato	30 g	6	0.27	1.08	0.06
Egg white	50 g	85	7	-	7
Papaya	100 g	32	0.6	7.2	0.1
Avocado	50 g	107.5	0.85	0.4	11.4
Apple	50 g	42.3	0.1	6.7	0.25
Honey	10 g	31.9	0.03	7.95	-
Rice	200 g	698	17	150.4	1.2
Potato	30 g	29.1	0.48	4.69	0.03
Pumpkin	30 g	7.5	0.42	1.38	0.03
Ridge gourd	70 g	11.9	0.35	2.38	0.07
Rohu	50 g	48.5	8.3	2.2	0.7
Oil	10 g	90	-	-	20
Samai	40 g	136.4	3.08	26.8	1.88
Skimmed milk	100 mL	29	2.5	4.6	0.1
Lentil	50 g	171.5	12.55	29.5	0.35
Paneer	40 g	106	7.32	0.48	8.32
Spinach	25 g	6.5	0.5	0.72	0.175
Mint leaves	10 g	4.8	0.48	0.58	0.06
Total		2000 kcal	77 g	300 g	66.0 g

Energy - 2000 kcal, Protein-77 g, CHO-300 g, Fat - 66.0 g

3. TO PLAN A DAY'S DIET FOR A PERSON AGE 65 YEARS SUFFERING FROM THROAT CANCER. PLAN A DIET AS TUBE FEEDING/LIQUID DIET

Nutritional Requirement

Energy: 1950 kcal acc. to RDA

Protein: 1g /kg/IBW = 55 gm

CHO: 50-55% = 268 gm

Fats: 20% of total energy = 43 gm

Menu

Meal timing	Menu
Early morning	Skimmed milk-250 mL Dates -20 g
Breakfast	Oatmeal + buttermilk • Oats -40 g • Tomato-30 g • Onion-30 g • Oil-10 g • Buttermilk -250 mL
Mid-morning	Mushroom broth • Mushroom-40 g • Garlic-5 g • Lemon-10 g • French beans-30 g • Oil-10 g
Lunch	Vegetable khichdi • Rice-100 g • Green gram dal-35 g • Carrot puree– 30 g • Tomato-30 g • Oil-10 g Coconut water-200 mL
Evening Snack	Banana smoothie • Banana-70 g • Milk-150 mL • Sugar-5 g
Dinner	Dal soup-1 katori • Green gram dal-40 g • Kale puree-100 g • Onion-30 g • Tomato-30 g • Oil-5 g
Bedtime	Kheer-1 katori • Rice flour-20 g • Milk-250 mL • Dates -20 g

Nutritive Value

Ingredients	Amount	Energy	Protein	CHO	Fats
Skimmed milk	250 mL	72.5	6.25	11.5	-
Dates	20 g	56.4	0.5	15	0.08
Oats	40 g	154	4.6	27.6	2.8
Tomato	30 g	12	0.54	2.16	0.12
Onion	30 g	15	0.36	3.33	0.03
Buttermilk	250 mL	72.5	2	10.75	2.75
Oil	10 g	90	-	-	10
Mushroom	40 g	6	0.88	0.92	0.08
Garlic	5 g	7.25	0.18	1.49	0.005
Lemon	10 g	5.7	0.1	1.11	0.09
French beans	30 g	15	1.08	2.13	0.24
Oil	10 g	90	-	-	10
Green gram dal	35 g	121.8	8.57	20.96	0.42
Rice	100 g	349	8.5	77.4	0.6
Tomato	30 g	12	0.54	2.16	0.12
Carrot	30 g	14.4	0.27	3.18	0.06
Oil	10 g	90	-	-	10
Coconut water	200 mL	48	2.8	8.8	0.2
Banana	70 g	81.2	0.84	19.04	0.21
Milk	150 mL	43.5	3.75	6.9	-
Sugar	5 g	19.9	0.005	4.97	-
Kale	100 g	35	5.24	4.42	3.9
Onion	30 g	15	0.36	3.33	0.03
Tomato	30 g	72.5	2	10.72	2.75
Oil	5 g	45	-	-	5
Green gram dal	40 g	139.2	10.2	23	0.48
Milk	250 mL	72.5	6.25	11.5	-
Rice flour	40 g	139	3.4	30	0.24
Dates	20 g	69.2	1.28	15.8	0.08
Total		1963	70.5	315 g	49.8 g

Energy – 1963 kcal, Protein-70.5 gm, CHO-315 gm, Fat – 49.8 gm.

QUESTIONS

1. Define Cancer. What are the different types of cancer?
2. Discuss about the role of dietary factors in the management of cancer.

3. What is oesophageal cancer? Discuss about its causes, symptoms and dietary modifications.
4. Define:
   (i) Hybernoma
   (ii) Leukaemia
5. Write briefly about rectosigmoid and rectal cancer. Discuss about their aetiology, symptoms and treatment.
6. Discuss about different types of oral cancers.
7. Write about different types of ovarian cancers, along with their dietary management.
8. Define leukaemia and discuss about its causes, symptoms and management.
9. Plan a day's diet for patient suffering from leukaemia.
10. Discuss about the dietary management of a patient suffering from oral cancer using a day's diet plan as reference.

11

Nutrition in Bone and Joint Disorders

11.1 GOUT

11.1.1 Introduction

Gout is an incessant, deforming disorder resulted from imbalance of purine metabolism and hence resulting in hyperuricemia, recurrent arthritis attacks, uric acid renal stones, deposition of monosodium urate. It is mainly developed due to increased excretion of uric acid. Gout is closely associated with hyperuricemia.

Default in dietary habits has always been primary, secondary or associated cause of many ailments. Similarly, in case of gout intake of purine-rich foods basically coming from animal and seafood sources can influence the development of gout. Allopurinol, is one of the potent anti-hyperuricemia drugs, being used for the treatment of gout for last many years. The mechanism of action of this drug involves the inhibition of enzyme xanthine oxidase. But long term use of allopurinol has already been associated with many side effects such as nephropathy, hepatitis and many other allergic reactions. There is a need of natural anti-hyperuricemicagents. Herbs and plants that show the properties of inhibition of uric acid biosynthesis through the inhibition of xanthine oxidasecanpreventhyperuricemia.Inconclusion,naturalantihyperuricemic agents need promotion.

11.1.2 Causes

Urate levels are exaggerated by the changes in lifestyle, diet, medications, over secretion in the body and insufficient emission by the kidneys. Increased production of uric acid as that is evident in people who have increased alcohol consumption, high protein diet, obesity, hypertriglyceridaemia or any genetically enzymatic defects.

Excessive production of uric acid develops from toxaemia of pregnancy, starvation, and glycogen storage disease. Genetic factor may also be the cause of gout.

Gout attack often occurs when macrophages in the joint space phagocytise urate crystals deposits and are very painful. Consumption of red meats and alcohol can lead to increase in free fatty acid congregations hence they are considered to be activators to acute gout attacks.

Notable causes are as follows:

- Severe dieting or starvation
- Excessive intake of high purine foods, i.e., shellfish,beans,red meats
- Heredity

Prevalence: It is common in men aged over 40. In women it is seen over 50 years of age. In males the condition begins at puberty and in females at menopause.

11.1.3 Types of Gout

- Asymptomatic hyperuricemia
- Acute gouty arthritis
- Intercritical gout
- Chronic tophaceous gout

11.1.3.1 Asymptomatic Hyperuricemia

It is a clinical manifestations of gout where there is elevation in uric acid levels. It is an accidental stage without any recognizable consequences and hence produced either due to cytotoxic chemotherapy indicating increased production or due to renal failure indicating decreased excretion. Only 5 per cent evidence is prevalent relating this to occurrence of gout.

Risk factors of this type are often related to kidney damage or renal stones

11.1.3.2 Acute Gouty Arthritis

It is signalized by acute inflammation of synovial membrane activated by precipitation of adequate amount of monosodium urate crystals. Synovitis mechanism includes crystal phagocytosis, activation of the complement and Kallikrein system. It usually eventuates in obese men with alcohol binging issue. In 90 per cent of acute attacks, only one joint is troubled. The troubled joint becomes inflammed, reddish kind of appearance and tender.

The affected zones of this stage includes majorly greater toe followed by instep, ankles, elbows, fingers, heels, knees, etc. In this stage, some degree of pain and discomfort is persistent in the joints. The first incidence of attack occurs usually after the sudden pain with varied intensity accompanied by shivering which makes the accused to wake up even after no significant symptoms seen while going to bed after a hearty meal.

Occurrence of fever around 102°F, chills, tachycardia, pruritus, anorexia, malaise. Possibilities of recurrent attacks cannot be denied in this stage.The duration of acute attacks may extend up to 2 weeks Colchicine, NSAIDS, oral steroids are the advised medications.

11.1.3.3 Intercritical Gout

During the varied time intervals of gout attacks, those in which the accused remains entirely non-emblematic is known as intercritical gout. It is claimed to be the asymptomatic phase of gout. In this stage the accused person is attacked by the second attack which is more prolonged and severe. Hence the patient progressively enters the chronic stage with no remissions.

11.1.3.4 Chronic Tophaceous Gout

The progressive evolution of acute attacks results in chronic gout. At least 10 years of gout suffering leads to the chronic stage. There are instances of synovial proliferation, pannus formation, progressive destruction of articular cartilage and bones. Chronic gout is mostly prevalent in metatarsophalangeal joints, mid foot and toe joints. It is characterized by the formation of firm, nodular swelling tophi on the walls of bursae, tendon sheath, ear lobules, ulnar surface of forearms, helix of ear, etc. Inflammation of tophi may lead to appearance of chalky white substance. 90 per cent of chronic cases may lead to renal dysfunction, renal failure, uric acid stones, etc.

It may be in the form of hyperuricaemic nephropathy nephrolithiasis and renal failure. Hypertension, isochaemic heart disease is also prevalent. Demonstration of birefringent crystals in synovial fluid under polarized light is gold standard for gout diagnosis. Restrictions relating to weight loss, alcohol consumption, high purine diets, and prevention of purine breakdown are important aspects of treatment.

11.1.4 Affected Areas of Gout

(a) Metatarsophalangeal joint of the big toe
(b) Tarsal area
(c) Ankle
(d) Knee
(e) Wrists, fingers, and elbows (may be)
(f) Joints of small toe (early injury)

11.1.5 Symptoms

(a) Swelling, unexpected pain in joint
(b) Tissue inflammation around tissues
(c) Hyperuricemia
(d) Uric acid crystals in joint fluid
(e) Acute arthritis attacks

11.1.6 Diagnosis

The doctor draws a sample of fluid from an inflamed joint to confirm the crystals associated with gout. Symptoms, medical history, genetic factors, lifestyle, and diet are factors related to diagnosis of gout.

11.1.7 Medical Management

Non steroidal anti-inflammatory drugs (NSAIDs).

11.1.8 Dietary Management

- Low purine foods recommended.
- Exclusion of red meats, organ meats, seafood, beans, peas, mushrooms, alcohol, etc., from diet.
- Increased intake of fluid.
- Low protein, low fat, high carbohydrate diet is recommended.
- Maintenance of normal body weight.
- Trauma, stress, alcohol are often said to be avoided due to inflammation and pain caused.

Gout is disorder of purine metabolism, directly related to uric acid being its end product. Increase in the level of uric acid which is present in form of urate in the body leads to the formation of crystals which with time deposit as monosodium urate crystals (MUC) in tissue mainly in and around joints, causing gout. Defaults in the metabolism of purines due to different factors - either due to overproduction of uric acid by increased xanthine oxidase enzyme or under excretion of uric acid in urine–can lead to hyperuricemia or even gout. There are abundant types of gifted spices and herbs, cultivated all around the world, with magical properties. From ancient times plants and there parts have been used, in treatment of many diseases, hyperuricemia being one of them. Therefore, many natural herbs and plants that show the properties of xanthine oxidase inhibition provide safe and effective alternative to allopathic drugs.

11.1.9 Case Studies: To Plan a Day's Diet for a Female, 65 Years Old Suffering from Gout

General Instructions

- Weight should not exceed expected ideal weight
- Regular exercise should be integral part of daily routine
- Drink plenty of water
- Avoid some, but not all, foods with purines

Include some foods that can control uric acid levels

- High fibre diet should be consumed

Foods allowed:

- High fibre foods like whole cereals, whole pulses, lentils and fruits
- Low fat substitutes like skimmed milk, curd
- Foods rich in soluble fibre like curry leaves, methi leaves

Foods to be avoided:

- Refined cereals like suji, maida
- Purine rich organ meats, seafoods and red meats
- Whole milk and its products
- Deep fried foods
- Bakery products as they contain baking soda

To make your food palatable use spices like cardamom, cinnamon, lemon juice, etc.

Dietary Allowances

Energy: 1500 kcal

CHO: 300 gm

Protein: 40 gm

Fat: 25 gm

Food Exchange List

Servings	No. of servings	Energy (kcal)	CHO (gm)	Proteins (gm)	Fats (gm)
Cereals	6	600	120	15	--
Pulses	2	200	50	12	2
Vegetables	5	150	50	5	1
Fruits	4	160	40	--	--
Milk and products	3	210	30	9	6
Fats and oils	3	135	--	--	15
Total		1455	290	41	24

Servings	Early morning	Breakfast	Mid-morning	Lunch	Evening snack	Dinner	Bed time
Cereals		1		2	1	2	
Pulses				1		1	
Vegetables		2		2		1	
Fruits	1	1	2				
Milk and products		1		1			1
Fats And Oils		1		1		1	
Sugars							

Diet Chart

Timing	Menu	Amount (g)	Energy (kcal)	Cho (g)	Protein (g)	Fats (g)
Early morning	Lemon water	50 g + 150 mL	40	10	--	--
Breakfast	Mix berries milkshake + Aloo ka paratha (1) + vegetable gravy	(30 g + 250 mL) + 100 g + 100 g	450	80	7	9
Mid-morning	Fruit + 1 cup of cherries	160 g	80	20	--	--
Lunch	Salad + 2 soft chapati (multigrain) + dal (lentils) + vegetable + low fat curd	100 g+ 50 g + 30 g + 100 g + 90 g	305	90	14	7
Evening snacks	Coffee + whole wheat biscuits	150 ml + 35 g	180	20	2.5	
Dinner	2 soft chapati (multi-grain) + vegetable dal	50 g + 35 g + 100 g	390	75	12	5
Bedtime	Milk (with pinch of turmeric)	150 mL	65	10	3	5

11.2 ARTHRITIS

11.2.1 Introduction

Arthritis is the inflammation of the joints and their painful effects all over the body. It can affect one part of the body or can involve the all joints. It is a disease of old age group but nowadays it is affecting the adolescents, Middle aged people as well as in some cases children.

Younger adults. It is most common in women.

11.2.2 Symptoms

- Stiffness and swelling
- Joint pain
- Redness of skin
- Loss of appetite
- Anaemia and fever

11.2.3 Causes

- A decrease in the usual quantity of cartilage results in development of arthritis.
- Cartilage is an unchangeable and elastic connective tissues in the joints saves them by absorbing the stress and jolts that are formed when we move and do daily chores.
- Autoimmune disorder can also cause arthritis.
- It is a disease which is born by the body immune system direct attack on the tissues of the body.

11.2.4 Treatment

Surgery

11.2.5 Lifestyle Changes

Eating balance and healthy diet is important factor for weight loss. Food rich in antioxidants properties such as fresh fruits, vegetables, and herbs can help reduce inflammation in body, for example, fish and nuts

One should minimize the foods like fried foods, processed foods, dairy products and high intake of meat.

Beside this regular exercise will keep joint flexible, swimming is also good for arthritis because it doesn't put pressure on joints.

11.2.6 Classification

People who have arthritis can also have risk of this disease

- Osteoarthritis
- Rheumatoid arthritis
- Reactive arthritis
- Hepatitis
- Celiac disease
- Inflammatory bowel disease
- Non-celiac gluten sensitivity

Lupus and rheumatoid arthritis are also responsible for further damage of organs in the body.

- Difficulty in using hands and walking
- Exhaustion
- Slenderize
- Difficulty in sleeping
- Muscle ache and also pain
- Tenderness
- Problem in working of joints
- Muscles fragility
- Dropping resilience/flexibility

11.2.7 Types of Arthritis

11.2.7.1 Osteoarthritis

- It is the most common form of arthritis.
- It can influence both larger and smaller junctions of the body, such as hands, wrists, feet, back, hip and also knee.
- It can also occur due to injury.
- Osteoarthritis starts in the cartilages and also eventually causes the two rival bones to abrade into each other.
- The condition includes minor discomfort during exercise but soon the pain continues and also even occurs during the state of rest.
- The discomfort prevents one from doing some or the other activity.
- It affects the joints which bear weight, such as back, knee and hip.
- It is most common in old people.
- Womens are more prone to osteoarthritis by the age of 65.
- Risk factors include prior joint injury, obesity and a dull lifestyle.

11.2.7.2 Rheumatoid Arthritis

- It is a disease in which immune system of body starts to attack on bodys tissues.
- The attack may not only directed to the joints but also to many other parts of the body.
- In rheumatoid arthritis injury occurs to the junction lining and cartilage which further results in erosion of two rival bones.
- It affects the articulation in the fingers, wrists, knees, elbows and can show severe deformity.

- It occurs mostly in people of age 20 and also above.
- In youngsters the disorder can present with a skin rash, high temperature, body ache, disability, and decrease in daily activities.
- More common in women than men at all ages and involvs all races, ethnic groups and also culture.

11.2.8 Diet in Arthritis

Mediterranean diet is recommended in arthritis

Food included:

- Fats and oils

  Quantity - 200-400 gm of fish twice a week

  Reason - Fishes are good source of omega-3 fatty acids which are known to reduce inflammation. Fish oil supplements help reduce joint swelling and pain, sources - Salmon, tuna
- Nuts and seeds

  Quantity - 1.5 ounces of nuts daily

  Reason - It acts as anti-inflammatory diet

  Origin- Walnuts, pine nuts, pistachios, and also almond
- Fruits and vegetable

  Quantity - Nine servings daily

  Reason - Fruits and veggies are rich in antioxidants and act as defense system

  Fruits - Orange, grape fruit, lime-rich in vitamin C

  Veggies of cruciferous family like broccoli, spinach, lettuce, cabbage

  Fruits like blue berries, cherries, spinach, kale and broccoli
- Olive oil

  Quantity - 10-15 g/ serving or one spoon daily

  Reason - It is heart healthy fat

  Sources - Extra virgin olive oils, avocado, safflower oil
- Beans

  Quantity - One cup twice a week

  Reason - It is rich in fibre and phytonutrient and it has abundant protein content.

  Sources - Small red beans, red kidney beans
- Whole grains

  Quantity - 6 ounce of grain per day from whole wheat

Reason – It contains large amount of fibre which help to maintain GI system and weight.

Sources – Whole wheat/dalia, rice.

11.3 OSTEOPOROSIS

11.3.1 Introduction

It is a condition where there is loss of bone minerals density due to increase in osteoclast bone a concomitant decrease in osteoblast mediated bone formation. As a result the bone become porous , lighter , and fragile leading to easy and frequent fractures. There is a generalized bone disease characterized by low bone density and deterioration of bone tissues.

Depression, poor diet, poor orientation and arrangement of furniture in the home can cause falls and fracture in elders. Osteoporosis is very common among women in the post-menopausal phase of life and the one who have a sedentary lifestyle.

In osteoporosis the total amount of bone is reduced but the remaining bone is of normal composition and quality.

There is decrease in thickness of cortex due to the reduction in number of cells a thinning of the trabecular and increased porosity of bone as a result fracture occur with a greater frequency.

Common fracture sites include the vertebrae , femur , and radius and often these occur in spite of little or no trauma.

It is a silent disease but found to be the major cause of high morbidity and disability particularly in elder population. Post-menopausal women are at higher risk than men of similar age group.

Elder persons are at greater risk and have chance of falls and fracture .There may be poor eyesight, diabetes, renal disorder.

11.3.2 Causes

The causes of osteoporosis may be age related such as decrease estrogen production associated with menopause.

The decline in circulating 17 beta estradiol is the predominant factor in the accelerated bone loss that begins after menopause and continues for 6 to 8 years.

Decreased intestinal absorption of calcium and production of vitamin D, reduced physical activity and increased parathyroid hormone secretion may also cause osteoporosis.

Inadequate protein intake may contribute to osteoporosis in the elderly.

The risk of fracture increases progressively with age and is associated with significant morbidity. Poor dietary habits, lack of exercise during the growing years limits the bone density even at younger age.

11.3.3 Common Cause of Osteoporosis

- Negative calcium balance
- Hyperthyroidism
- Diabetes
- Chronic renal failure
- Gastrointestinal malabsorption
- High PTH level
- Family history
- Age above 60 years
- Menstrual status, menopause
- Smoking
- Fibre intake
- Race/ethnicity
- Excessive weight loss
- Immobility increases bone loss

11.3.4 Risk Factors for Osteoporosis

11.3.4.1 Nutritional Factors

Energy and protein intake is directly proportional to the bone mass density, during bone formation, there is secretion of collagen and formation of hydroxyapatite, which requires adequate supply of calcium, phosphorus, protein, vitamin C and vitamin K. Deficiency of any of these nutrients leads to osteoporosis

11.3.4.2 Calcium

Parathyroid hormone and calcium level in blood are critical in maintaining bone density. Low blood calcium leads to osteoclast (eating away the bone).

Calcium is withdrawn from bone bank in order to maintain the blood calcium level which leads to weak and porous bone. Calcium (500 mg) and vitamin D (700 d) supplement can reduce the risk of fracture.

11.3.4.3 Phosphorus

Thus it is disturbance in the calcium-phosphorus ratio. Phosphorus stimulates PTH secretion. It is important to have the balance between calcium and phosphorus. If necessary, consume calcium rich foods such as milk or curd with meals or other foods to maintain a good bone health.

11.3.4.4 Magnesium

50 per cent and above magnesium is found in bone tissues. It serves as a cofactor for several enzymes and useful in bone cellular functioning and bone fluids.

11.3.4.5 Vitamin K

Formation of osteocalcin is regulated by vitamin K, which is a bone specific protein made by osteoblasts and needed for maturation of bones. Optimal intake reduce the risk of fracture.

11.3.4.6 Protein

1 gm per day intake of protein intake is required for bone formation. Fluoride increases the hardness of bone. Cross-linking of collagen and elastin is regulated by copper. Magnesium is required for biosynthesis of mucopolysaccharides in bone matrix formation.

11.3.4.7 Physical Activity

High sodium intake along with low calcium intake increases the risk of osteoporosis. Weight bearing exercises increase bone remodelling and strength.

11.3.4.8 Lifestyle Factor

The people who indulge in alcohol and smoking have adverse effects on bone. High intake of caffeine like cola and coffee has deleterious effects on bones because they limit the intestinal absorption of calcium.

11.3.5 Prevention and Control of Osteoporosis

Estrogen treatment results in increased parathyroid hormone and synthesizes which may explain the observed improvement in the intestinal absorption and renal reabsorption of calcium. Ensuring additional calcium intake of about 200 mg per day with a total intake of 800 mg per day. It is necessary to have ample amount of calcium and to drink 2 to 3 glasses of milk regularly.

Adequate exercise and physical fitness is necessary. The more you are on your feet the less is the risk of pathological fracture of the femur and spine. Exercise combined with adequate calcium and vitamin D intake may have a modest effect on slowing the decrease in bone mineral density in post-menopausal women. Milk and sardines are good sources of vitamin D.

These may also be helpful in dealing with osteoporosis:

- Regular intake of food rich in calcium, protein, vitamin K.
- Regular consumption of milk and milk products.
- Avoid smoking and cola drinks.
- Regular exposure to sun to ensure adequate vitamin D status.
- Regular exercise to maintain integrity of bone tissues and BMD.
- Regular checkup of BMD after the age of 50 to 60 years.

QUESTIONS

1. Define gout. Write about its causes, symptoms and management.
2. Discuss about different types of gout along with their dietary modifications.
3. Discuss the role of high purine diet in the disease of gout.
4. Plan a day's diet for a diabetic male of 65 years suffering from gout.
5. Define arthritis. Discuss their types and causes.
6. What is osteoarthritis? Write about its causes, symptoms, prevention and management.
7. What is the dietary management for rheumatoid arthritis? Discuss with a day's diet plan.
8. Differentiate between osteopenia and osteoporosis.
9. What is osteoporosis? Write abouts its diagnosis criteria, types, causes and symptoms.
10. Discuss the dietary management of a patient suffering from osteoporosis. What precaution they need to take?

12

Nutrition in Febrile Conditions

12.1 INTRODUCTION

Due to imbalance between the heat produced in the body and the amount of heat eliminated from the body, there is an elevation or sudden change in the levels of temperature in the body. Due to this whenever the body temperature elevates and reaches above the normal range, such a condition is known as fever. Fever can occur due to the several reasons. Some of the reasons are mentioned below.

- Fever may occur in the body whenever the body responses or reacts against an infection.
- Several antigen-antibody reactions may also cause inflammation accompanied by fevers.
- Bacteria or fungi or viral exogenous agents may induce fever in the body.

Fevers can be classified into two categories based on their duration and severity.

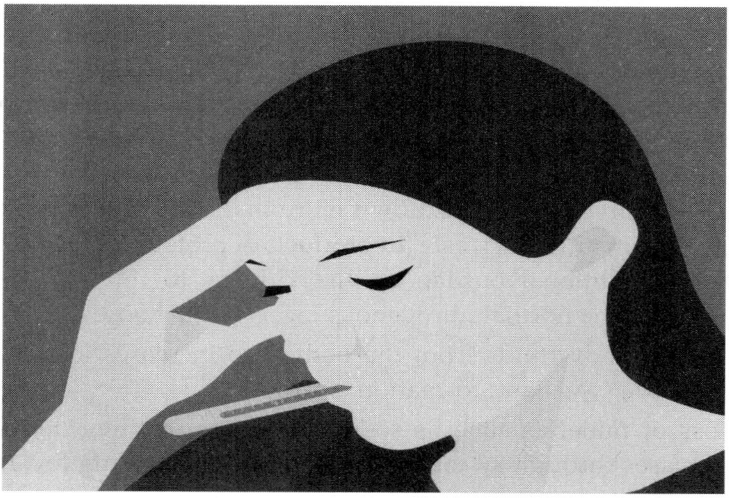

12.1.1 Acute Fever

As the name suggests, acute means small. Thus, acute fever is a fever that is for a short duration, but it can be highly severe. The body temperature may rise above 104°F. Chicken pox, tonsillitis, influenza, pneumonia, typhoid, malaria are some examples of infections that are accompanied by acute fevers. Malaria is an acute fever but can also be considered a recurrent fever because it is accompanied by repeated episodes of high fever.

12.1.2 Chronic Fever

Chronic fevers are those fevers that persist for a long duration of time with less severity as compared to acute fever. The temperature can be high but usually remains low and persists for a longer duration of time. In some cases, chronic fever may remain up to several months as in the case of tuberculosis.

12.2 METABOLISM IN FEVERS

Normal body temperature is 98.4°F or 37°C. Whenever there is a rise in the body temperature, following are the metabolic changes that are seen in the body during fevers:

(a) With every 1°F increase in the body temperature, basal metabolic rate increases by 7 per cent or with every 1°C increase in the body temperature, basal metabolic rate increases by 13 per cent.

(b) As the energy expenditure increases, the glycogen and adipose tissue stores decrease drastically. Therefore, high energy is required to maintain energy balance.

(c) With the severity of infection and increase in duration of fever, the rate of protein catabolism (breakdown of proteins) increases. Protein loss is highly seen in long duration chronic fevers as compared to short duration acute fevers. Protein breakdown is highly seen in fevers such as typhoid, malaria, poliomyelitis and tuberculosis. Increase in protein breakdown more than the normal rate leads to increase in nitrogen waste (byproducts of protein catabolism) which exerts additional burden on the kidneys to filter the waste to maintain the normal nitrogenous levels in the body.

(d) Loss of body fluids from the body also increases in the form of excessive sweat and formation of urine.

(e) Loss of minerals such as sodium, potassium, chloride, etc., also increases through sweat, urine and vomiting during fevers which also leads to water and electrolyte balance.

(f) The absorption of various nutrients such as proteins, minerals and vitamins also decreases during fevers.

(g) The above changes result in the loss of appetite. Loss of appetite results in the low intake of food which causes weight loss and nutritional deficiencies.

12.3 ROLE OF VARIOUS NUTRIENTS DURING INFECTIONS

An inadequate dietary intake or malnutrition during or before infections leads to various problems such as:

- Weight loss
- Resistance to infections is lowered
- Damage to mucosal lining
- Invasion by pathogens
- Impaired growth and development in children
- Diarrhoea
- Malabsorption of nutrients
- Loss of appetite
- Urinary nitrogen loss
- Damage to defense mechanism of the body

12.3.1 Protein

Proteins are very essential for adequate immune function. The deficiency of proteins alters the immune response of the body and makes it more prone to infections because immune responses in the body are completely dependent on cell replication and the production of proteins with biological activities. Proteins play a different role in all kinds of immune responses in the body.

12.3.2 Vitamin A

The integrity of the epithelium layer in the gastrointestinal tract and respiratory tract is mainly maintained by vitamin A. The deficiency of vitamin A increases the risk of diarrhoea, malaria, measles and mortality. The chances of developing respiratory diseases and chronic gut infections increases due to the deficiency of vitamin A. Vitamin A plays an important role in enhancing immunity.

12.3.3 Vitamin E

Vitamin E is a fat soluble vitamin and is also an antioxidant. Deficiency of vitamin E impairs B and T cells that play an important role in immune response of the body. Vitamin E reduces prostaglandin synthesis and prevents oxidation of PUFA in cell membranes. It can be consumed more than the recommended doses.

12.3.4 Vitamin C

Vitamin C is a water soluble antioxidant which is found in blood fluids. Vitamin C is very important for the proper functioning of phagocytes. Improper functioning of phagocytes causes an impairment of the immune response to infection. That is why immunity is highly affected due to vitamin C deficiency. Deficiency of vitamin C causes pathological changes in the epithelial cells which further decreases the resistance of the tissues to infections.

12.3.5 Zinc

Cells of the immune system require a large number of enzymes that need zinc to function. Hence, zinc is indirectly very essential for immune health. Zinc deficiency leads to:

- Reduced neutrophils.
- Reduced natural kill cell function.
- Decreased number of T and B lymphocytes.
- Suppressed hypersensitivity, cytotonic activity.
- Suppressed antibody production.
- Increased chances of HIV disease.

12.3.6 Iron

Deficiency of iron impairs cell mediated immunity and also reduces neutrophil action.

12.3.7 Selenium

Selenium plays an indirect role in immune function by protecting macrophages and other cells from pro-oxidants.

12.3.8 Vitamin B6

These are essential for the synthesis and metabolism of amino acids and antibodies that are highly important in resisting infection and enhancing immunity. Deficiency of vitamin B6 impairs lymphocyte growth and maturation and impairs the activity of T cells.

12.3.9 PUFA

N-3 plays an important role in immunity by inhibiting the macrophase and other cell functions. N-6 PUFAs enhance immune function and promote inflammatory response. Hence, ratio of N-3 and N-6 have an important effect on immune function.

12.4 ACUTE FEVER TYPHOID

Bacteria *salmonella typhi* causes an infectious disease called typhoid. Typhoid infection is transmitted through the faecal-oral route such as consumption of contaminated food, water or milk contaminated with intestinal contents, raw vegetables and fruits grown on or near sewage also contain infectious bacteria. Typhoid disease begins in the small intestine. Bacteria attach themselves to the epithelium of small intestine and penetrate the layer where it multiplies in the mesenteric lymph nodes and finally reaches in the blood stream. In blood, antibodies lysis the bacteria and endotoxins are liberated which causes fever. Some bacteria pass from the liver to the gall bladder and bile ducts and are secreted into the intestine where diarrhoea can also be caused.

12.4.1 Body Changes in Typhoid Fever

- Loss of tissue protein.
- Drastic depletion of glycogen stores.
- Disturbed water and electrolyte balance
- Irritable, inflamed intestinal tract with diarrhoea which also interferes with the absorption of nutrients.
- Ulcers in the intestines may also occur. Peyer's patches are seen which can be highly severe that haemorrhage and even perforation of intestine may also occur.

12.4.2 Treatment

- Bed rest is important.
- Patient should be kept warm.
- Antibiotics are needed to cure the infection.
- Appropriate modified diet for the patient to enhance recovery, treat symptoms and maintain good health to avoid nutritional deficiencies.

12.4.3 Objectives of Dietary Management

(a) Maintain adequate nutrition.
(b) Restore positive nitrogen balance and reduce the burden on kidneys.
(c) Provide relief to symptoms.
(d) Correct and maintain water and electrolyte balance.
(e) Avoid irritation of intestinal tract.

12.4.4 Energy

Due to rise in body temperature, the basal metabolic rate may increase upto 50 per cent . Hence, energy requirement by the body also increases as the energy expenditure is increased. So, to maintain the energy balance the right amount of energy is needed. Energy intake should be increased by 10-20 per cent. If the patient cannot consume or tolerate enough energy, then the energy intake should be increased gradually with recovery and improved level of tolerance.

12.4.5 Protein

Due to increased protein catabolism and tissue protein breakdown, protein intake should be increased up to 1.5-2 times the normal, that is 1.5-2 gm protein/kg/bw/day. To minimize the tissue loss, the protein rich foods of high biological value such as milk and eggs should be included in the diet.

12.4.6 Carbohydrates

A good amount of carbohydrate is necessary to replenish the glycogen stores. Easily digestible carbohydrates should be consumed so that there is less load on digestive tract to digest food. Simple starches, glucose, honey, sugarcane can be included.

12.4.7 Fats

Fats are the macronutrients that provide the highest amount of calories as compared to other macronutrients. 1 gm of fat provides 9 kcal. When the fevers are accompanied by diarrhoea, fats are given in emulsified form only. Examples of emulsified fats include cream, butter, whole milk, and egg yolk. Emulsified form of fats is easy to digest and are easily tolerated by the patients.

12.4.8 Minerals

During fevers the loss of electrolytes is increased in excess. Salty soups, broths, fruit juices, milk, foods rich in sodium, potassium, chloride should be included in diet to compensate the imbalance of electrolytes in the body.

12.4.9 Vitamins

During infections the vitamin C stored in the tissues deplete highly. Hence, the intake of vitamin C and vitamin A is also essential during infections as they enhance the process of healing and enhance recovery. Vitamin B is also essential for recovery. Hence, supplements are recommended to prevent deficiency to enhance recovery.

12.4.10 Fibre

Due to inflammation and improper functioning of GI tract, the irritating foods should be avoided. Irritating and insoluble fibres are considered mechanical irritants and cause discomfort and pain.

12.4.11 Fluid

Fluids are lost from the body through sweat and urine. Hence, to compensate for the water loss and to ensure that all the excretory wastes are excreted through urine, daily intake of 2.5-5 litres/day is necessary. Fluids can be water, soups, juices, and beverages.

12.4.12 Dietary Recommendations

- High energy.
- High protein.
- Full fluid in the beginning.
- Small frequent meals after every 2-3 hours.
- Sufficient intake of fluids and electrolytes.
- When fever comes down, a low fibre, bland, soft, easy to digest, easy to absorb kind of diet is recommended.
- During recovery, well cooked, well mashed, sieved, bland, semisolid foods like khichdi, rice with curd, kheer, custard are some of the options to consider.
- Readily digested food that provides physiological rest to the alimentary tract.

Foods to be avoided

- High fibre foods like whole grain cereals and related products, e.g., whole wheat flour, whole pulses, pulses with husk.
- Raw fruits and vegetables.
- Fried fatty foods such as samosas, pakoras, halwas, laddoos.
- Thermally irritating foods such as ice cream, chilled shakes, etc.
- Mechanically irritating foods such as foods containing high fibre.
- Chemically irritating foods such as condiments, spices, pickles, relishes, chutneys, strongly flavoured vegetables such as onions, capsicum, radish, turnip, cabbage, garlic.

Foods to be included

- Fluids such as juices and soups.
- Milk and milk based beverages.

- Low fibre foods such as refined cereals and their products, dehusked pulses, pureed vegetables, mashed fruits.
- High biological value proteins, e.g., eggs, cheeses, tender meats, fish, poultry.
- Plain gelatin based desserts, sugar, honey, jam.

DIET PLAN

Case Study 1: To plan a day's diet for the patient suffering from typhoid

Category	Exchanges	Energy	Carbohydrates	Proteins	Fats
Milk and milk products	4	680	48	32	40
Meat category 1	1	97	-	7	7
Meat category 2	1	26	-	7	-
Pulses	2	200	34	14	-
Cereals	5	350	75	10	-
Vegetable A	5	100	17.5	5	-
Vegetable B	7	280	70	14	-
Fruit	6	270	60	-	-
Fats	3	135	-	-	15
Sugars	3	60	15	-	-
Others	1	400	-	-	-
Total		2400	319.5	89	62

Category	Breakfast	Mid-morning	Lunch	Evening	Dinner
Milk and milk products	1		1	1	1
Meat category 1	1		-	-	-
Meat category 2	1		-	-	-
Pulses	-		1	-	1
Cereals	1		2	-	2
Vegetable A	-		1	3	1
Vegetable B	2		2	3	-
Fruit	2	1	-	2	1
Fats	1		1	-	1
Sugars	1		-	1	1
Others	-		-	-	1

Time	Amount	Menu
Breakfast	1 bowl	Vegetable (peas+carrot) upma
	1	Egg whole
	1	Egg white
	1 glass	Orange juice
Mid-morning	1 glass	Coconut water
	1 bowl	Papaya chat
Lunch	1 bowl	Rice pudding
	1 bowl	Vegetable khichdi (beans + carrot)
	1 cup	Curd
Evening	1 bowl	Vegetable soup (drumstick, parwal, ridge gourd, fenugreek leaves, pumpkin, beans)
	1 cup	Mashed paneer, banana,papaya
Dinner	1	Chapati
	1 cup	Rice
	1 bowl	Dal
	1 bowl small	Spinach curry
	1 cup	Custard

12.5 TUBERCULOSIS

Tuberculosis comes under the category of chronic fevers. It is one of the major causes of illness and death in the underdeveloped countries as well as the deprived sections of developed countries. Malnutrition due to poverty or lack of knowledge, Ignorance, unhygienic living conditions, poor sanitation make a person more prone to infections. Tuberculosis is caused by a bacteria *Mycobacterium tuberculosis*. This bacteria highly affects the lungs, leading to pulmonary tuberculosis (Srilakshmi; 2014).

12.5.1 Symptoms of Tuberculosis

- Wasting of tissues
- Exhaustion
- Cough
- Expectoration
- Fever
- High fever in the beginning
- Flushed face
- Increased circulation and respiration
- Constant fatigue
- Loss of weight

- If body temperature rises above 39°C, the metabolic rate increases by 20 - 30 per cent above the normal levels.
- In acute phase, this disease is similar to acute fevers.
- In the chronic phase, low grade fever, increase in metabolic rate is seen.
- Loss of muscle tissues and body wasting is the major symptom of tuberculosis.

12.5.2 Treatment

- Rest
- Antibiotics
- Fresh air
- Nourishing food
- Sanitation and hygiene

12.5.3 Objectives of Diet Therapy

- Reduce mortality by providing enough nutrients that are required by body's immune mechanism.
- Prevent or control weakness.
- Prevent weight loss and muscle loss.
- Accelerate convalescence.

12.5.4 Energy

Energy is necessary to prevent weight loss and to compensate energy needs for proper functioning of the body. Energy should be increased by 300-500 kcal/day above the normal intake.

12.5.5 Protein

During fever severe muscle wasting is seen accompanied by low serum albumin levels. However, proteins of high biological value are recommended to be included in the diet. 1.2-1.5 g/kg bw/day.

12.5.6 Carbohydrates and Fats

Due to high energy needs in the body the metabolism is also increased. So to meet the energy requirements for the proper functioning of the body, adequate energy intake should be there. Adequate amount of carbohydrates also helps in sparing proteins for tissue building. Excess of fats should also be avoided.

12.5.7 Minerals

A good amount of calcium should be included in the diet.

12.5.8 Vitamins

A diet should be planned such that all vitamins are provided. Beta carotene is converted to retinol in the intestines. During fevers this conversion is highly affected and beta carotene is not converted to retinol. So, the diet should provide high amounts of retinol. This can be achieved by including milk and milk products, egg, and meat in the diet. During tuberculosis ascorbic acid is excreted in urine in excess. Hence, to prevent the deficiency of ascorbic acid, foods rich in ascorbic acid are given. Ascorbic acid also plays an important role in healing. Calcium intake is increased to prevent bone mineral loss, and to enhance absorption of calcium, vitamin D. Utilization of B group vitamins is adversely affected due to the use of chemotherapeutic agents in the treatment of tuberculosis.

12.5.9 Dietary Recommendations

- High fever
  - ◊ A high protein
  - ◊ High energy
  - ◊ Full fluid diet
- Recovery
  - ◊ Soft diet
  - ◊ Normal diet
  - ◊ Simple meals
  - ◊ Easily digestible
  - ◊ Well prepared
  - ◊ Food should be tempting to encourage the patient to eat, as during this phase the patient experiences loss of appetite. Cereal-pulse combination with some amount of animal protein, e.g., khichdi with curd, sweet dalia with milk, vitamin C sources such as guava, sprouted pulses, seasonal vegetables should also be provided.

12.5.10 Tuberculosis

One of the most chronic infectious disease, that human kind has ever known since the past centuries is tuberculosis (TB).

TB is caused mainly by two organisms:

- *Mycobacterium tuberculosis.*
- *Mycobacterium bovis.*

The bacteria often infect lungs, leading to a deadly condition, pulmonary tuberculosis. The infections may be localised in other organs such as lymph nodules, kidneys, bones or may be generalised.

12.5.11 Symptoms of Tuberculosis

Initially the symptoms of TB are very similar to viral fever and are thus hardly considered seriously. Symptoms such as:

- Unusual loss of weight.
- Fatigue.
- Poor appetite.
- Fever.
- Continuous or increasing cough.
- Sweat during night.

Severe symptoms include:

- Cough with unusual increase in production of mucus.
- Blood in cough.
- Certain initial and major tests are performed for diagnosing tuberculosis. The patient is generally not hospitalised during the test processes or initial days of treatment.
- X-ray of the chest is the most common test performed.
- Tuberculin skin test (TST or PPD test) is generally carried out when people are infected with *M. tuberculosis* bacteria but no visible symptoms are present.
- QuantiFERON-TB. Gold test is an advanced test using blood sample. It can detect both active and latent tuberculosis.

12.5.12 Dietary Management

To fight against TB huge sources of vitamins, certain minerals and specific nutrients are required.

- Leafy and dark coloured green vegetable such as spinach and kale, which are rich in iron and vitamin B.
- Intake of whole grains like cereals and bread should be increased.
- Bright coloured vegetables rich in antioxidants are a must for daily meal. Example, carrots, tomatoes, blueberries.
- Concentrate more on unsaturated fat sources such as vegetable oils, virgin olive oil.
- Avoid tobacco.
- Say no to alcohol.

- Coffee and caffeinated drinks should be limited.
- Restrict intake of all sorts of refined products such as white bread, sugar.
- Also, try to avoid high-cholesterol food items such as red meat.

12.5.13 Nutritional Management

Energy: In most of the cases a higher energy intake is prescribed. 2000-2300 kcal are suggested for women and 2700-2900 kcal for men, respectively. Plan diet 30-35 kcal/kg body weight.

Protein: An adequate supply of protein is needed for disease management. Protein requirement varies according to severity of the disease. In general conditions 1.2-1.5 gm/kg protein daily is recommended, emphasise on high biological proteins.

Fat: Fats make the food more palatable and increase the calorie intake. In severe case 20 gm while in mild case 30-40 gm is allowed. Emphasise on MCT instead of LCTs.

Carbohydrate: High carb diet is prescribed, it comprises 55-60% the diet; so that tissue proteins are not broken down for energy purpose. Simple carbohydrates like potato, jaggery are given not only to provide carbs but also to supply adequate electrolytes.

Vitamins: They are essential to regenerate body metabolism. Deficiencies in water-soluble vitamins (particularly the vitamin B complex) are common. Thus, vitamin supplements can be given to meet the daily needs.

Fluids: Adequate amount of fluids should be taken in the form of water, coconut water, clear soups, veg broths, stocks, lemon water, rose water, etc.

Case Study 2: To plan a day's diet for a boy, 10 years old suffering from tuberculosis and constipation.

Nutrition plays a vital role in the management of patients with tuberculosis and constipation. Diet is an important part of the treatment plan, along with medications. The diet must provide enough calories to ensure that muscles are not wasted. This becomes a challenge as most patients have very poor appetite. Depending on the conditions and age, diet should be planned.

General instructions:

- Drink plenty of water.
- Fibre rich diet should be consumed.
- Diet should be rich in carbohydrates and proteins.
- The electrolyte balance should be maintained.

Foods allowed:

- High fibre foods like whole cereals, whole pulses, sprouts and fruits.
- Milk and milk products.
- Foods rich in soluble fibre like curry leaves, methi leaves.
- Food items rich in Omega-3-fatty acids.

Foods to be avoided:

- Refined cereals like suji, maida.
- Spicy foods.
- Deep fried foods.
- Bakery products as they contain baking soda.

Dietary Allowances

Energy: 1650 kcal

CHO: 300 gm

Protein: 55 gm

Fat: 25 gm

Food Exchange List

Servings	No. of servings	Energy (kcal)	CHO (gm)	Proteins (gm)	Fats (gm)
Cereals	8	800	160	17	2
Pulses	2	200	50	12	--
Meat	1	90	--	12	--
Vegetables	4	120	40	4	1
Fruits	2	80	20	--	--
Milk and products	3	210	30	9	8
Fats and oils	3	135	--	--	15
Sugar	2	40	10	--	--
Total		1685	300	54	26

Servings	Early morning	Breakfast	Mid-morning	Lunch	Evening snack	Dinner	Bed-time
Cereals		2		3	1	2	
Pulses				1		1	
Meat			1				
Vegetables		2		2			
Fruits		1		1			

Milk and products		1		1			1
Fats and oils		1		1		1	
Sugars				1	1		

Diet Chart

Timing	Menu	Amount (g)	Energy (kcal)	Cho (g)	Protein (g)	Fats (g)
Early morning	Jeera water	200 mL	--	--	--	--
Breakfast	Milk + Multi-grain soft paratha roll with stuffed vegies + apple	200 mL + 60 g + 160 g + 80 g + 5 g	385	80	9	9
Mid-morning	Chicken stew	200 mL + 30 g	90	--	12	--
Lunch	Jeera-rice + mix vegetable saute+ fruit custard	75 g + 100 g + 5 g + 80 g + 150 mL	570	130	19	5
Evening snacks	Coconut water + oats and multiseed balls	200 mL + 30 g + 5 g	150	50	--	--
Dinner	Rice+ dal makhani	60 g + 30 g	360	70	9	5
Bedtime	Curd	150 g	70	10	3	6

QUESTIONS

1. What is typhoid? Discuss its diagnosis, causes, symptoms, complications and treatment.
2. Plan a day's diet for patient suffering from typhoid fever.
3. Discuss about different types of tuberculosis and their diagnosis.
4. Name the bacteria responsible for tuberculosis. What are the causes, symptoms, risk factors, and dietary management of tuberculosis disease?
5. Plan a day's diet for a male patient of 55 years suffering from tuberculosis.

References

- Kumud Khanna (2016) *Textbook of Nutrition & Dietetics* (Second edition). Elite Publishing House Pvt. Ltd.
- Y.K. Joshi (2014) *Basics of Clinical Nutrition*. Chaukhamba Auriyantalia.
- Krause & Mahan (2020) *Krause's Food & the Nutrition Care Process* (Krause's Food & Nutrition Therapy) (15th edition). Saunders.
- F.P. Antia & Philip Abraham (2002) *Clinical Dietetics and Nutrition* (4th edition). Oxford University Press.
- C. Gopalan, B.V. Rama Sastri and S.C. Balasubramanian (2018) National Institute of Nutrition (India), *Nutritive Value of Indian Foods*. Indian Council of Medical Research.

Index

A

Acute diarrhoea 158
Acute fever 388
Acute fever typhoid 391
Acute glomerulonephritis 236
Acute gouty arthritis 374
Acute myeloid leukaemia (AML) 359
Acute renal failure 225
  clinical features 226
  complications associated with 231
  dietary management of 226
  enteral nutrition in 227
  nutritional administration 232
  pathophysiology of 230
  stages of 229
Adeno-carcinoma 355
Adequate electrolyte diet 10
Adiposity 24
Adjustable gastric band (AGB) 217
Alcohol cirrhosis 285
Aldosterone 251
Alpha glucosidase inhibitors 112
Alpha linolenic acid (ALA) 78
Amino acid diet 11
Android obesity 27
Angina pectoris 63
Angiotensin II 251
Anorexia nervosa 46, 47
Antacids 144
Anthropometric assessment 15
Antibiotics 144
Antioxidant activity 353
Arachidonic acid 77
Arthritis 378
  causes 379
  classification of 379
  diet in 381
  symptoms 379
  treatment 379
  types of 380
Asymptomatic diverticulosis 198
Asymptomatic hyperuricemia 374
Atherosclerosis 62
Atherosclerotic lesions, stages of development in 62
Atkins diet 41
Azotaemia 231

B

Balanced diet 3
Bariatric operations 216
  groups of 214
Bariatric surgery 163
Behaviour therapy 38
Bicarbonate deficiency 252
Biliopancreatic bypass with duodenal switch (BPDS) 218
Binge eating 46
Biochemical assessment 16
Biological carcinogens 353
Blenderized feeding 11
Body composition, concept of 24
Body mass index 26
  assessment for children 28
  classification of 27
Bone marrow 359
Bulimia nervosa 48
Bulimia nervosa laxative 49

C

Calcium oxalate 238
Cancer (malignant tumours) 362
Cancers 30, 351
  aetiology of 352
  definition 351
  development of 351
  dietary factors, role of 353
  dietary management 351, 354
  stages of 351
  types of 351, 355
Carbohydrates 35
Carbohydrate metabolism 97
Carcinoma in situ 352
Cardiac oedema 65
Cardiovascular disease, definition 61
Cardiovascular disorder 29
  aetiology of 67
  dietary management of 69
Carifate 143
Celiac disease 169
Cerebrovascular disease 66
Chemical carcinogens 353
Cholestyramine 195
Chronic diarrhoea 159
Chronic fever 388
Chronic glomerulonephritis 237
Chronic kidney failure 227
  aetiology 228
Chronic obstructive pulmonary disease 32
Chronic renal failure, dietary management of 232
Chronic tophaceous gout 375
Classic and clinical variant galactosemia 312
Classical PKU 300
Clear fluid diets 5
Clinical assessment 16
Coffee 71
Colonic neuromusculature, adjustments in 199
Congestive heart failure 64
Constipation 149
  clinical signs and symptoms 151
  dietary management 157
  pathophysiology 151
  prevention and management of 155
Continuous renal replacement therapy (CRRT) 247
Corticosteroids 195
Crohn's disease 189
  dietary recommendations for 194
Cystic fibrosis 332
  causes/aetiology 332
  diagnosis 333
  nutritional management 334
Cystic stones 241
Cyto protective agents 145

D

Diabetes mellitus 89
  assessment of 102
  cause 95
  complications of 97, 101
  diets for 112, 115, 117, 120
  emergencies of 97
  factors 95
  main symptoms of 89
  management of 112
  metabolism of carbohydrates, proteins and fats 97
  signs and symptoms 96
  types of 90
Dialysis patients, dietary recommendations for 247
Dialysis, types of 246
Diarrhoea
  causes of 163
  classification of 163
  complications 165
  dehydration of 160
  dietary deficiencies 166
  dietary management of 159
  dumping syndrome 162
  management of 161, 165
  nutritional care for 166
  symptoms of 164
  types of 158

Dietary assessment 16, 29
Dietary modifications 9
Diet-liquid diet, principle of 360
Digestion
  foods which improve 185
  problems in 165
Digestive system, foods to improve 183
Diuretics 257
Diverticulitis 196, 198
  nutrition and 202
  pathophysiology of 198
  risk factors 201
  segmental colitis associated with 197
Docosahexaenoic acid (DHA) 78
Drug interactions 112
Duarte variant galactosemia 314
Dumping syndrome 162
  causes of 163
  classification of 163
  complications of 165
  management of 165
  nutritional care for 166
  surgeries for 163
  symptoms of 164
Duodenal ulcer 137, 141, 143
Dyspepsia 180
  medication 181
  treatment 182
Dysplasia 352

E

Early dumping syndrome 163
Eating disorders 45
Eicosapentaenoic acid (EPA) 78
Electrolytes, importance of 249
Enteral nutrition 11
Essential fat 24

F

Fat metabolism 100
Fatty acid diet 12
Febrile conditions, nutrition in 387
Fevers, metabolism in 388
Fibre 71
Flatulence 182
Fluid and electrolyte balance 248
Food allergy diet 11
Food frequency questionnaire 17
Food group questionnaire 17
Full fluid diet 6

G

Galactitol reduction 319
Galactokinase deficiency 315
Galactose accumulation 317
Galactose metabolism 317
  metabolic pathway of 319
Galactosemia 312, 317
Gall bladder disease 31
Gamma linoleic acid 76
Gastric obstruction 143
Gastric ulcer 137
Gastroesophageal reflux disease (GORD) 174
  diagnosis of 177
  management and treatment of 177
  mechanics of 176
Gastrointestinal disorders, dietary management in 137
Gastrointestinal disturbances 31
Gastrointestinal surgeries 163
  dietary management in 206
Gastroscopy 139
Gestational diabetes 93, 132
Glomerulonephritis 233, 253
  aetiology 234
Glossectomy surgery 361
Glucose regulation 103
Gluten 169, 173
Gluten intolerance (celiac disease) 168, 169
  diagnosis and clinical features 170
  medical treatment 170
  nutrition therapy for 171
  signs and symptoms 170
Gluten-free diet 172
Glycaemic index 122
Glycaemic load 122
  components influencing 128
  digestion and 129
  usefulness 129

Glycaemic load 127
Glycemic index 36
Glycogen storage disease 330
  aetiology 331
  complications 331
  dietary management in 331
  management and treatment of 331
  symptoms of 331
  types of 330
Gout 373
  affected areas of 375
  causes 373
  diagnosis 376
  dietary management 376
  medical management 376
  symptoms 376
  types of 374
Grave's disease 347
  management of 348
  symptoms 348
Gynoid obesity 27

H

Haemmorhoids
  management of 207
  precautions 209
Head and chest circumference 28
Heart attack 65
Heart stroke 65
Helicobacter pylori 140
Hepatitis 286
Herbs, role of 291
Hernia 206
  possible complications and risks 206
  post-operative complications 206
Hiatus hernia
  diagnosis of 179
  dietary management of 180
Hibernoma 357
High blood pressure 72
High fibre diet 9, 35
High GI/GL diet 131
High protein diet 10
Histamine2 receptor antagonist 144
Human kidney 223
  disorders of 224
  functions of 224
  microscopic structure of 224
Hyperkalemia 230
Hyperlipidemia 29, 64
Hyperliproproteinemias 64
Hyperphosphatemia 252
Hyperplasia 352
Hypertension 72
  aetiology of 73
  nutritional management 74
  risk factors 73
  symptoms 73
Hyperthyroidism 347
Hyperuricemia 231
Hypervolemia 251
Hypocalcaemia 252
Hypocaloric diets 39
Hypoglycaemia 109
Hypoglycaemic drugs 107
Hyponatremia 252
  treatment of 255
Hypothyroidism 345-346
Hyperthyroidism 345, 347

I

Immunogenicity 104
Increased free-cell potassium 65
Individual nutrients, laboratory
  assessment for 19
Inflammatory bowel disease 188, 191
  complications of 196
  role of medication 195
Inhaled insulin 106
Inositol 341
Insulin dependent diabetes mellitus
  (IDDM) 91
Insulin
  absorption 105
  adverse effect of 107
  characteristics of 103
  concentration of 105
  elimination of 105
  formation of 104

sources of 104
storage of 107
types of 102
Intercritical gout 375
Intermediate acting insulins 106
Intermittent hemodialysis 246
Internal bleeding 142
Intestinal medicines 157
Iodine and nutritional management 347
Irritable bowel disease, dietary management of 193
Irritable bowel syndrome 153

J

Jaundice 284
Joints, stress and strain on 29

K

Ketogenic diets 40
Kidney disorders
electrolyte imbalances in 251
water and electrolyte balance in 248
Kidney stones 237
classification of 238
dietary management in 244
pathophysiology 237
sizes of 242
surgical methods for removing 243
symptoms of 242
Kidneys
maintenance of calcium and phosphate balance by 251
maintenance of water balance by 250

L

Laboratory assessment 19
Laboratory evaluations 19
Lactic acid accumulation 111
Lactose intolerance 219
management of 220
Larger calculi 242
Late dumping syndrome 164
Latent autoimmune diabetes of adults 94
Left ventricular hypertrophy (LVH) 72
Leloir pathway 317
Leukaemias 359
Linoleic acid 76
Liver disorders 283, 284
background and causes of 285
dietary management 290
signs and symptoms 284
Long acting (basal) insulin analogs 106
Low calorie diet 9
Low fat diet 10
Low fibre diet 10
Low GI/GL diet 131
Low oxalate foods 244
Low protein diet 10
Low residue diets 7
Low sodium diet 11

M

Maple syrup urine disease 323
causes/etiology 325
characteristics 324
classification of 324
clinical features and manifestation 326
dietary management 326, 327
manifestation/symptoms 325
pathology 324
possible complications 326, 329
prevention 329
Maturity onset diabetes of the young (MODY) 94
Medical and laboratory data, nutritional interpretation of 17
Mediterranean diet 43
Metabolic acidosis 231
Metabolic disorders 30
Metabolism, inborn errors of 299
Metformin 110
Minerals 20
Mixed insulins along with short or rapid acting insulins 106
Modified diets 5
Modified microbiomes 201
Myocardial infarction 65

N

Natiglinide 110
Natural liquid foods 11

Nephron 223
Nephrotic syndrome 233
Non-cleansing bulimia nervosa 48
Non-insulin dependent diabetes mellitus (NIDDM) 91
Normal diet 5
changes in 2
therapeutic adaptation of 2
therapeutic modifications of 1
NPO (nil per oral) 358
Nutritional assessment, techniques of 12
Nutritional contraindications 218
Nutritional status 13

O

Obesity 210
aetiology of 25
and bariatric surgery 212
assessment of 26
complications during 29
definition 23
diet and feeding 36
diets of 39
diet therapy 33
energy requirements 34
fats 34
fluid 35
management of 33
minerals 35
protein 34
treatment 33
very low calorie diet <800 kcal 33
vitamins 35
Obstetrical risks 30
Oesophageal cancer 355
Oesophageal ulcer 137
Oesophagitis 175
Oesophagus, anatomy of 175
Omega six fatty acids 76
Omega three fatty acids 77
Omega-3 polyunsaturated fatty acids 71, 76
Omega-6 polyunsaturated fatty acids 70, 76
Omeprazole 144
Open and the laproscopic bariatric surgery 216
Oral cancer (tongue cancer) 360
Oral hypoglycaemic drugs 108
Ornish diet 42, 54
Osteoarthritis 30, 38, 380
Osteoporosis 382
causes 382-383
prevention and control of 384
risk factors for 383
Ovarian cancer 362
aetiology/causes 363
manifestations/symptoms 362
risk factors 263

P

Painkillers, use of 140
Paleo diet 44
Pancreas 102
Parenteral nutrition 12
Peptic ulcer 135
causes of 139
complications of 141, 142
diagnosis 139
management of 143, 145
menu planning for 147
pathophysiology 138
Perforations 142
Peripheral vascular disease 66
Peritoneal dialysis 247
Pharmacokinetics 109
Pharmacotherapy 38
Phenylketonuria 299
biosynthetic pathway of 302
development of 301
dietary management of 311
in infants 303
management of 305
pathophysiology of 301
phenylalanine- free formulas for 307
pregnancy and 304
screening 303
sources of 304
stages of 300
variations of 300

Phosphorous 250
Physical carcinogens 353
Physical disabilities 29
Physical exercise 37
Polyarthritis 236
  granulomatosis with 236
Polycystic ovarian disease 31
Polycystic ovarian syndrome (PCOS) 337
  causes/aetiology 337
  clinical indications of 338
  complications related to 339
  diagnosis 340
  dietary management 341
  pathophysiology 338
  symptoms and complications 339
Polyunsaturated fatty acids 70
Potassium 249
Potassium lowering medications 257
Prediabetes 94
Prednisone 196
Primary glomerular pathologies 228
Pritikin diet 42
Protein 20
Protein metabolism 99
Proton pump inhibitors 144
Purging subtype 46

R

Ranitidine 145
Rapid acting insulin analog 106
Rectosigmoid and rectum cancer 364
Renal calculi 237
  management 243
  treatment of 243
Renal disorders 223
Repaglinide 110
Respiratory disorders 32
Rheumatoid arthritis 380
Roux-en-Y gastric bypass (RYGB) 216

S

Saturated fatty acids (SFAs) 70
Shock wave lithotripsy 243
Short (prandial or bolus) acting regular insulin 105
Silybum marianum 292
Skinfold thickness 28
Sleep apnea 29
Sleeve gastrectomy 218
Small calculi 242
Sodium 249
  and water imbalance 231
Soft diets 7, 146
Squamous cell carcinoma 355
Starlix 110
Storage fat 24
Stress management 37
Struvite stones, treatment and causes for 240
Sulfasalazine 196
Sulphonylureas 108
Surgery 38
Systemic glomerular pathology 229

T

Therapeutics diets
  objectives of 1
  planning 1
  types of 4
Thyroid disorders 345
  management of 346
  symptoms of 346
Trans fatty acids 71
Transient lower oesophageal sphincter relax 176
Tuberculosis 395, 397
  dietary management 398
  symptoms of 398
  treatment 396
Tubulointerstitial pathology, diseases causing 229
Type IV galactosemia 316
Typhoid fever, body changes in 391

U

Ulcerative colitis 189
  dietary recommendations for 194
Uric acid stone 241

V

Vasculitis 236
Vitamin D 341
Vitamins 20

W
Waist circumference 28
Waist-hip ratio 28
Water and electrolyte imbalances
  management of 255
  symptoms of 254
Weight loss 165
Weight reducing diets, criteria for 36
White-wheat bread 124
Wilson's disease 289

Z
Zollinger Ellison syndrome 140